Nineteenth Century American Asylums

Nineteenth Century American Asylums

A History in Postcards

Alma Wynelle Deese and Cathy Faye, editors

Drs. Nicholas and Dorothy Cummings
CENTER FOR THE HISTORY OF PSYCHOLOGY
AT THE UNIVERSITY OF AKRON

ISBN 978-1-937378-73-8

The paper used in this publication meets the minimum requirements of American National Standard for Information Sciences—Permanence of Paper for Printed Library Materials, ANSI Z39.48–1984. ∞

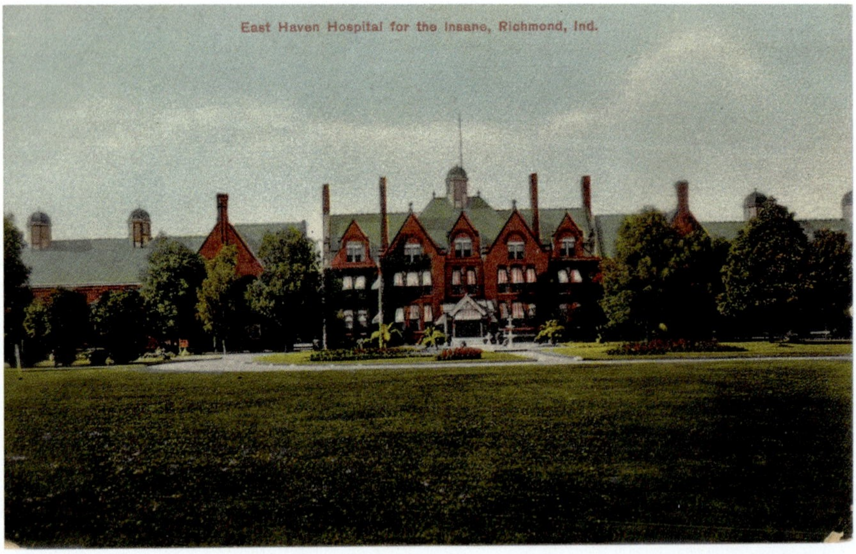

Cover photo (original photo pictured above): Archives of the History of American Psychology, The Drs. Nicholas and Dorothy Cummings Center for the History of Psychology, The University of Akron, A. Wynelle Deese Postcard Collection. The image shows the Administrative Building of the Southern Indiana Hospital for the Insane and can found on page 239 of this manuscript. The image has been cropped and repairs have been made for use on the cover. Cover by Tyler Krusinski

Contents

Introduction 1

Part One

Eastern State Hospital 7
Kentucky Lunatic Asylum 10
Western Lunatic Asylum 14
South Carolina Lunatic Asylum 16
Worcester Lunatic Asylum 18
Lunatic Asylum of Ohio 24
Tennessee Lunatic Asylum 27
Maine Insane Hospital 29
New Hampshire Asylum for the Insane 32
Georgia State Sanitarium 36
Utica State Hospital 39
Indiana Hospital for the Insane 41
New Jersey State Lunatic Asylum 44
State Insane Asylum 45
Pennsylvania State Lunatic Hospital and Union Asylum for the Insane 47
Missouri State Lunatic Asylum 51
Illinois State Hospital for the Insane 53
Insane Asylum of California 54
Taunton Insane Hospital 57
Western Lunatic Asylum 59
Northern Ohio Lunatic Asylum 61

Ohio State Insane Asylum 63
Mississippi State Lunatic Asylum 65
Insane Hospital of North Carolina 68
State Lunatic Hospital 70
Michigan Asylum for the Insane 72
State Lunatic Asylum for Insane Convicts 75
Trans-Allegheny Lunatic Asylum 78
Alabama Insane Asylum 81
Wisconsin Hospital for the Insane 83
Mount Pleasant State Hospital 86
Texas State Lunatic Asylum 88
Kansas Insane Asylum 91
St. Peter Asylum for the Insane 93
Tewksbury Almshouse 96
Connecticut General Hospital for the Insane 101
Willard State Hospital 104
Central Lunatic Asylum 108
Hudson River State Hospital for the Insane 109
Insane Asylum of Washington Territory 111
Lincoln State Hospital 113
Danville State Hospital 115
Northern Illinois Hospital and Asylum 118
Iowa Hospital for the Insane 121
Illinois Southern Hospital for the Insane 123
Northern Hospital for the Insane 126
Central Kentucky Lunatic Asylum 128
Athens Lunatic Asylum 131
State Homeopathic Asylum for the Insane 135
State Hospital for the Insane No. 2 138
State Hospital for the Insane 140
New Jersey State Hospital for the Insane 142
Florida State Hospital for the Insane 144
Grafton State Hospital 146
State Lunatic Hospital 148
Eastern Michigan Asylum 151

Topeka Insane Asylum	153
Illinois Eastern Hospital for the Insane	156
Second Minnesota Hospital for the Insane	158
Dakota Hospital for the Insane	162
Buffalo State Asylum for the Insane	169
State Hospital for the Insane	171
State Hospital for the Insane of the Southeastern District of Pennsylvania	173
Asylum for Colored Insane	177
New York State Inebriate Asylum	178
Nevada Insane Asylum	181
Western North Carolina Insane Asylum	182
Colorado State Insane Asylum	184
Oregon State Insane Asylum	186
Arkansas Lunatic Asylum	189
Territorial Insane Asylum	190
Northern Michigan Asylum	193
East Mississippi Insane Asylum	195
Michigan Asylum for Insane Criminals	197
North Dakota State Hospital for the Insane	200
North Texas Lunatic Asylum	203
Toledo Asylum for the Insane	206
East Tennessee Asylum for the Insane	209
Idaho Insane Asylum	211
Westborough Insane Hospital	213
Southwestern Lunatic Asylum	215
Lunatic Asylum No. 3	217
Territorial Insane Asylum	219
Northern Indiana Hospital for the Insane	221
Iowa State Hospital for the Insane	224
California Hospital for the Chronically Insane	226
Insane Asylum	227
Department for Insane, Anamosa Penitentiary	229
West Tennessee Hospital for the Insane	230
Hospital for the Incurably Insane	232

Wyoming Insane Asylum 235
Insane Department and Hospital of New Castle County 236
Southern Indiana Hospital for the Insane 238
Eastern Indiana Hospital for the Insane 240
Fergus Falls State Hospital 242
St. Lawrence State Asylum 244
Vermont State Hospital for the Insane 246
Asylum for Insane Criminals 248
Eastern State Hospital for the Insane 249
New Mexico Insane Asylum 251
Southwestern Insane Asylum 253
Second Hospital for the Insane 255
Mendocino State Asylum for the Insane 257
Southern California State Asylum for the Insane and Inebriates 258
Asylum for the Chronic Insane of Pennsylvania 260
Asylum for Insane Criminals 263
Upper Peninsula Hospital for the Insane 264
Medfield Insane Asylum 266
Springfield State Hospital 268
Eastern Ohio Asylum for the Insane 269
Gowanda State Homeopathic Hospital 273

Part Two

Pennsylvania Hospital 277
Asylum on Blackwell Island 280
County Asylums in Wisconsin 282
Asylum for Insane Indians 284
Battle Creek Sanitarium 286
Asylums in Attleboro, Massachusetts 291
The New England Sanitarium and Hospital 293

Conclusion 296
References 299

Introduction

Throughout the nineteenth century and into the beginning of the twentieth century, state hospitals, private asylums, and other institutions for housing and treating the mentally ill slowly became a common sight in the landscape of the United States. In 1773, the Public House for Persons of Insane and Disordered Minds opened in Williamsburg, Virginia as the first public institution in the United States created for this purpose. Beginning in the nineteenth century, each of the 48 states approved the construction of at least one institution per year designated specifically to care for the mentally ill (Zwelling, 1985). By 1880, there were nearly 140 public and private asylums and state hospitals in operation (Grob, 1983). This period represents the golden age of institutionalized treatment in the history of mental health care; although additional facilities opened in the twentieth century, their sheer numbers and their prominence as the sole sites of psychiatric treatment would never again reach the same heights.

The institutions of this period—often called insane asylums, lunatic asylums, insane hospitals, and later state hospitals—were grand architectural feats, frequently standing as the largest or tallest buildings in their respective states (Yanni, 2007). The buildings were often designed by leading, well-known architects and tended to be ornate and sprawling, occupying vast expanses of land, set on manicured grounds with extensive gardens, lawns, and farms. Leaders of the facility placed great emphasis on the beauty and expansiveness of the grounds and buildings, since relaxation, fresh air, proximity to nature, and opportunities for exercise were considered necessary for treating mental illness (Morissey & Goldman, 1986). It was therefore common to find these grand buildings nestled back on extensive lawns, marked by ponds and rivers, flower gardens, and walking paths. Indeed, these institutions and the grounds they occupied would have been quite a sight for a passerby.

These institutions were of great interest to the general public, becoming a highlighted destination for tourists eager to see them up close (Miron, 2011). State hospitals and asylums were frequently discussed in newspapers and magazines, drawing public attention to their physical appearance as well as the treatment practices and activities that occurred within them. This kind of attention prompted considerable institutional tourism, when local residents and touring visitors arrived at these institutions to get a firsthand look at their facilities and operations.

However, an in-person visit to the asylum was clearly not an option for everyone. For those who could not travel to see the asylums in person, a new option arose for experiencing these institutions: the picture postcard. First introduced in the 1860s, postcards were at the peak of their popularity in the United States from approximately 1890 to 1919 (Hook, 2005; Rogan, 2005). During this period, an estimated 200 to 300 billion postcards were manufactured, rendering the postcard fad second only to postage stamp collecting (Rogan, 2005). The appeal of the postcard was widespread, crossing both age and gender boundaries. While some cards served the purpose of communicating a short message through the mail, the majority served as a means of photographically commemorating events or trips (Bogdan & Weseloh, 2006). Postcards of this period featured drawings or photographs, showcasing scenes from towns, cities, and countrysides across the globe. Hook (2005, p. 386) has noted that postcards were "a matter of civic pride during the early 1900s. At that time, even the smallest town used postcards as a way to market itself as a "good place to work, live, and visit".

Asylums and state hospitals, as well as other public and private institutions of the period, were commonly featured on such postcards (Bogdan & Marshall, 1997; Hook, 2005). These cards sometimes featured a "real photo" view of the facility, while most provided an artist's rendering of it. These postcards provide a look at the grounds and buildings of each institution, often from a distance. They also frequently show the gates or entrances of the institution, and less frequently, the interior rooms. Such cards may have been produced by the hospitals to publicize the modernity and innovativeness of their treatment facilities. The height of postcard popularity in fact coincided with increased criticism surrounding the institutional treatment of the mentally ill (Grob, 1983) and postcards portraying the asylum as an idyllic and peaceful place may have served as a way of counteracting such critiques. Despite the fact that such facilities were often overcrowded and underfunded, the cards portray the asylum in an idealized fashion, as a place that is both inviting and benign (Hooks, 2005).

Regardless of the originally intended purpose of these picture postcards, they now provide a unique way of exploring and experiencing many aspects of the history of mental health care in America. This book features one of the largest and most diverse collections of postcards depicting American asylums and state hospitals. The product of years of collecting by the first author, Alma Wynelle Deese, the collection includes 572 postcards of different state institutions from 47 states and 82 private facilities. Displayed together for the first time, this unique visual collection reveals a novel and intimate look at the ways in which asylums were presented to the public on postcards. The first section of this book provides images of public asylums and state hospitals in the United States opened before 1900. The institutions are presented in the order in which they appear on the list of hospitals provided by the American Psychiatric Association (1944). The next section features private and county facilities, run without assistance from the state or government. In both sections a brief account of each institution's history is given to provide some context for the images.

The architecture of these institutions, so frequently depicted on the postcards, is reflective of changing ideas about mental illness and its treatment. In the late eighteenth century, physicians emphasized *moral treatment* in the care of the mentally ill (Rosenberg, 1985). This type of treatment included the provision of rest, relaxation, engagement in occupational tasks, good nutrition, a regimented schedule, a change of environment and, more generally, a removal from the chaos of city life. The importance of this treatment is reflected in the expansive grounds of the asylums and the prevalence of dairy farms, gardens, and greenhouses which were tended to by the patients. It is also reflected in the open corridors and vast windows, which were intended to let in restorative light and fresh air. In this way, the history of treatment practices can be explored through the places and spaces occupied by patients and their caregivers.

In this same vein, postcards also provide viewers with a look at two central kinds of asylum architecture that reflect treatment practices: the Kirkbride plan for asylums and the cottage plan. In the 1850s, physician Thomas Story Kirkbride (1809–1883) advocated for the careful and conscientious design of asylums that would support the ideas and practices behind moral treatment. The Kirkbride plan, as it came to be known in asylum architecture, included a central administration building that housed offices for physicians and staff, flanked by wings extending to either side. The wings allowed for the successful separation of patients by gender and severity of illness and also permitted light and air to enter the building. Kirkbride asylums were often very large and impressive, visible from considerable distances. By 1866, more than thirty Kirkbride asylums had been built (Yanni, 2007).

The postcards in this book also show a smaller number of institutions built on another popular plan: the cottage plan. Around 1850, physicians and architects began experimenting with and advocating a new architectural plan for asylums that established institutions as a series of scattered cottages, rather than one large building, each housing a smaller number of patients. Some physicians believed that the sheer size of Kirkbride asylums was a detriment, impeding patient progress. The cottage plan was thought to be particularly useful for calmer patients with chronic rather than acute cases of mental illness. It was believed that such patients would find relaxation in the community-like atmosphere engendered by the cottage system and would benefit from being physically separated from more agitated patients (Yanni, 2007). The first institution built on the cottage plan was the Illinois Eastern Hospital for the Insane, opened in 1877.

The postcards in this work present not one but rather many images of the American asylum, from the vast countryside Kirkbrides, to the small cottages dotting green grounds, to public and private buildings repurposed to house a growing number of individuals diagnosed with mental illness. The images also provide readers with a sense of what day-to-day life involved in a nineteenth-century asylum, showing images of the asylum greenhouses, dairy farms, dormitories, theaters, entertainment halls, and gymnasiums. They show images of buildings that were built, expanded and renovated, and often, destroyed by fire. They also show images of buildings that have been significantly altered in recent years to be used for modern residential housing, commercial shopping centers, or educational institutions. More frequently, these postcards provide a lasting record of buildings that have long since been demolished. In this way, this magnificent collection serves not just as a source of visual information about the history of mental health care and its institutions or the history of picture postcards; it also serves as a lasting visual image of unique architectural creations that have long since disappeared.

Part I

Early American State Hospitals

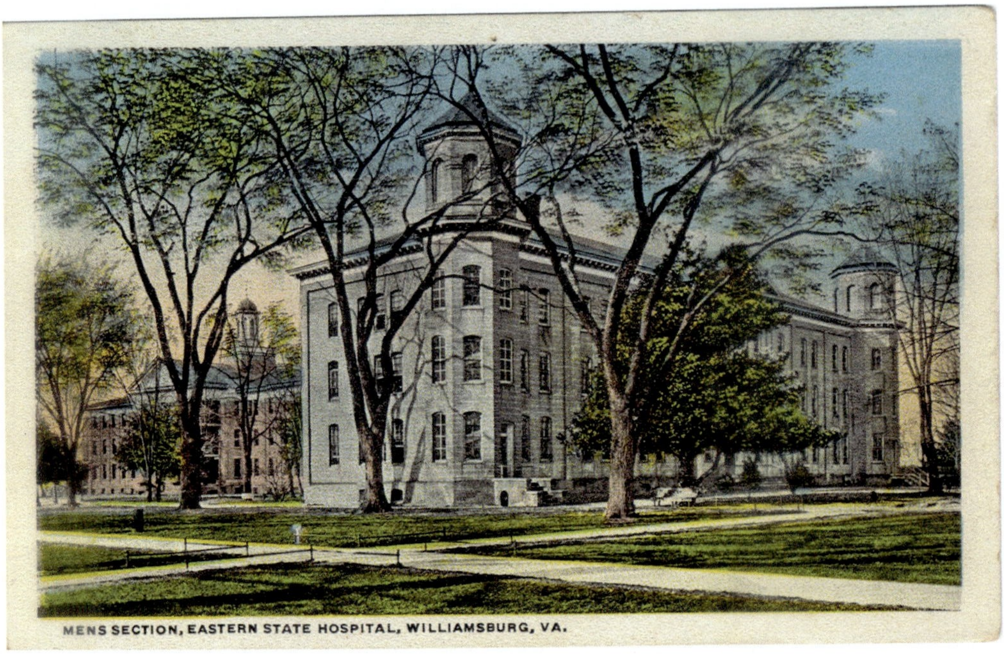

Figure 1

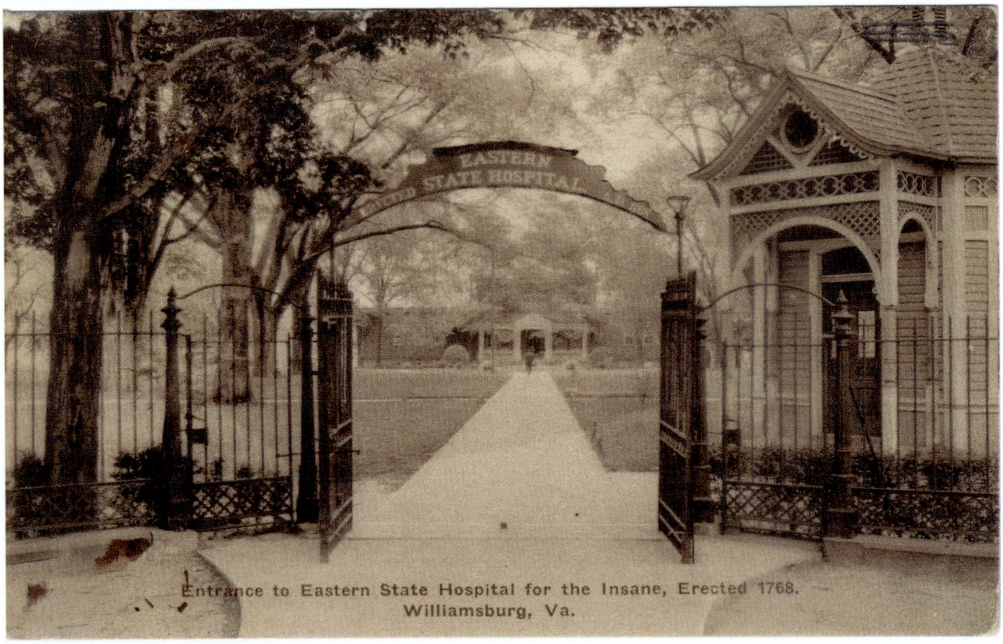

Figure 2

Eastern State Hospital
Williamsburg, Virginia, 1773

Eastern State Hospital opened in Williamsburg, Virginia in 1773 as the Public Hospital for Persons of Insane and Disordered Minds. The hospital was the first state hospital in the United States and the first in the country to admit black patients. By 1820, the population included approximately 43 patients and in 1841, the institution's name was changed to the Eastern Lunatic Asylum. By 1900, the number of patients had increased to 563 and by 1914, the facility was known as the Eastern State Hospital, attended by two physicians, one male and one female. Tubercular patients were segregated in two colonies, one for men and one for women.

The original building was destroyed by fires in 1876 and 1885. The structures that replaced them were built a convenient distance apart to reduce the spread of any fires in the future.

The postcard in figure 1, dated about 1915, shows the center of the asylum and the men's ward. The building on the right, frequently referred to as the "Tower Building," was built in 1844. In 1902, the Tower Building was destroyed by fire, years before this postcard was produced. However, it was common practice for postcard publishers to use pictures that were up to a decade old.

The postcard in figure 2 shows the gates to the hospital. Iron fences and gates became a common sight at these early facilities. This postcard lists 1768 as the date the hospital was erected. According to Hurd (1916) this facility was incorporated in 1768, the land was purchased in 1770, and the buildings were completed in 1772. The first patients were admitted in 1773.

Physical illnesses and ailments were common among the patients at the hospital and in the nineteenth century, separating individuals requiring medical care from the rest of the patients was not a common practice. However, housing these patients together was inconvenient, requiring physicians and the superintendent to check in on their patients on the wards. Therefore, in 1897, an infirmary (shown in figure 3) was opened, equipped with modern surgical appliances and an operating room.

The hospital infirmary is again pictured on the left of the card in figure 4 and the men's building is shown on the right. The opening date of 1758 on this card also appears to be incorrect. By 1935, the original Eastern State Hospital housed approximately 2,000 patients and there was no more room for expansion. The restoration of Colonial Williamsburg meant the hospital had no room to grow and the Williamsburg Inn surrounded the facility with a thriving tourist trade. Therefore, in order to expand the facility, the hospital was moved to a new facility on the outskirts of Williamsburg in 1960. That facility continues to operate today while the original buildings were demolished.

This reproduction of the original building stands on the site of the original hospital and serves as a museum (figure 5).

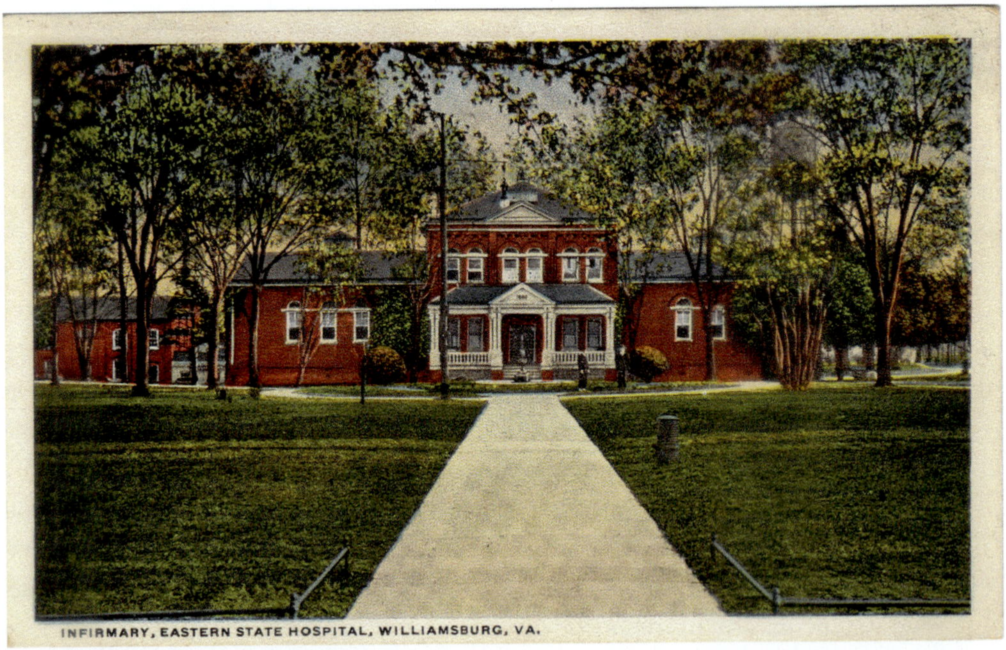

Figure 3

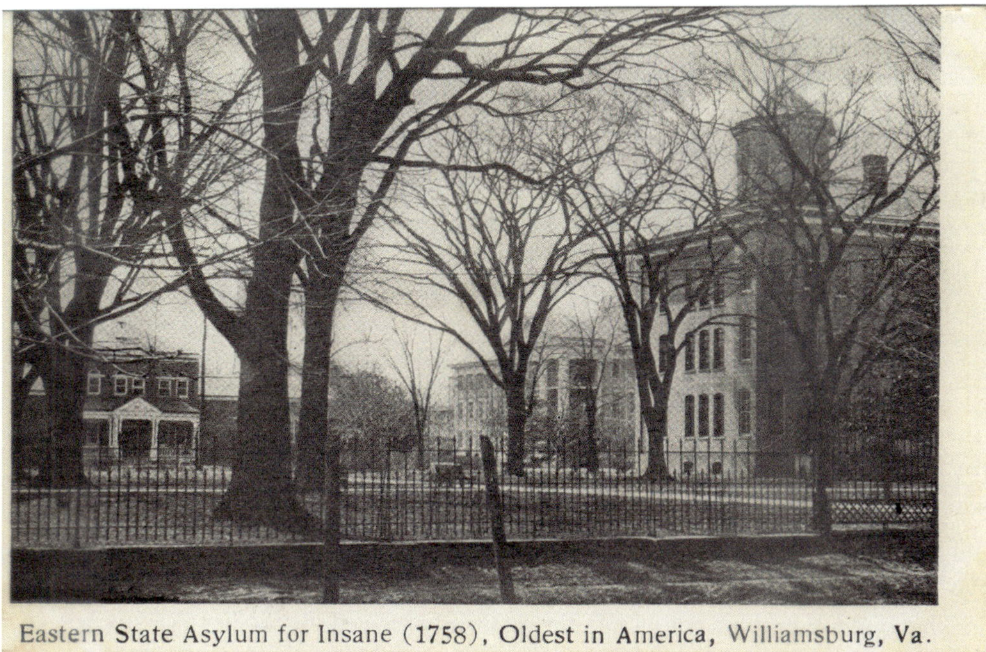

Figure 4

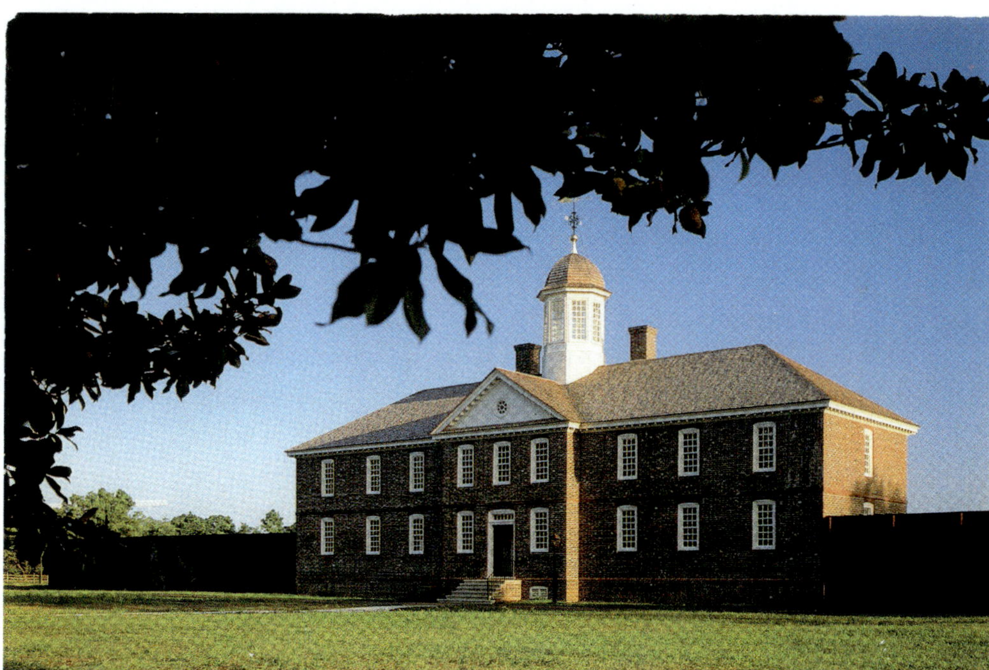

Figure 5

Kentucky Lunatic Asylum
Lexington, Kentucky, 1824

The second state hospital in the United States was opened in Lexington, Kentucky in 1824. The cornerstone for a private institution was laid in 1817, but adequate funds were never secured to complete the building. The state of Kentucky took over the unfinished building and the Kentucky Lunatic Asylum began accepting patients on May 1, 1824.

The founders of the Kentucky Lunatic Asylum viewed the facility as an early leader in the field of state care. Dr. Chipley, superintendent from 1855 to 1869, opposed the county system which he claimed provided lower quality care for patients deemed incurable. Kentucky followed his leadership to avoid county asylums, while states such as Iowa provided them.

The postcard in figure 6 is the original building, begun in 1817 and completed in 1824, shown on the right. It consisted of three stories and a basement. The building on the left was completed in the early 1900s as an administration building. The location of the asylum was chosen in part because of its proximity to a water source. However, by the 1850s, that water source was later found to be contaminated and the fence pictured here was built to protect patients from contamination. City water had to be temporarily brought into the facility.

As the number of patients increased, additions were made to the facility. After the Civil War, the original building became a building for male patients, while female patients were housed in a newer building. This separation of sexes was a common practice into the 1900s.

The 1905 postcard (figure 7) shows the administration building. An amusement hall or ballroom on the third floor was used for dances and parties with patients and local community members. Reports of these festivities were often found in the local newspapers with stories of citizens who attended.

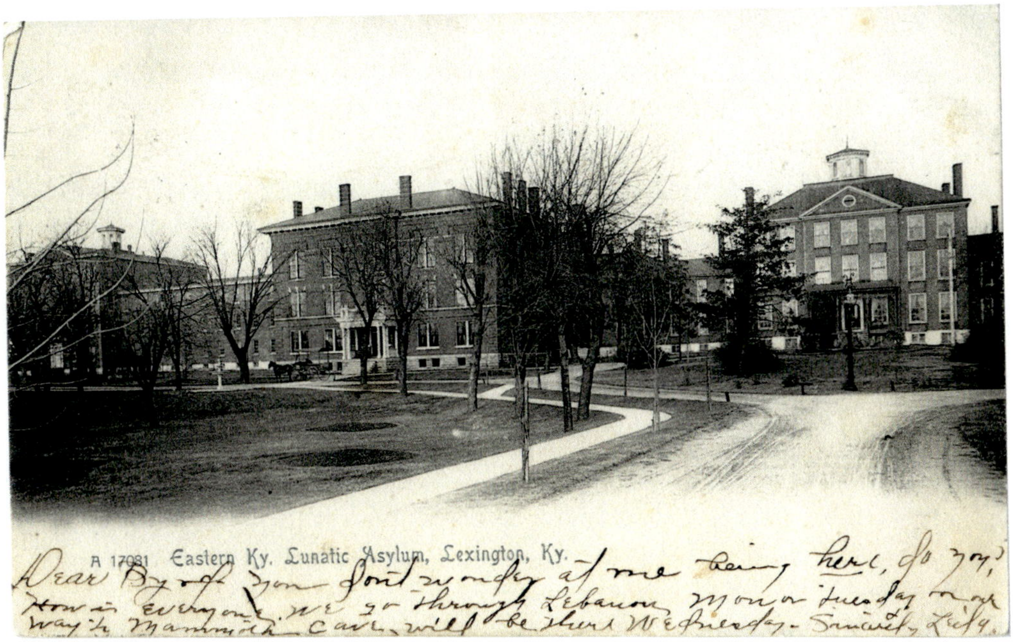

Figure 6

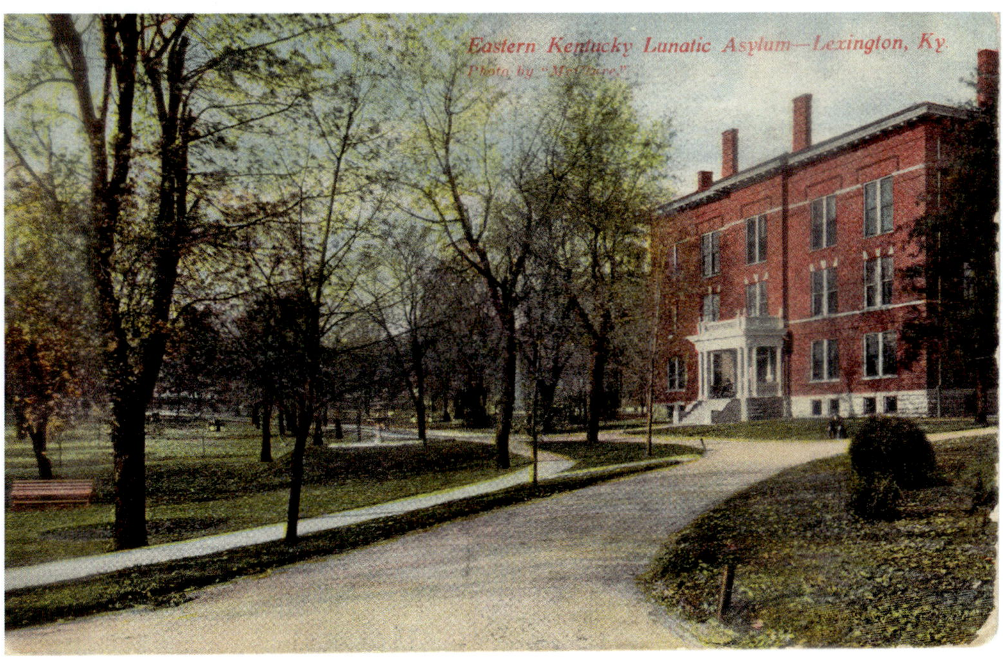

Figure 7

The opposite view of the administration building (figure 8) shows that it was not originally connected to the other buildings in the early 1900s. A connecting corridor was added later. In addition, the road in this image is unpaved and the building for female patients—erected after the Civil War—is visible on the left side.

A small wood structure pictured between the two buildings is a nativity scene made by the patients and employees. During the Christmas season, they used the stable and animals from the asylum farm to reenact the nativity scene for the staff, patients, and the local community. Local newspapers often showed this nativity scene during the holidays.

The black-and-white postcard (figure 9) shows all three of the main buildings: from left to right, these include the female ward, the administration building, and the male ward.

By 1917, the facility included a separate two-story infirmary, a tuberculosis shack, two buildings for black patients, and a 260-acre farm where patients worked.

By 1944, the institution housed more than 1,975 patients with only 140 employees. The large farm that provided years of support and work was sold in the middle 1950s.

In 2013, plans were established to build a replacement facility for the hospital at a new location. The original hospital grounds and buildings were demolished or renovated to serve as a campus for the Bluegrass Community and Technical College in Lexington. The Eastern State Hospital Cemetery Preservation Project was started several years ago to identify patients buried on the grounds with the goal to improve the cemeteries and honor the patients.

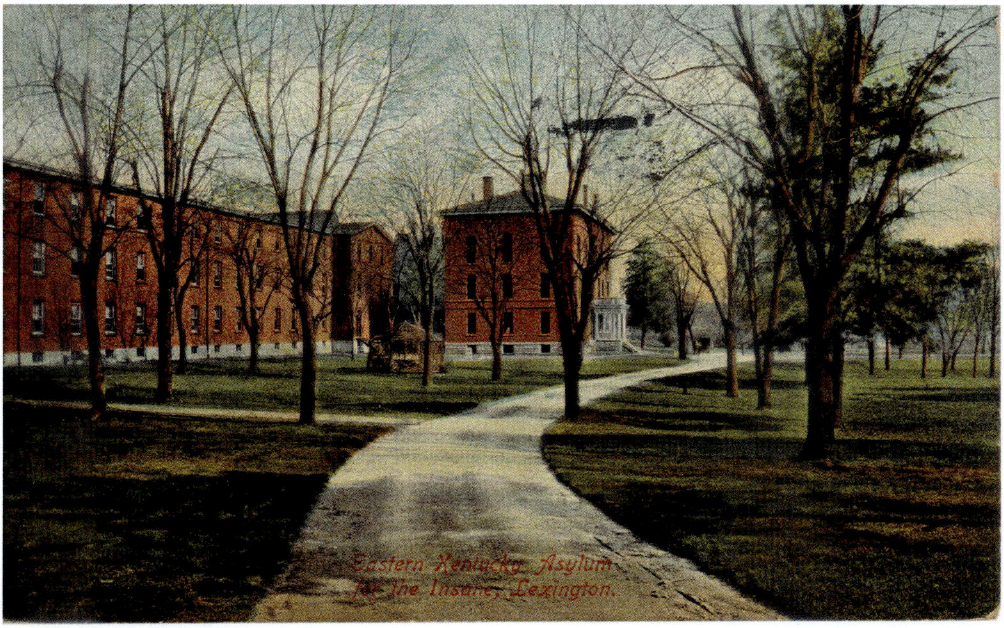
Eastern Kentucky Asylum
for the Insane, Lexington.

Figure 8

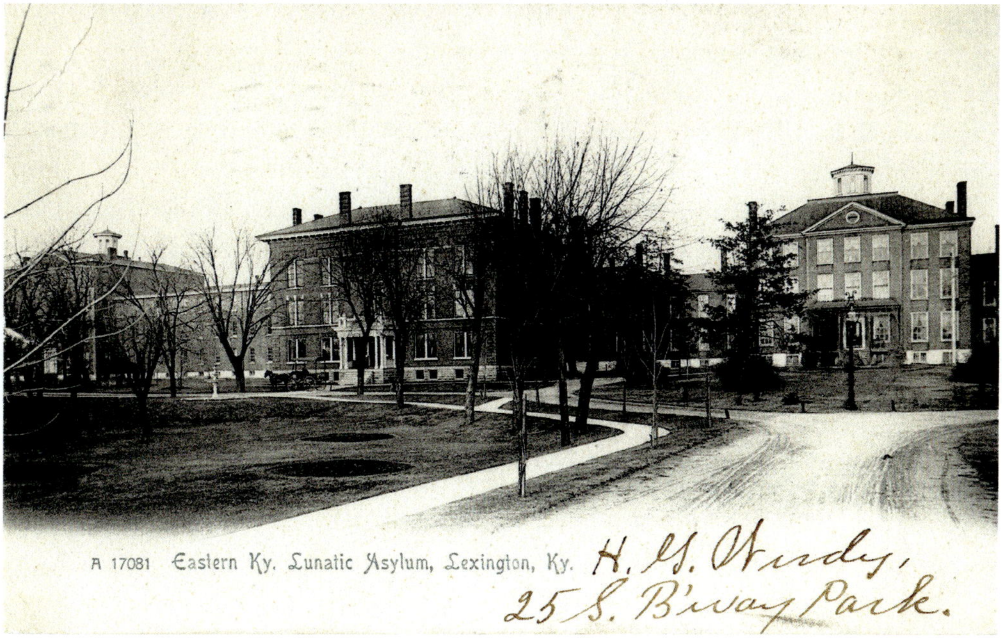
A 17081 Eastern Ky. Lunatic Asylum, Lexington, Ky.

Figure 9

Western Lunatic Asylum
Staunton, Virginia, 1828

Western State Hospital opened as the Western Lunatic Asylum in 1828 in Staunton, Virginia. The facility was intended to provide relief from crowded conditions at the first state asylum located in Williamsburg.

This original building was quite beautiful, designed with a French architectural style. However, as the number of patients increased, the appearance changed dramatically, with more and more additions being made to the original structure. The original buildings were planned with a central, imposing main building with adjoining wings for wards. The early administration building is pictured in figure 10.

A more distant view of the asylum on the following postcard (figure 11) misidentifies the structure as Eastern State Hospital. However, a magnified look at the building in the center of image suggests it is the same facility.

In 1894, the name of the facility was changed to Western State Hospital, the name under which it still operates. In the 1960s, a newer facility was built and patients were slowly transferred there. The hospital continues to operate under the Virginia Department of Behavioral Health and Developmental Services at a new site in Staunton.

Many of the original buildings have survived and are still visible at the original site. The site eventually became the home of a Correctional Center and was closed in 2002.

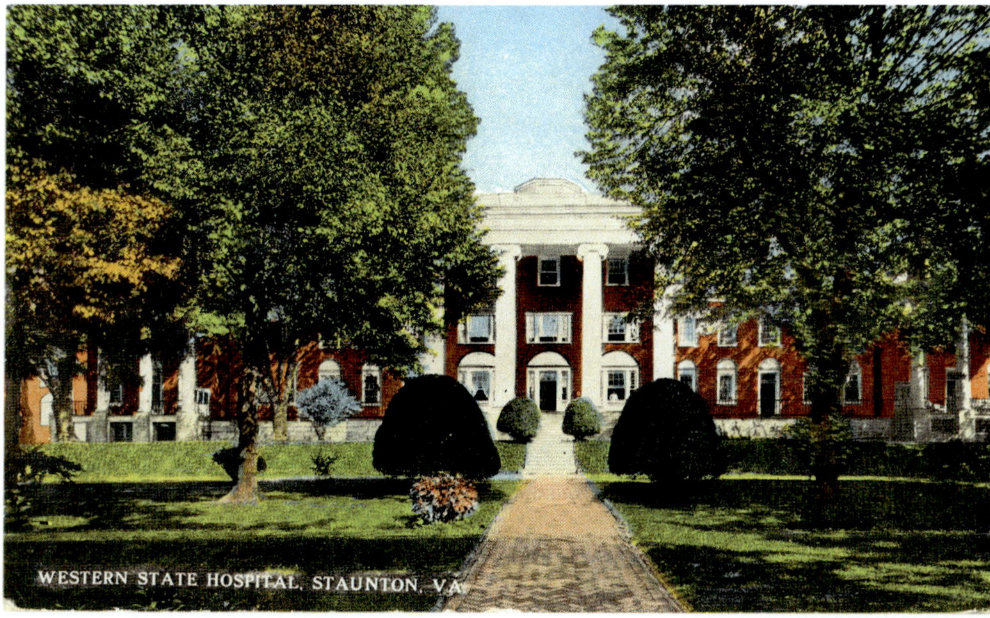
WESTERN STATE HOSPITAL, STAUNTON, VA.

Figure 10

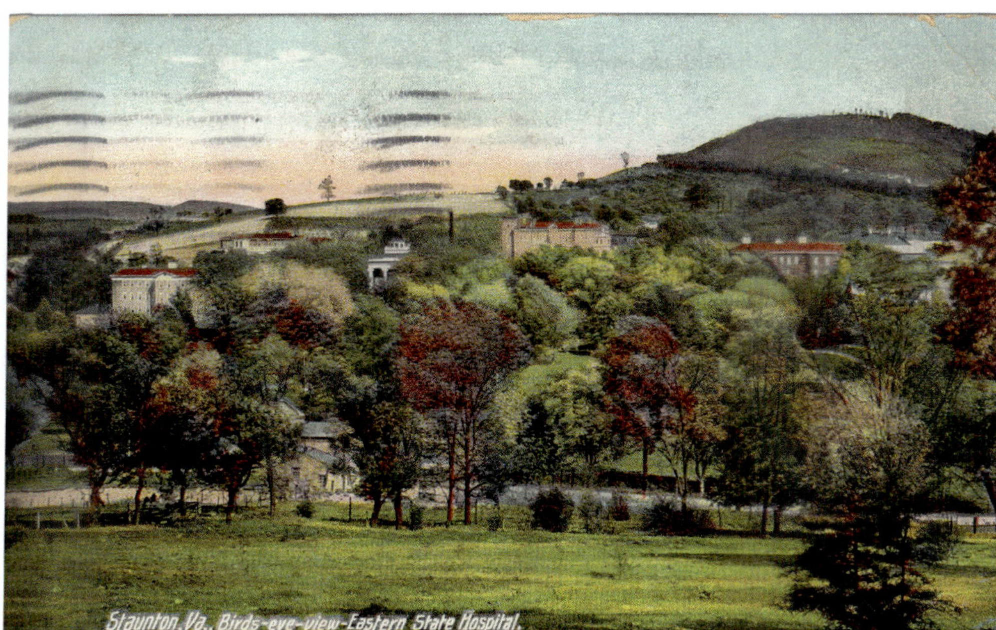
Staunton, Va., Birds-eye-view-Eastern State Hospital.

Figure 11

South Carolina Lunatic Asylum
Columbia, South Carolina, 1828

The South Carolina Lunatic Asylum first accepted patients on December 12, 1828, six years after the building foundations had been laid. It was expected to admit 100 patients. Thirty acres were to be cultivated by the patients, which was in line with treatment philosophies of the time that emphasized exercise and recreation as curative.

Entrance to the center building was built under a grand portico of six massive Greek Doric columns, with wings on either side. The postcard in figure 12 shows the hospital entrance.

In 1896, the name of the facility was changed to the South Carolina State Hospital for the Insane and in 1920, it became known as the South Carolina State Hospital. The hospital had about 200 patients during the Civil War. During that time, the state could not provide the necessary financial support and the Board of Regents borrowed money in order to sustain the facility.

Next is a 1910 postcard (figure 13) showing a more distant view of the entryway. During this time, the facility housed over 1,000 patients, a significant increase from the 750 that lived there in 1890.

In 1964, the facility was absorbed into the larger operation of the South Carolina Department of Mental Health. Many of the original buildings remain standing and some are listed in the National Register of Historic Places. The property and the majority of the buildings on the original site were sold to a developer in 2011.

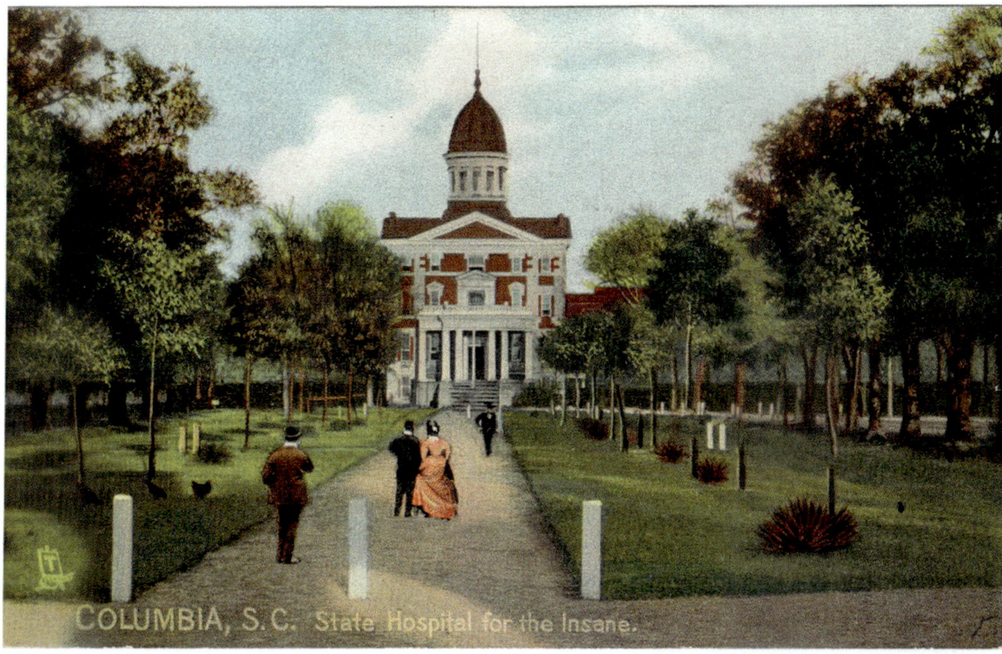

Figure 12

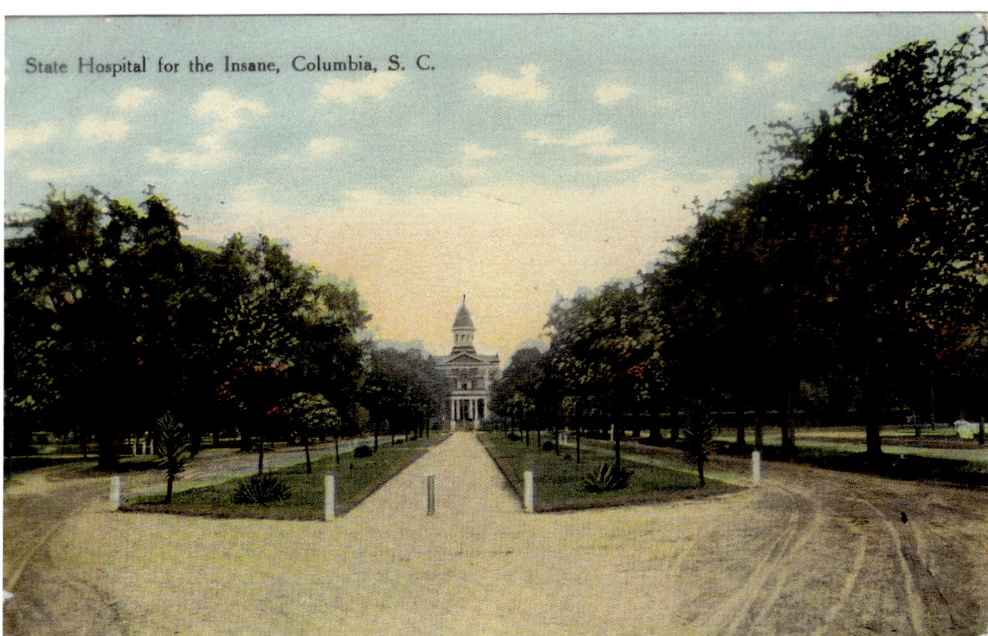

Figure 13

Worcester Lunatic Asylum
Worcester, Massachusetts, 1833

The Worcester State Hospital, originally named the Worcester Lunatic Asylum, first accepted patients on January 19, 1833. It included accommodations for a superintendent and extended wings sufficient for 120 patients. Ten years later, quarters for 150 more patients were added. However, admissions continued to rise; by 1846, the patient census had reached 359. Despite additions to the building on the original site, the institution quickly became too small for the influx of patients.

To accommodate this growth, a new facility overlooking Quinsigamond Lake was opened in 1877. The building at the old location was repurposed as the Temporary Asylum for the Chronic Insane, taking patients with chronic mental illness from the new location as well as from other surrounding state institutions. Many superintendents opposed the separation of chronic and acute patients, but the Massachusetts State Board of Charities favored it as a way of saving funds.

The 1915 postcard (figure 14) shows the main building sometime after 1877.

The 1910 postcard on the top of page 21 (figure 15) shows a distant view of the facility. Such distant views are among the most common in asylum postcards. Postcard collectors and historians surmise that this type of card was published with greatest frequency.

The Worcester Asylum operated until the early 1900s. A separate farm colony was established in 1877 and later was made into a separate facility named Grafton State Hospital in 1915. Figure 16 shows the administration building at Grafton State Hospital.

The image on the top of page 22 (figure 17) shows a different view of the hospital, providing a look at the expansive size of the facility.

The following postcard on the bottom of page 22 (figure 18), postmarked 1915, shows the wood fence and entrance to the facility.

A 1930 postcard on the top of page 23 (figure 19) highlights newer buildings of the hospital.

A fire in 1991 destroyed or damaged many of the original structures and the majority of them were demolished shortly thereafter. In 2012, the Worcester Recovery Center and Hospital opened on the same site. The original administration building was demolished in 2013, but materials from the original clock tower were preserved and the tower was rebuilt as part of the new hospital.

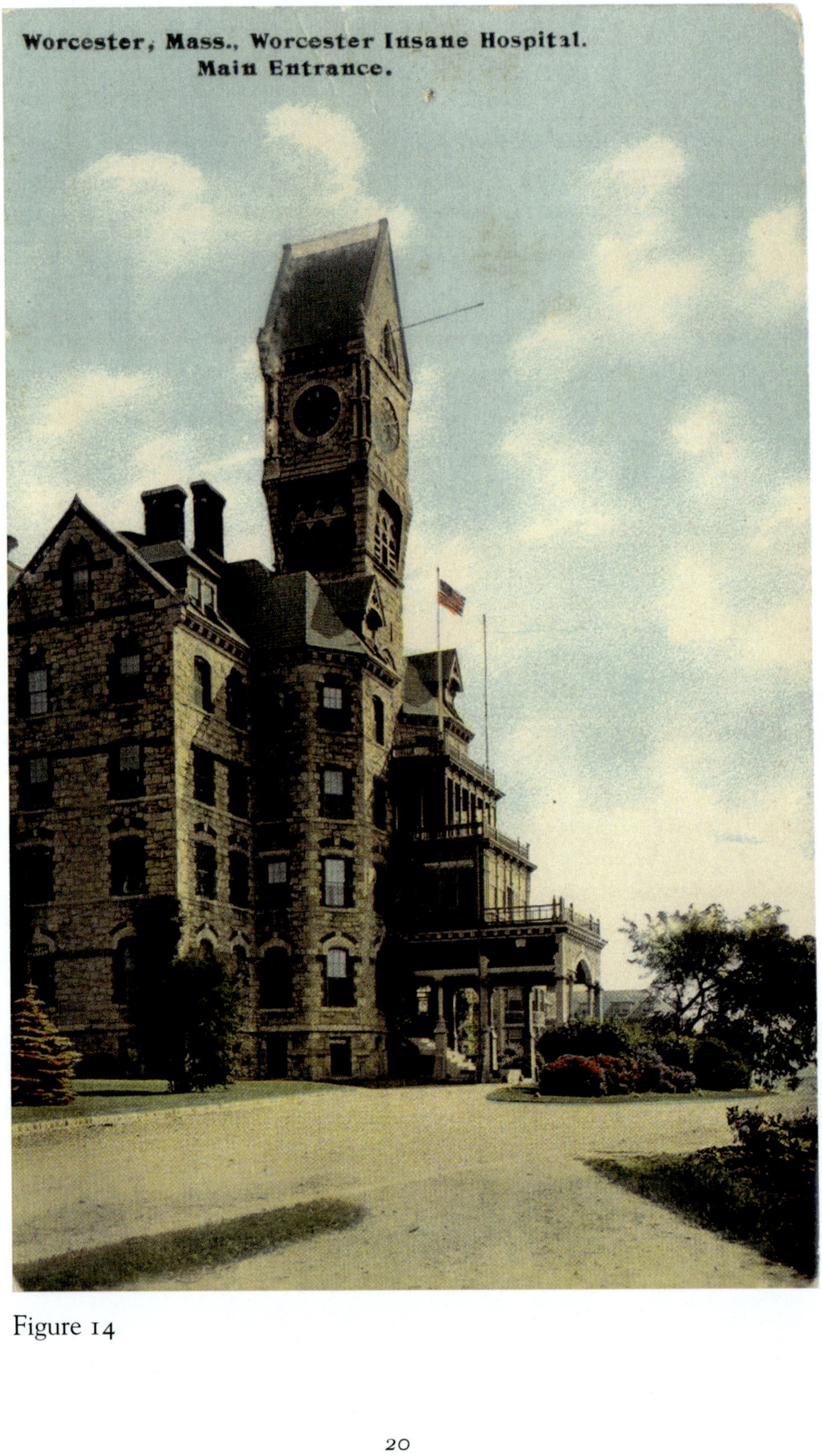

Figure 14

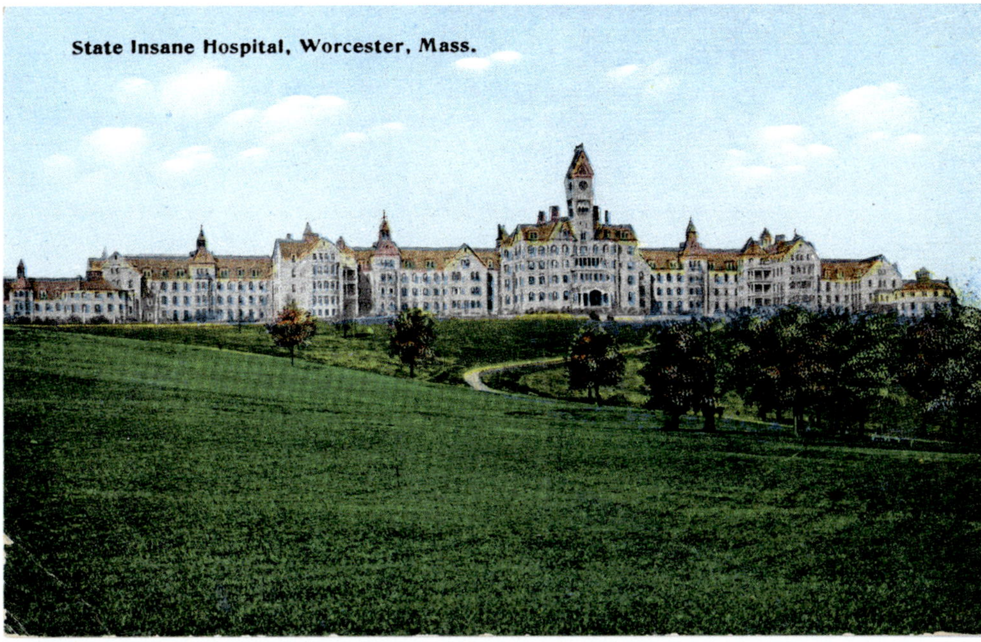
State Insane Hospital, Worcester, Mass.

Figure 15

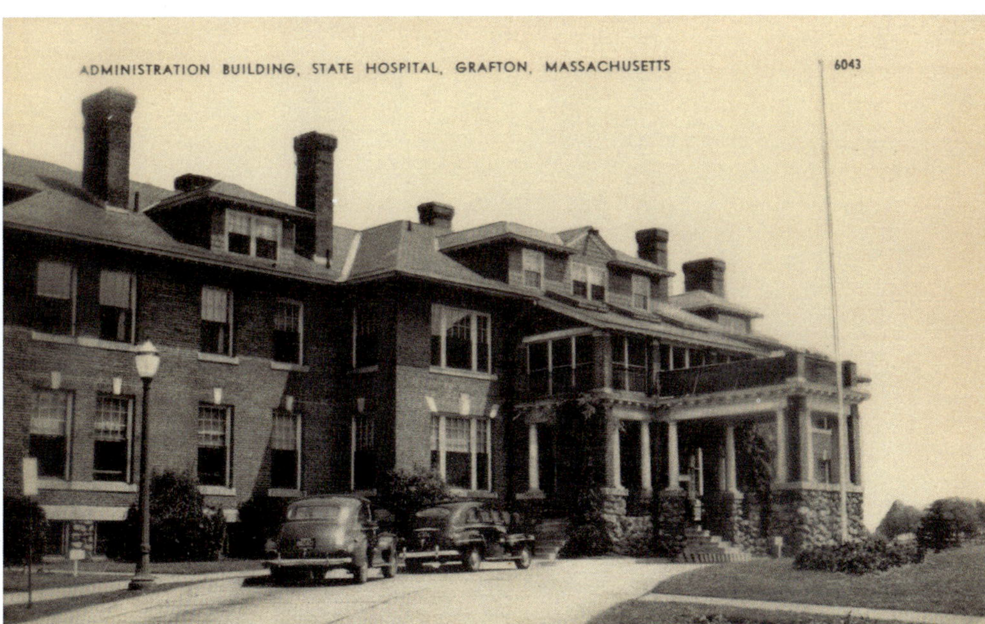
ADMINISTRATION BUILDING, STATE HOSPITAL, GRAFTON, MASSACHUSETTS
6043

Figure 16

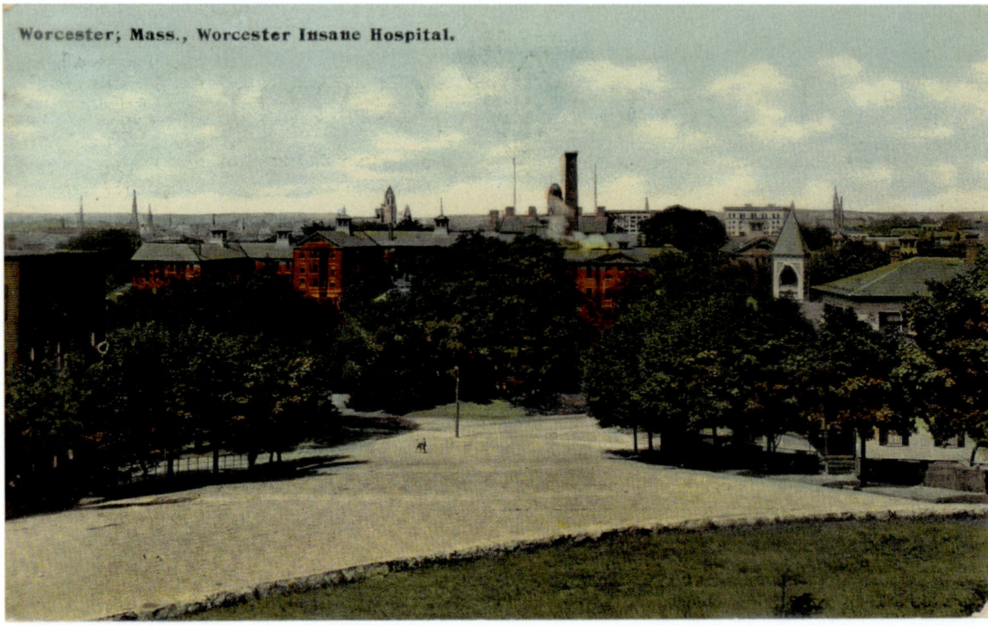

Figure 17

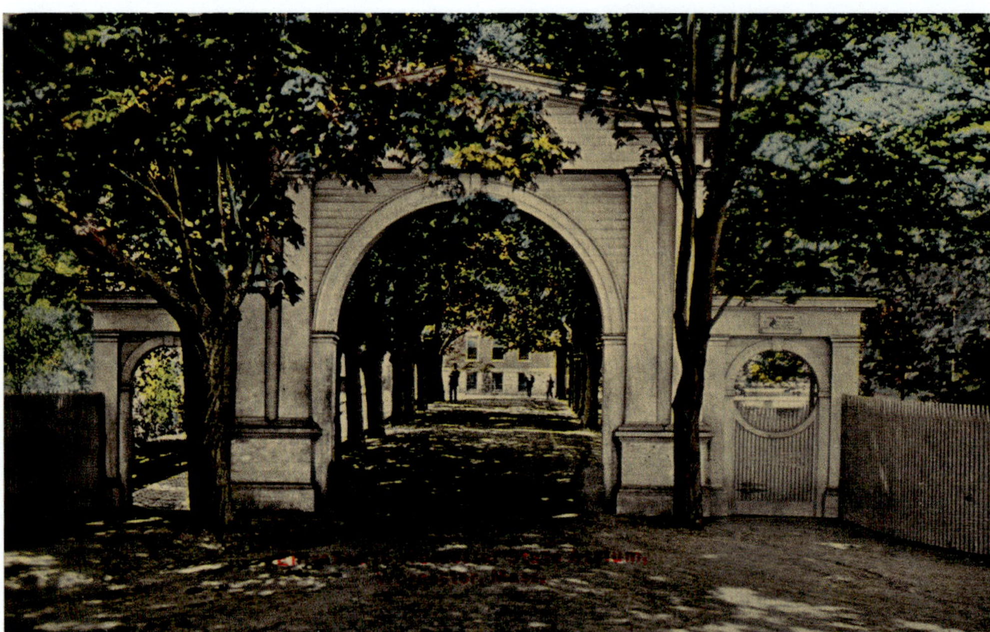

Figure 18

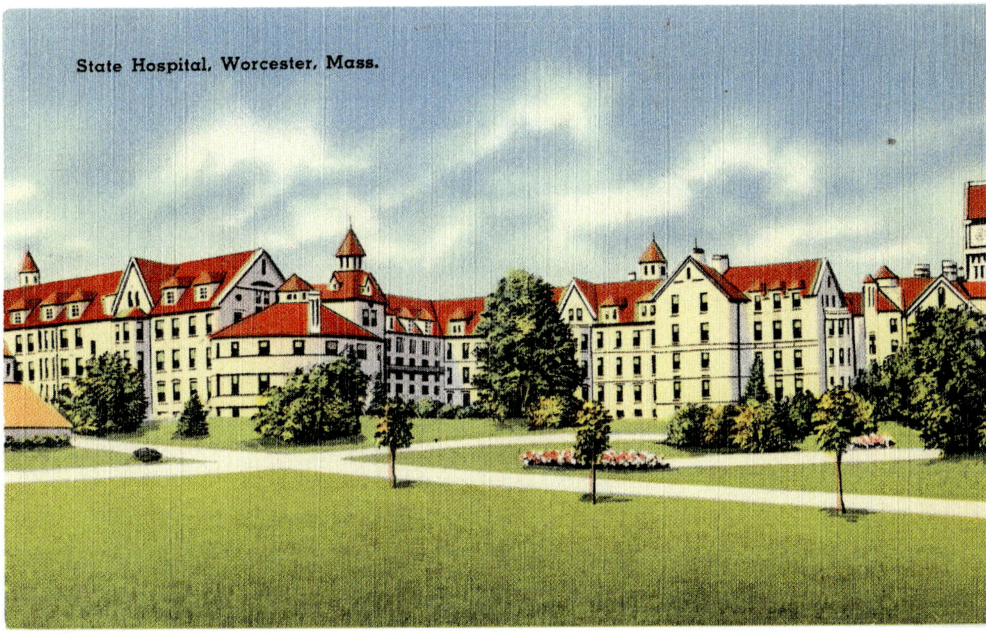
State Hospital, Worcester, Mass.

Figure 19

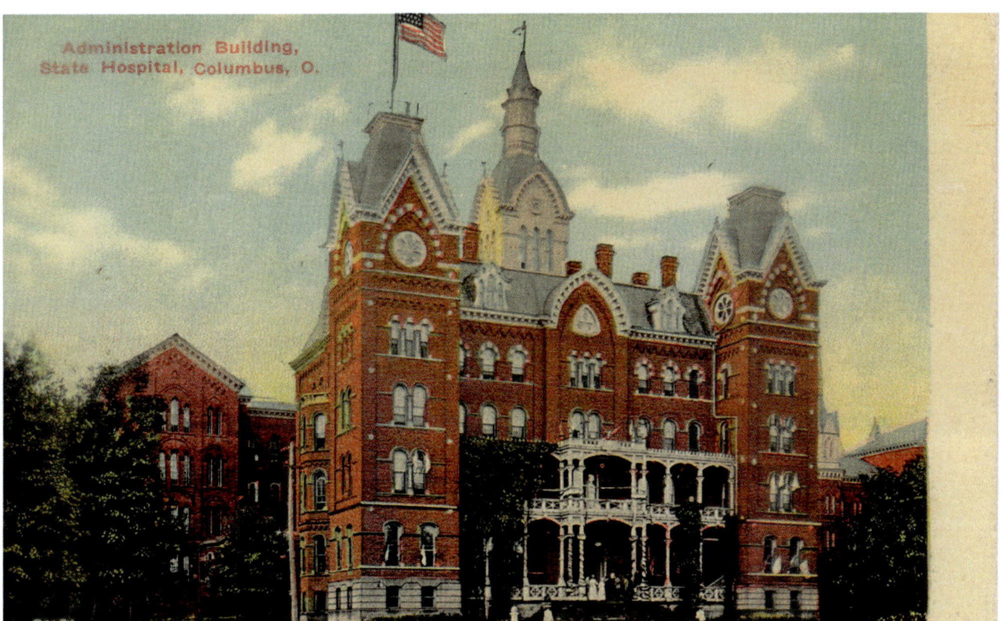
Administration Building,
State Hospital, Columbus, O.
21161

Figure 20

Lunatic Asylum of Ohio
Columbus, Ohio, 1838

The Lunatic Asylum of Ohio first accepted patients on November 30, 1838. The facility was destroyed by fire just 11 years after its opening. It was then rebuilt on a new, much larger site in 1877.

A postcard on the previous page (figure 20), postmarked 1907, shows the second generation of buildings.

The buildings covered one acre, with an area enclosed by the quadrangular buildings. The center building was built on the Kirkbride plan with three stories, a basement, and an attic. The wings were each three stories high and the building was extensive; the distance covered when walking through all of the wards exceeded a mile.

Postcards (figures 21 and 22) from the period show the size of the facility.

The building pictured in the postcard on the top of page 26 (figure 23) is unidentified. It may be one of the cottages built in 1907 to house patients that were less disturbed and capable of working on the grounds.

In 1915, the state of Ohio displayed images of all of the state's facilities on one postcard (figure 24). The administration building of this state hospital was displayed with other state facilities on the postcard below. Such postcards were mass produced for the general public to buy to show their pride in the state's facilities.

Attempts at preserving the Kirkbride building failed and it was demolished in the 1990s. The hospital merged with other mental health care institutions in 1997 to form Twin Valley Behavioral Healthcare.

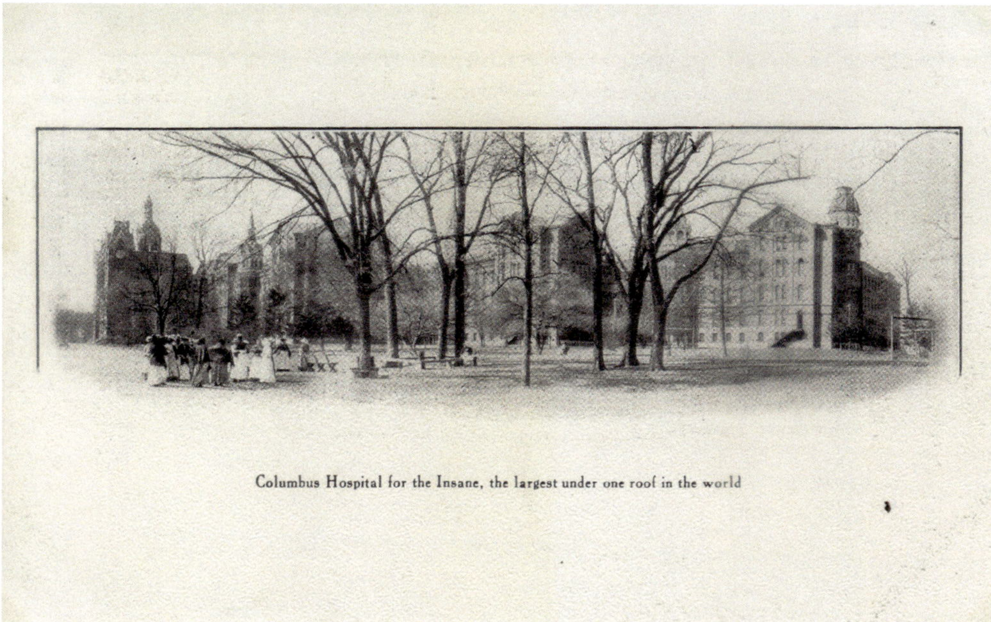
Columbus Hospital for the Insane, the largest under one roof in the world

Figure 21

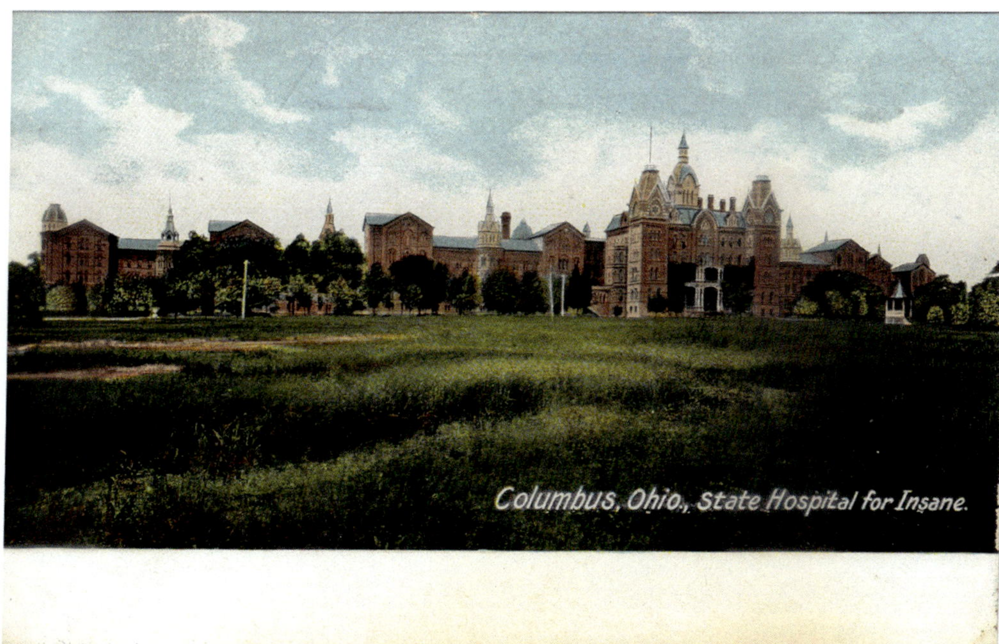
Columbus, Ohio., State Hospital for Insane.

Figure 22

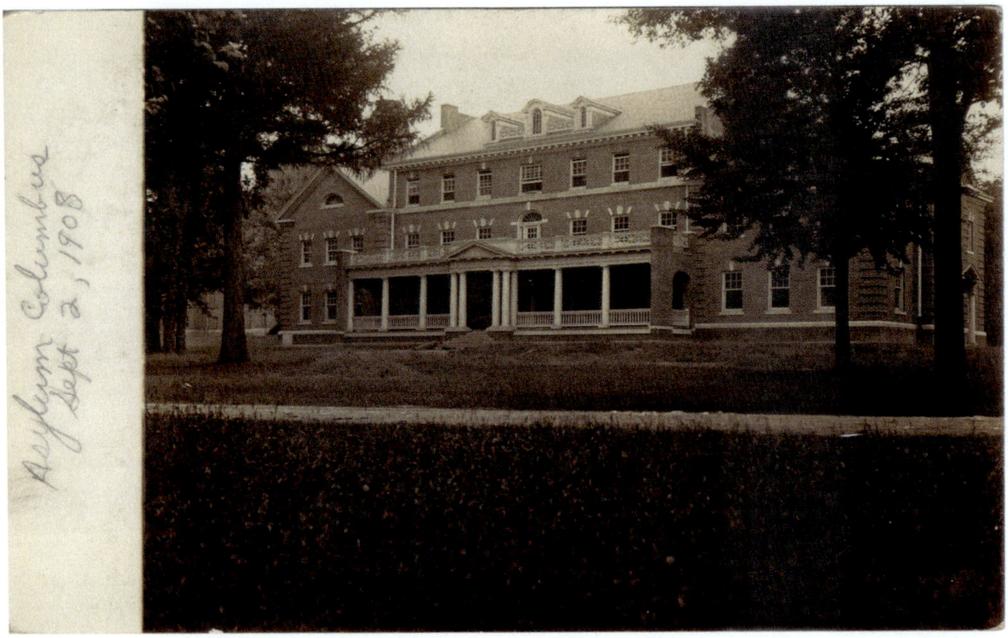

Figure 23

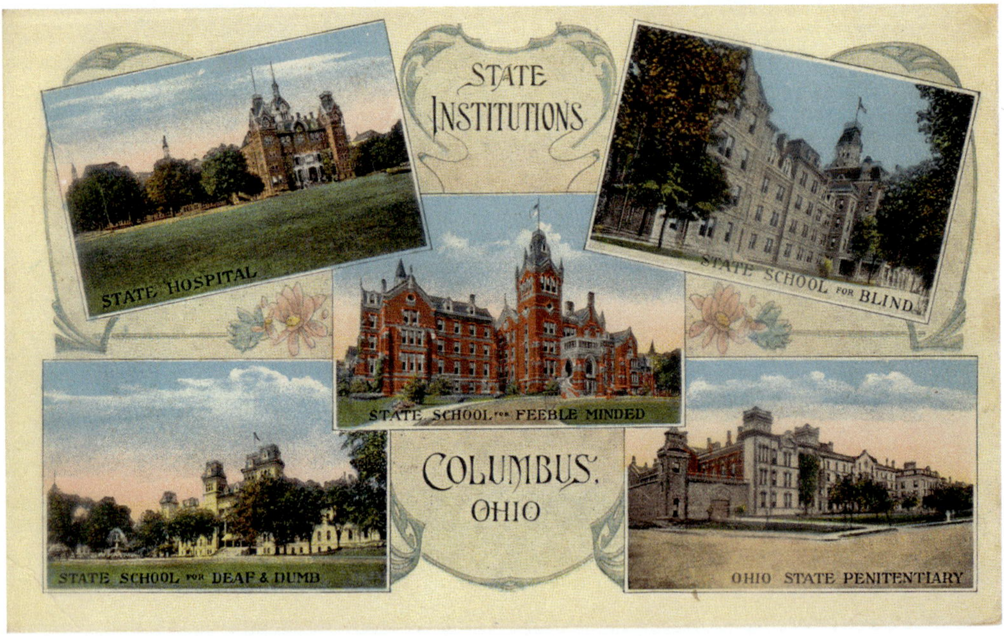

Figure 24

Tennessee Lunatic Asylum
Nashville, Tennessee, 1840

The Tennessee Lunatic Asylum was established in 1832 and first accepted patients on March 1, 1840. The facility was built on a few acres near the Nashville city limits. The small stone building provided room for only a small number of patients and proved to be inadequate within 12 years. More expansive facilities were built in 1852 on 225 acres about six miles from Nashville on Murfreesboro Pike. Renamed the Tennessee Hospital for the Insane, the new building could accommodate 138 patients, but by 1862, it too was overcrowded.

The design of the new building was influenced by an asylum in Maidstone, England which was also the inspiration for Butler Asylum in Providence, Rhode Island. It had a massive flat roof, octagonal towers, and castellated style of architecture. Wings were added to each side of the original building in 1871. In 1891, the west wing was destroyed by fire and 11 patients died. It was rebuilt and by 1912, the hospital housed 690 patients.

The postcard on the next page (figure 25) is postmarked 1907.

The institution was later renamed the Central Hospital for the Insane and is now known as the Middle Tennessee Mental Health Institute in its new location. The 1840 building no longer existed by 1992. The 1852 buildings were demolished in the 1990s when the site was sold to the Dell assembly plant.

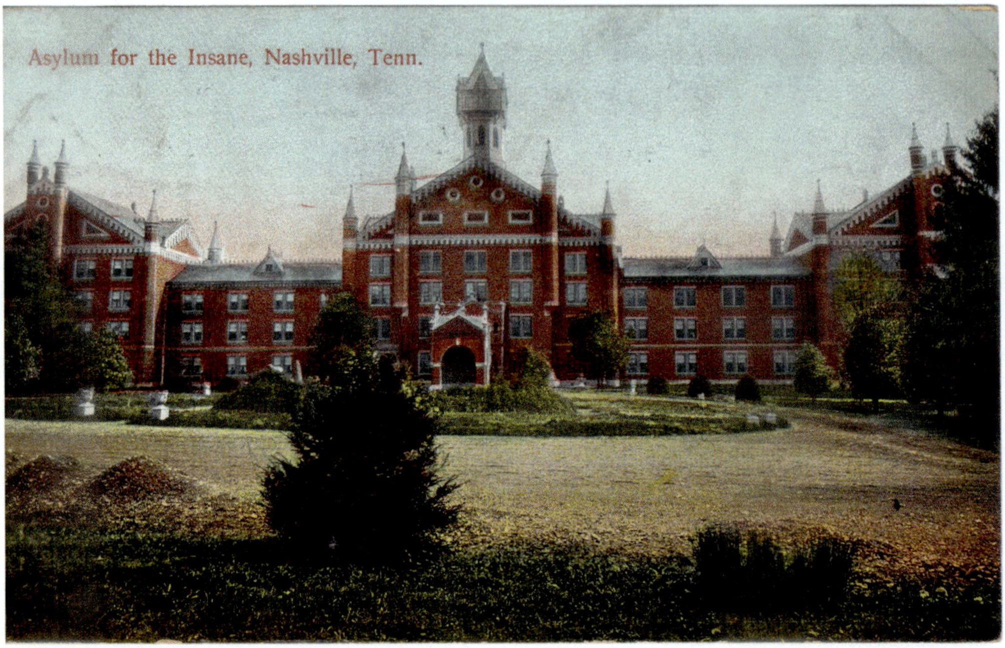
Asylum for the Insane, Nashville, Tenn.

Figure 25

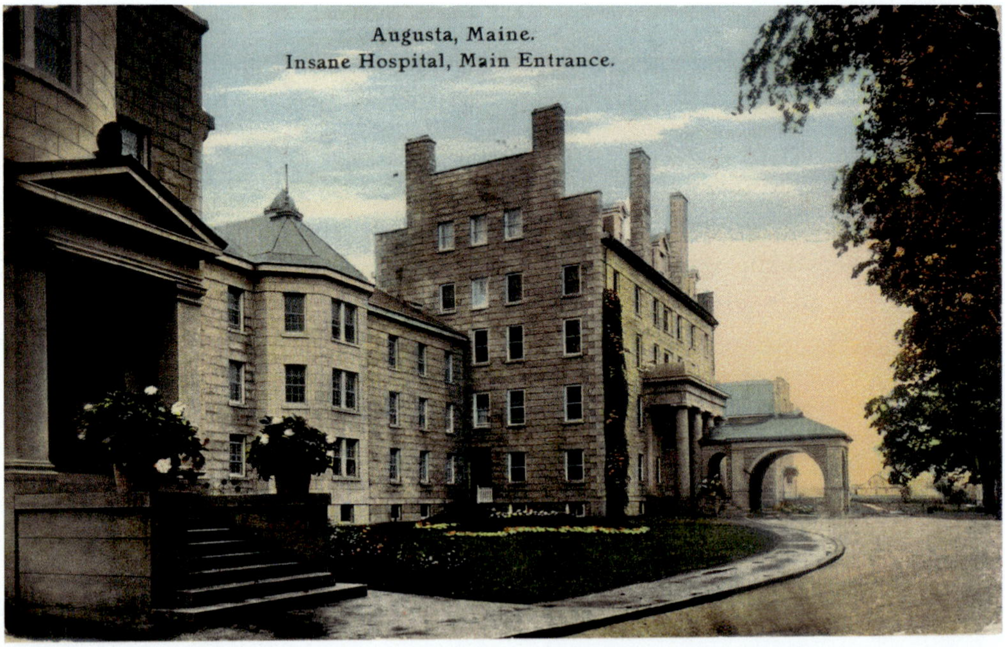
Augusta, Maine.
Insane Hospital, Main Entrance.

Figure 26

Maine Insane Hospital
Augusta, Maine, 1840

The Maine Insane Hospital in Augusta, Maine first accepted patients on October 14, 1840. The institution originally consisted of a main building and two south wings, which were almost completely destroyed by fire in 1851. The fire originated in the hot air chamber and spread rapidly. The flues leading from the hot air chamber filled the rooms with smoke. Twenty-seven patients and one attendant died.

Following the fire, some patients were placed in private dwellings and in county jails until a new facility was established the following year. The facility established a unique summer colony, the Summer Hospital at Chase Island, which provided outings for recovering patients or working patients who desired a vacation. In 1909, an additional building, accommodating 30 patients, was also constructed on the original grounds of the hospital to house the criminally insane.

The postcard on the bottom of the previous page (figure 26), postmarked 1912, shows the center building of the asylum.

Several additional postcards (figures 27–29) provide alternative views of the buildings and grounds.

Britt House, pictured in figure 30, was one of the oldest homes in Maine and is pictured next to the State Hospital in Augusta. The river pictured here may be the Kennebec River that ran behind the hospital.

The hospital which was later renamed the Augusta Mental Health Institute, closed in 2004 and was replaced by the Riverview Psychiatric Center. The original buildings have survived.

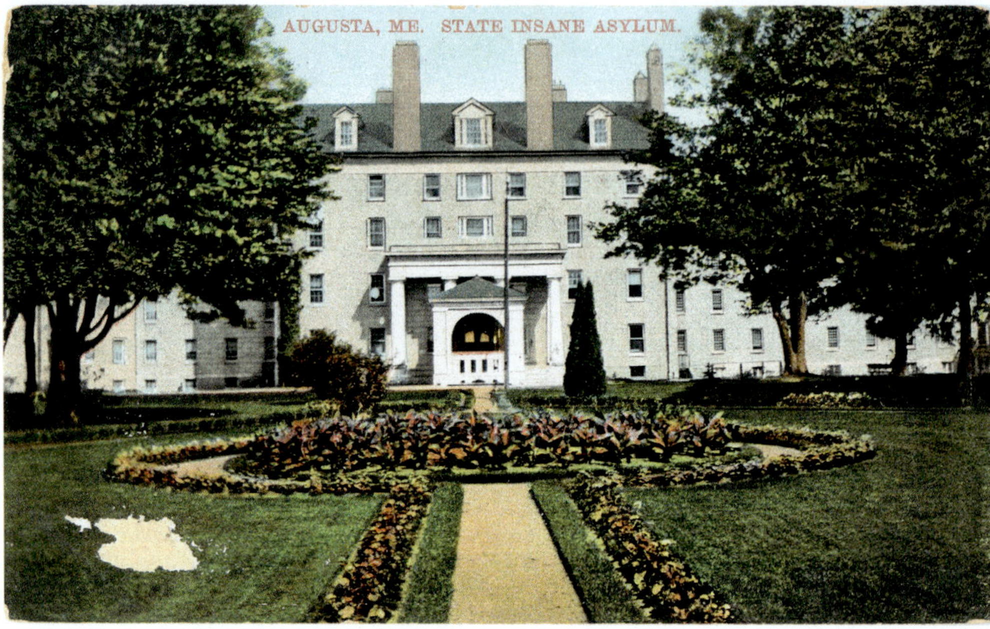

Figure 27

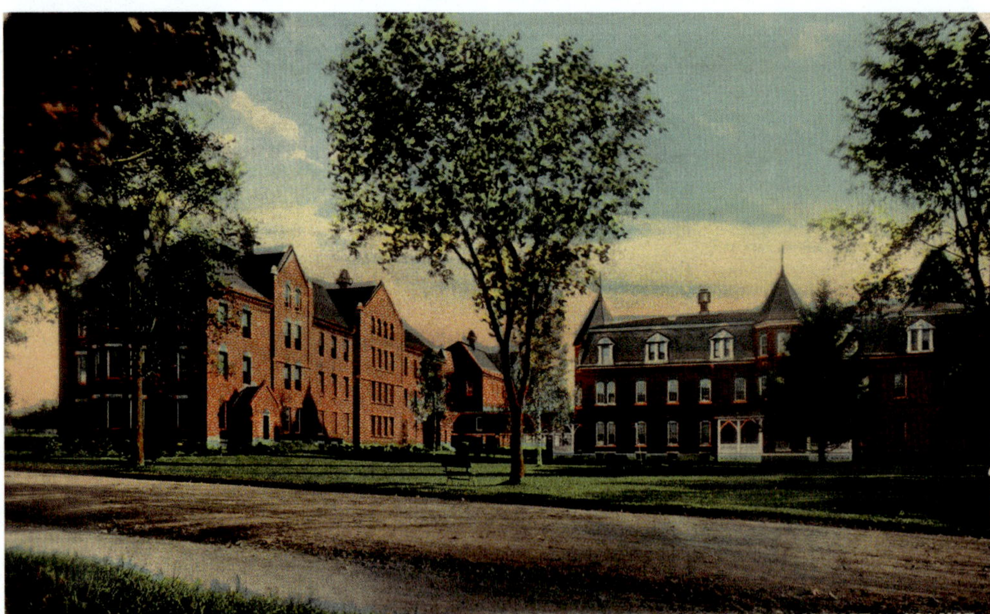

Figure 28

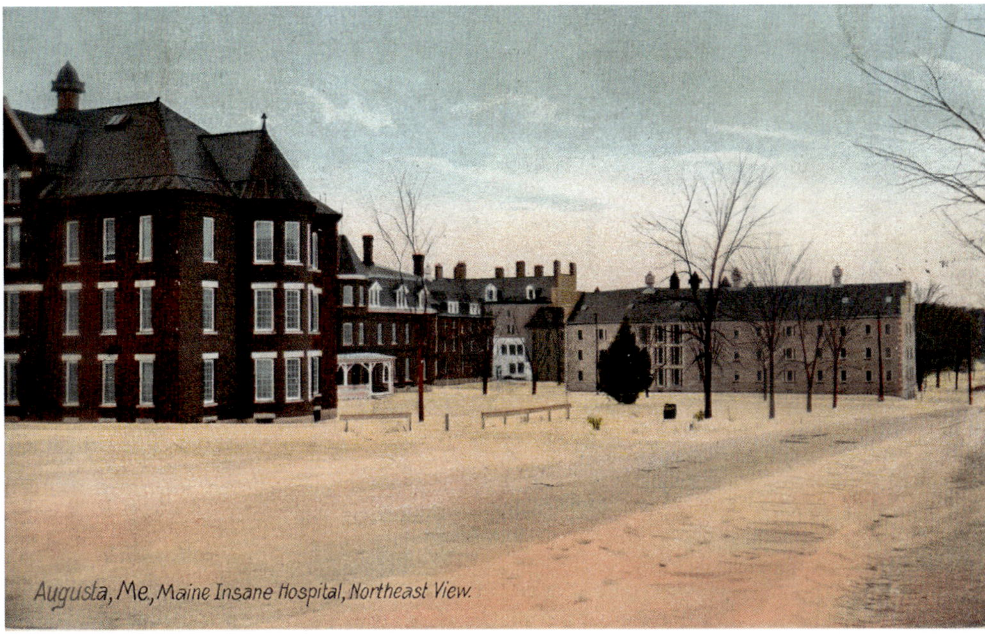
Augusta, Me., Maine Insane Hospital, Northeast View.

Figure 29

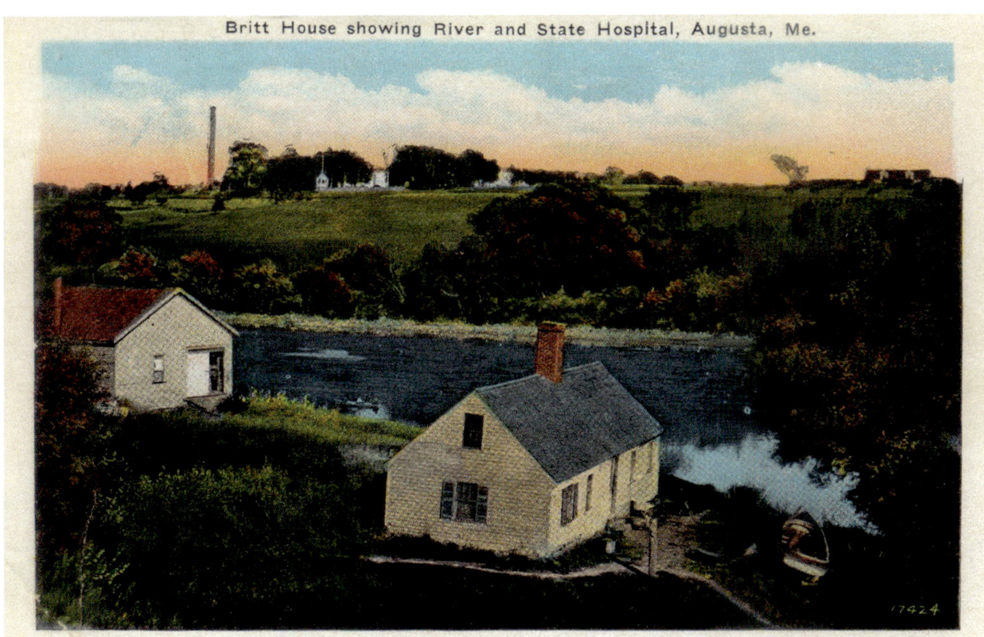
Britt House showing River and State Hospital, Augusta, Me.
17424

Figure 30

New Hampshire Asylum for the Insane
Concord, New Hampshire, 1842

The New Hampshire Asylum for the Insane at Concord, New Hampshire first accepted patients in 1842.

The center building pictured in figure 31 was completed to house 96 patients on a farm with 121 acres. A first wing was added in 1849 and a second one in 1854, providing space for 225 patients. By 1914, this facility housed 960 patients.

The facility was affiliated with a nearby general hospital in 1888 and included a training school for nurses. The name was changed from New Hampshire Asylum for the Insane to the New Hampshire Hospital in 1901.

The hospital was unique in that it relied on both public and private donations and was managed both publically and privately as well. The state was represented by a board of management that assisted in leading and managing the facility.

The comments on the postcard in figure 32 depict a casualness, suggesting that such postcards were used and circulated by travelers and tourists in the same way as any other postcard featuring local sites.

Throughout the life of the hospital, other buildings were added, including the Peaslee building in 1854, the Bancroft building in 1882, and the Twitchell building in 1894. All of these buildings were attached to the main building by a long corridor. In 1907, a new building was opened to serve as both a psychopathic hospital (responsible for the reception of new cases and separation of short-term cases from long-term cases) and as an infirmary for patients who were physically ill. The Walker building was added in 1913 to house 212 patients who were engaged in various kinds of work.

The Bancroft Building was constructed to house patients who were recovering and did not require restraint. The postcard in figure 33 shows the greenhouse on the grounds in front of the Bancroft Building. The greenhouse was used to grow flowers for the wards and vegetables for the patients and staff.

In 1886, 230 acres of land located four miles from the original buildings at Lake Penacock were added to the facilities and three cottages were constructed. There, male patients engaged in various work tasks, including raising crops and chopping wood.

The postcard in figure 34 shows another unnamed building.

The facility, still called New Hampshire Hospital, continues to occupy the same grounds. Several of the original buildings, including the majority of the main buildings, have survived and have been renovated and repurposed.

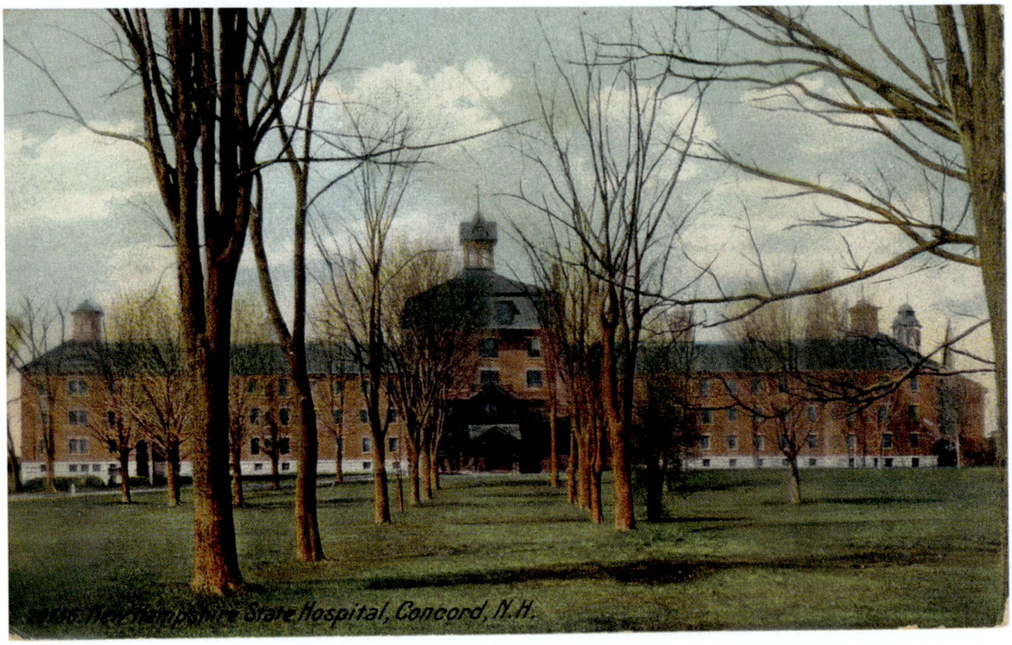

Figure 31

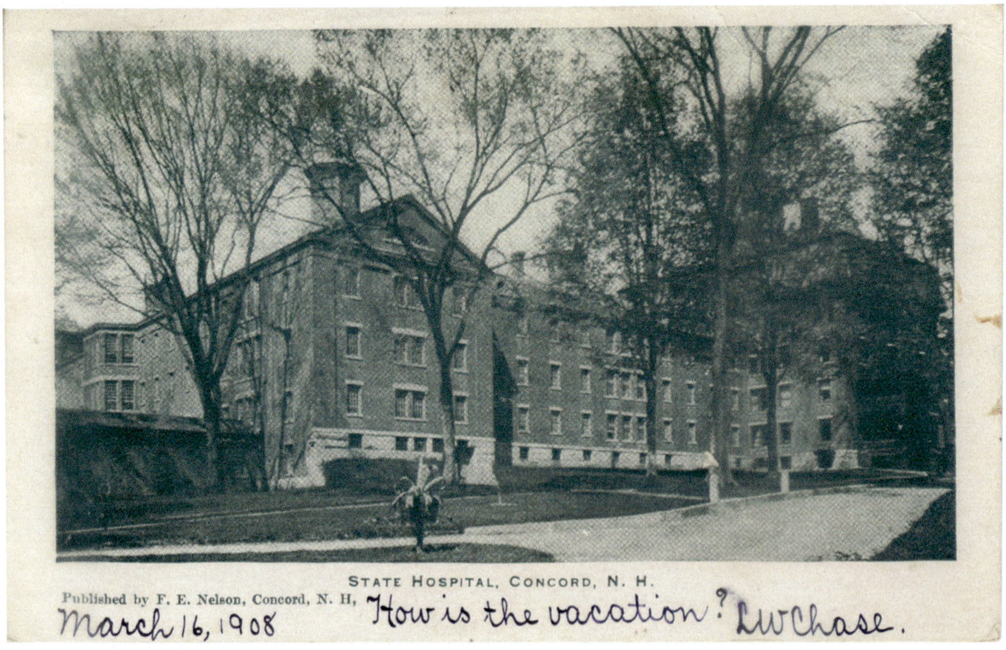

Figure 32

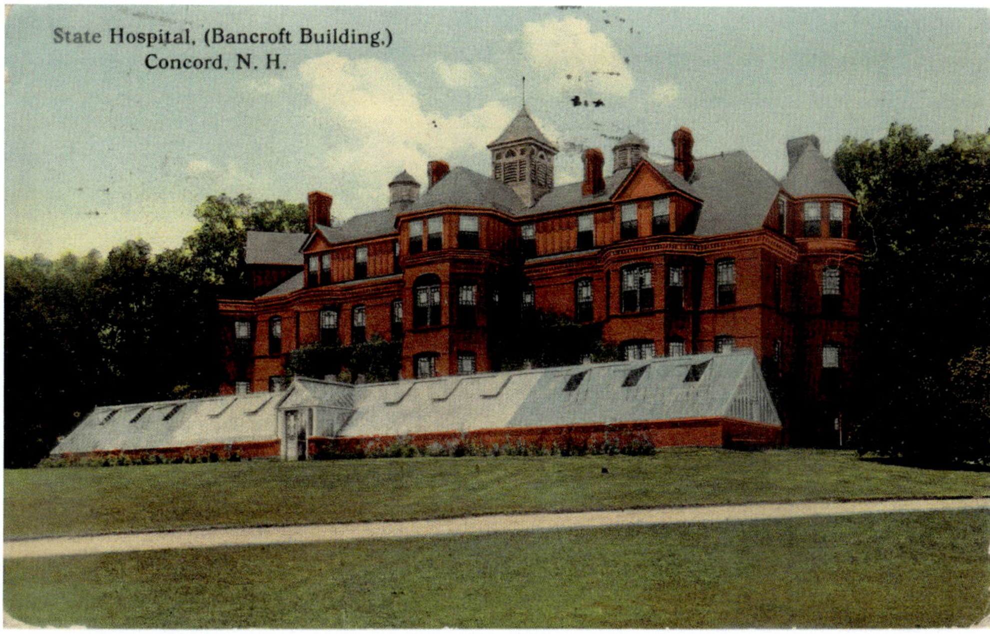
State Hospital, (Bancroft Building.)
Concord, N. H.

Figure 33

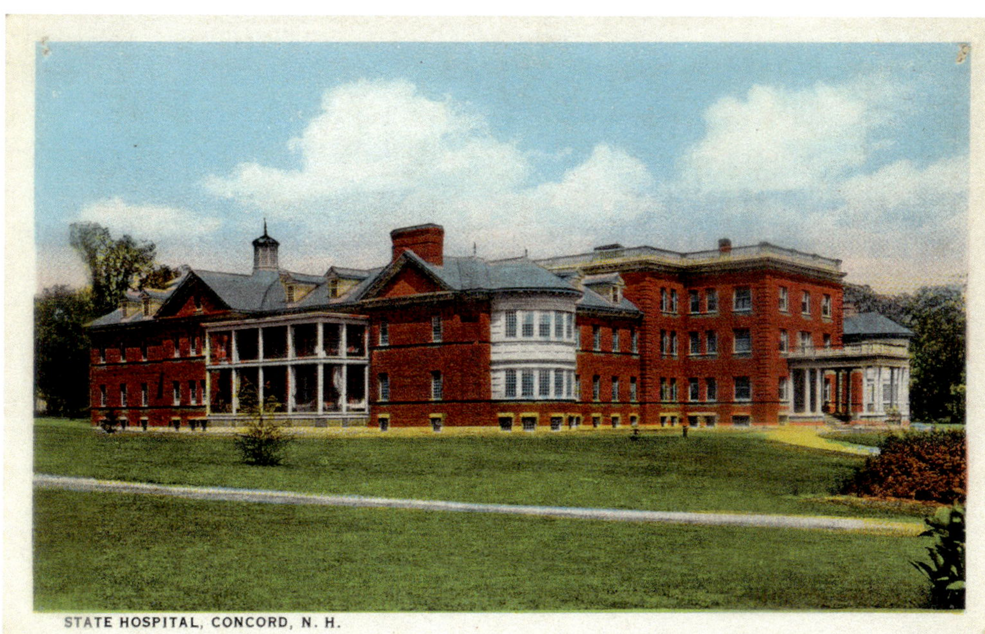
STATE HOSPITAL, CONCORD, N. H.

Figure 34

Georgia State Sanitarium
Milledgeville, Georgia, 1842

The Georgia State Sanitarium at Milledgeville first accepted patients in 1842. Initially, each county in the state was expected to financially support poor patients, but in 1846, the state began providing support for all patients.

The main building was built in 1858 and was considered to be one of the most handsome buildings in Georgia. Following the Kirkbride plan, it provided accommodations for asylum officials, individual rooms for a large number of patients in wings, and administrative offices.

Figure 35, postmarked 1907, provides a rare message from a patient. The patient notes that she has marked her cell with an "x", visible in the dome of the building. She then noted, "I am so bad at times, they had to put me off to myself. I can get the beautiful views. I'm not improving as rapidly as I expected. My visit will be prolonged." She wrote only on the front, leaving the reverse side of the card blank.

Other buildings were added to the facility over the years, including a building erected in 1898 for 40 patients to do farm work on a colony plan. In 1901, rooms for surgical operations were built as an annex to the infirmary. The postcards in figures 36 and 37 show newer buildings added. By 1929, the sanitarium was renamed Milledgeville State Hospital.

The hospital had a training school for nurses with a laboratory that opened in 1912 when there were 2,100 patients. By the mid-1900s, electroshock therapy became a common practice in many state hospitals. In 1952 a Milledgeville doctor, Peter Gordon Cranford, described the overuse of the therapy at the hospital in a book titled *But for the Grace of God*.

The hospital closed in 2012 and plans for restoration, demolition, and repurposing of several of the original buildings continue. A museum in Milledgeville houses original artifacts and documents from the hospital.

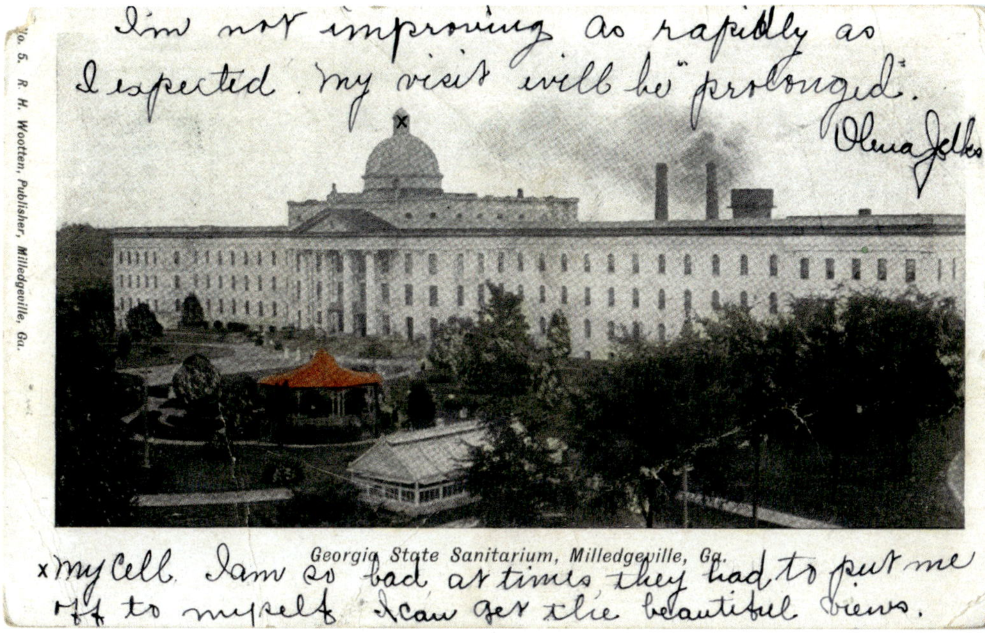

Figure 35

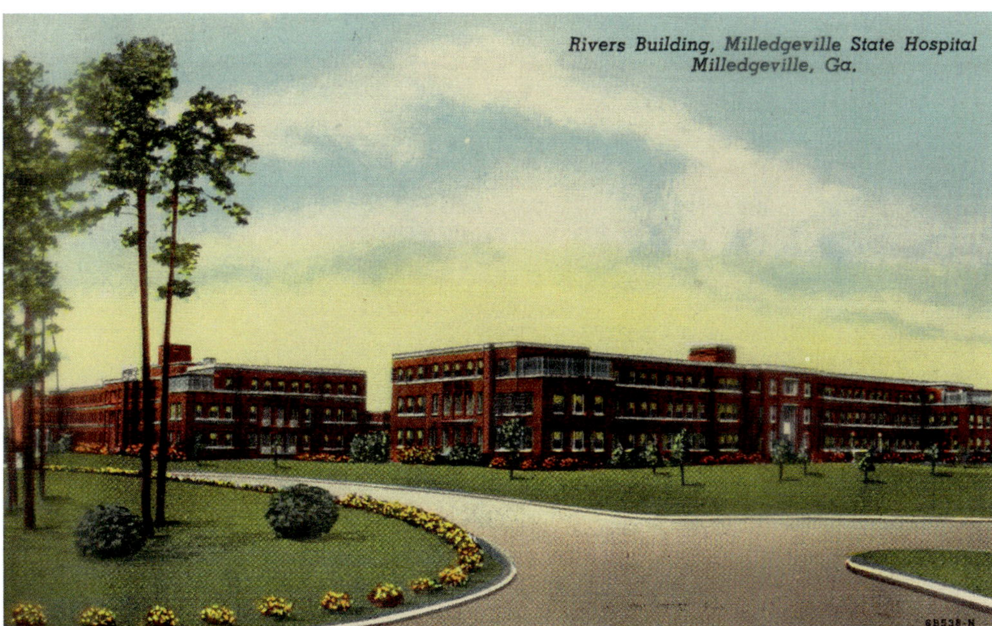

Figure 36

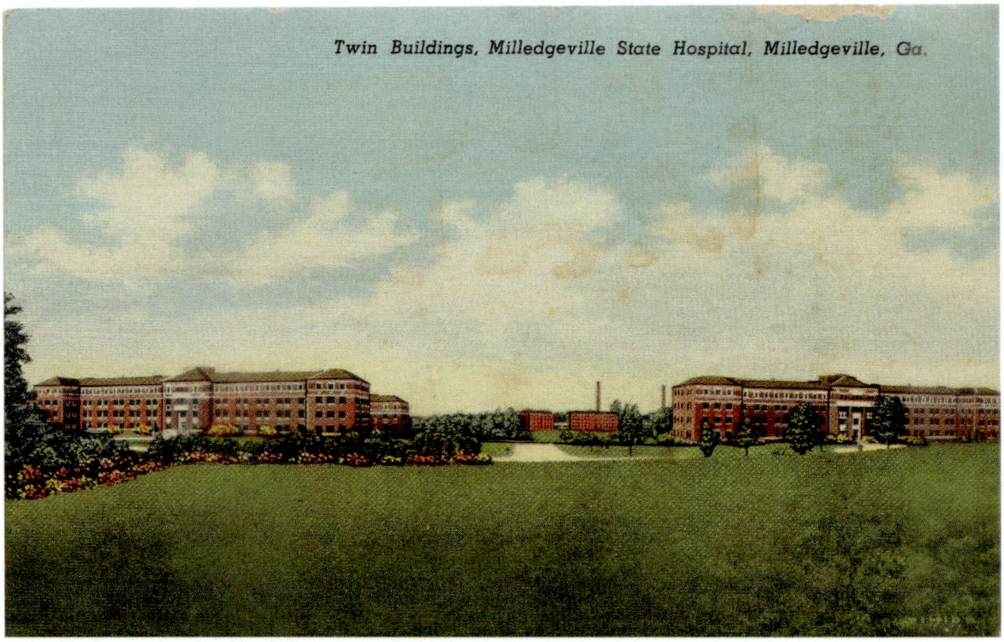
Twin Buildings, Milledgeville State Hospital, Milledgeville, Ga.

Figure 37

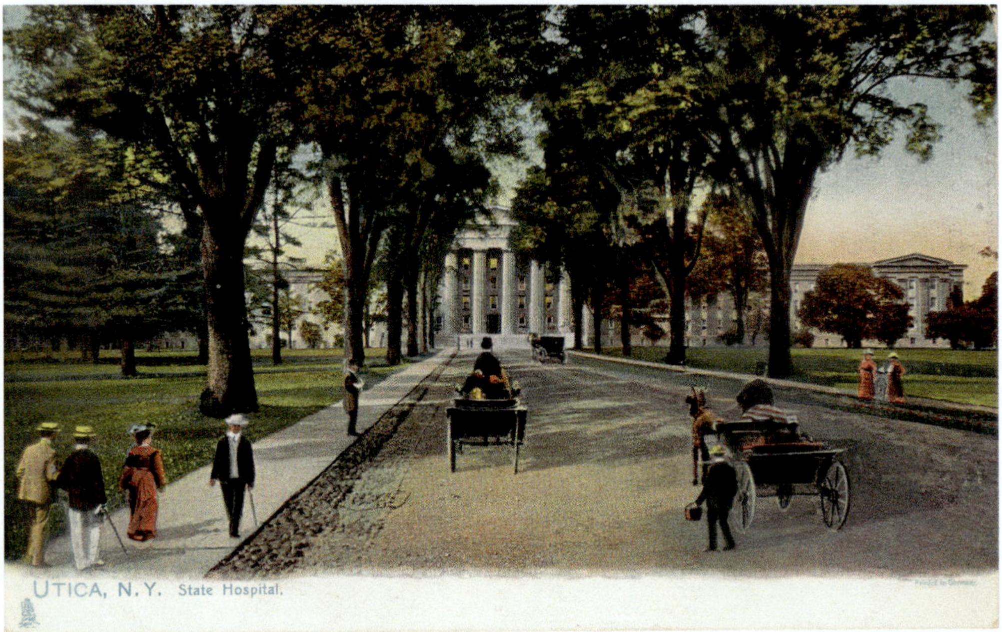
UTICA, N.Y. State Hospital.

Figure 38

Utica State Hospital
Utica, New York, 1843

Utica State Hospital first accepted patients in 1843. The act under which this hospital was organized served as a model for similar American institutions and was an important example for developing state care for the mentally ill. Citizens suffering from mental illness were to be taken out of almshouses and jails where they were frequently housed and placed instead in state hospitals. This new system of care was not achieved until 1895.

The postcard on the previous page (figure 38) provides a view of Utica's main building and entryway. The building was set on expansive grounds that included a farm and schools for both male and female patients.

The image on the top of the next page (figure 39) shows one of the original buildings. This building, characterized by Greek revival architecture, was closed in 1987. Although renovation was considered, it was replaced with a modern 250 bed facility in 1985.

Marcy State Hospital at Utica was opened in 1911 with the expectation that it would replace Utica State Hospital. However, Marcy grew to be larger than Utica. By 1985, deinstitutionalization had decreased the populations of these two institutions considerably and they were combined into one facility.

The 1920s postcard (figure 40) shows the Marcy Building. In 1983, Marcy Psychiatric Center became a medium security prison.

Utica State Hospital now operates as Mohawk Valley Psychiatric Center. The original main building, opened in 1843, has been renovated and currently serves as the home for the New York State Office of Mental Health Record and Artifact Center.

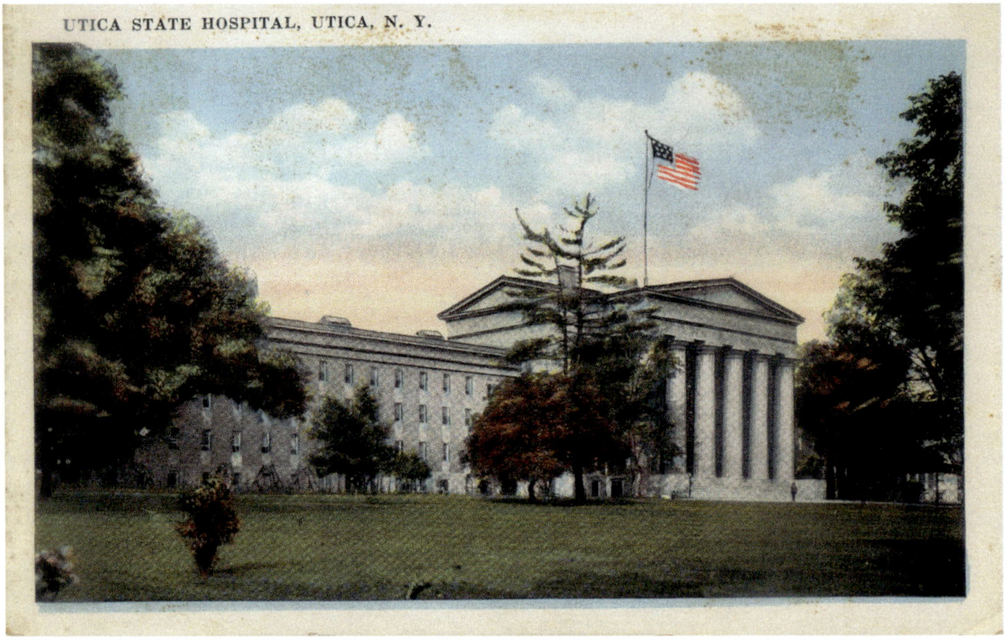

Figure 39

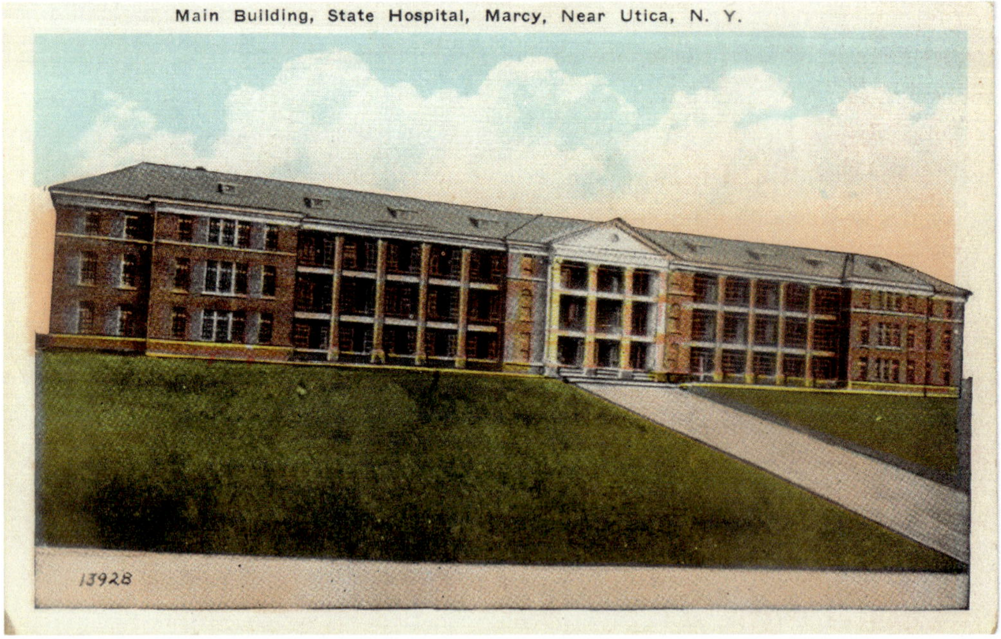

Figure 40

Indiana Hospital for the Insane
Indianapolis, Indiana, 1848

The Indiana Hospital for the Insane at Indianapolis (figure 41) first accepted patients on November 21, 1848, with a capacity of 225. Less than 10 years later, the hospital housed 300 patients.

The original buildings consisted of two main wings, one for men and one for women. In 1857, the state legislature failed to provide sufficient funds for the facility and it was closed. Patients were sent back to their counties, some to prisons and some to the poorhouse. By October, the facility was reopened.

A building for the pathological department was added in 1896 and dining rooms were added in 1899. An amusement hall and chapel were built in 1912. By 1916, the hospital (figure 42) consisted of five distinct buildings connected by corridors.

The next postcard (figure 43) shows the entrance with a guard house rather than a gate. One guard usually lived in the house.

In 1994, Central State Hospital closed. While many of the original buildings were demolished, some buildings continue to exist, including the original pathology building which has been restored and serves as a museum.

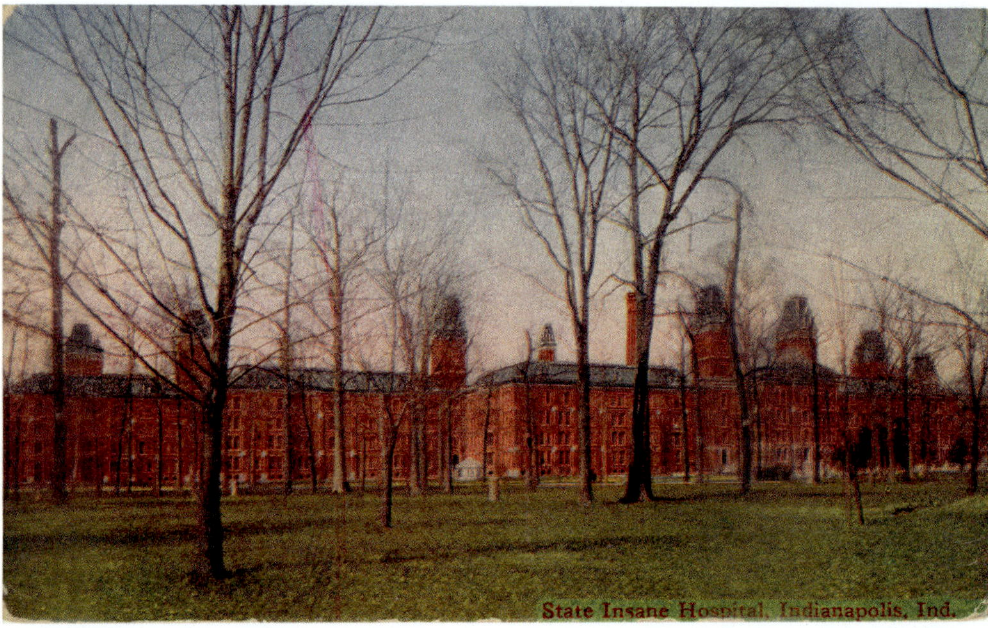

Figure 41

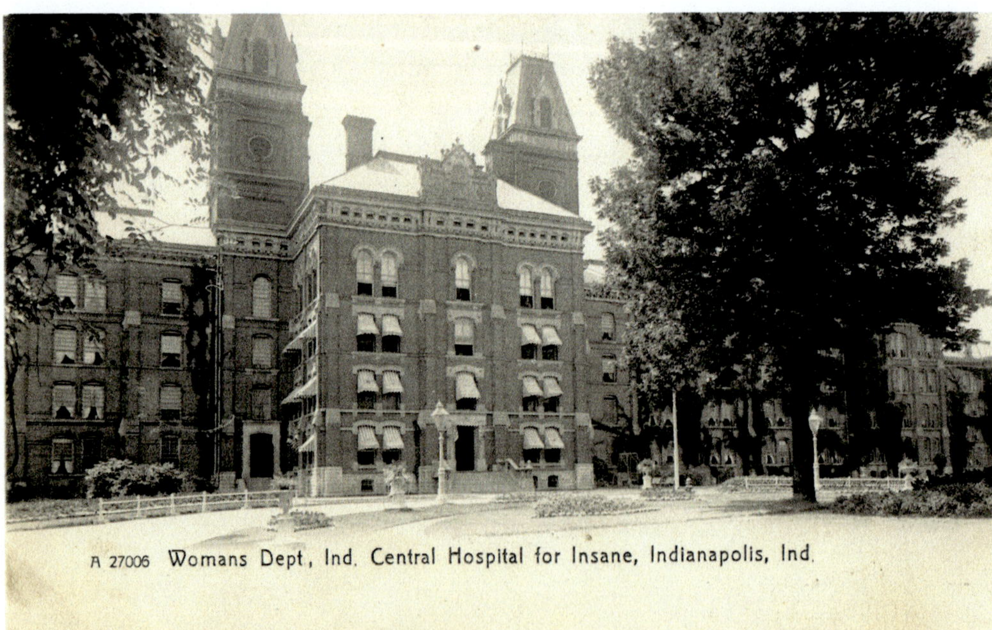

Figure 42

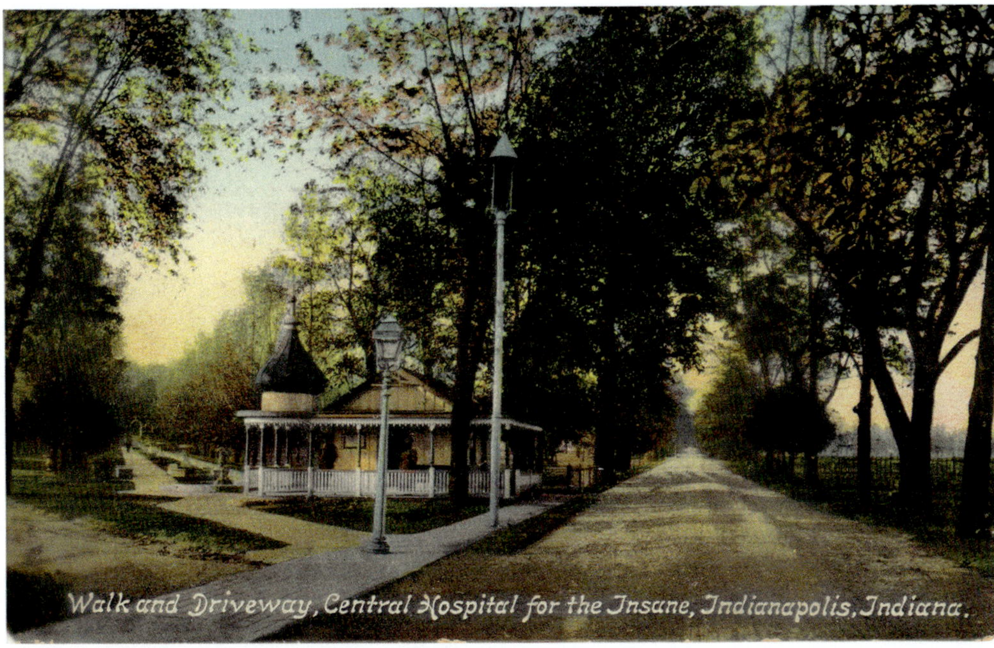
Walk and Driveway, Central Hospital for the Insane, Indianapolis, Indiana.

Figure 43

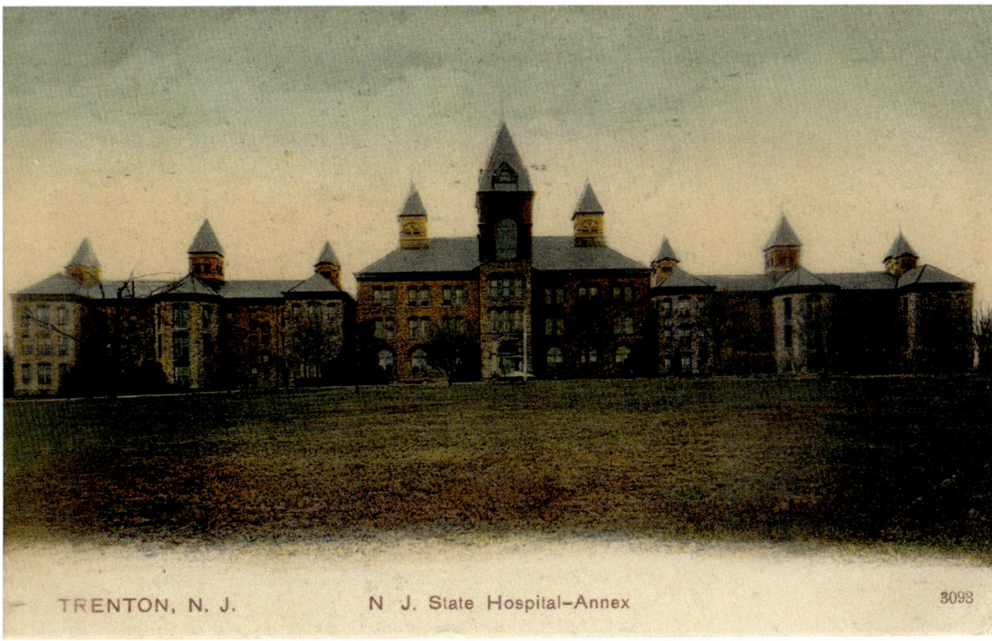
TRENTON, N. J.
N J. State Hospital-Annex
3093

Figure 44

New Jersey State Lunatic Asylum
Trenton, New Jersey, 1848

This New Jersey State Lunatic Asylum at Trenton, New Jersey started accepting patients on May 15, 1848. Dorothea Dix, an influential activist in asylum reform, was instrumental in establishing this hospital. While she influenced 22 state legislatures to establish such hospitals, she viewed this facility as her "first born child."

The postcard in figure 44 shows the main building erected to house the physicians, officers, chapel, kitchens, and six wards for 200 male and female patients. Various additions were made to accommodate more patients. Two wings were added in 1855 with room for 250 more patients. In 1893, two additions to the main building allowed a segregation of more difficult patients. By 1913, there were 1,547 patients.

For years, the criminally insane of New Jersey were confined in two state institutions: Morris Plains and Trenton. At Trenton, a detention building was opened in 1913 for the care for prisoners. The state developed a systematic program for classifying and distinguishing between criminally insane patients and mentally ill patients. An annex was added to the building for admission and classification of new cases.

A female psychopathic building for cases requiring more acute care was opened in 1914 and the male psychopathic building was added eight years later.

The postcard at the bottom of the previous page (figure 44), postmarked 1907, shows a view of the hospital.

The facility currently operates as the Trenton Psychiatric Hospital, where many of the original buildings—including a cafeteria, a firehouse, and the gatehouse—remain standing.

State Insane Asylum
Jackson, Louisiana, 1848

The original State Insane Asylum in Jackson, Louisiana consisted of a central building (figure 45) with wings extended in a linear direction on each side. The facility suffered from overcrowded conditions that were expected to be relieved as other state facilities were built. While the facility was designed to house 1,000 patients, the population had reached 1,378 by 1910.

A female physician was added to the medical staff located in the women's area of the facility. The grounds were carefully laid out in a beautiful park with exercise and baseball grounds on the west side. Additions were made to improve the facility's farm which, along with the gardens, provided patient employment. The farm supplied all of the required vegetables for the facility.

By 1912, the facility consisted of 30 brick structures on 323 acres. There were beds for 830 patients, with about 794 being occupied on a daily basis.

The facility (figure 46) included twenty cottages arranged in the form of a quadrangle and connected by covered porches or cloisters. These cottages could accommodate 1,000 patients. The general kitchen and dining rooms were included in the quadrangle while the heating plant, laundry, storerooms, and other industrial buildings were situated in the rear. The hospital had separate receiving wards for men and women that included hydrotherapy and electrical apparatus, a laboratory, and operating rooms.

The facility currently operates as the East Louisiana State Hospital. The Center Building, with its large columns characteristic of Greek revival architecture, remains and was added to the National Register of Historic Places in 1980.

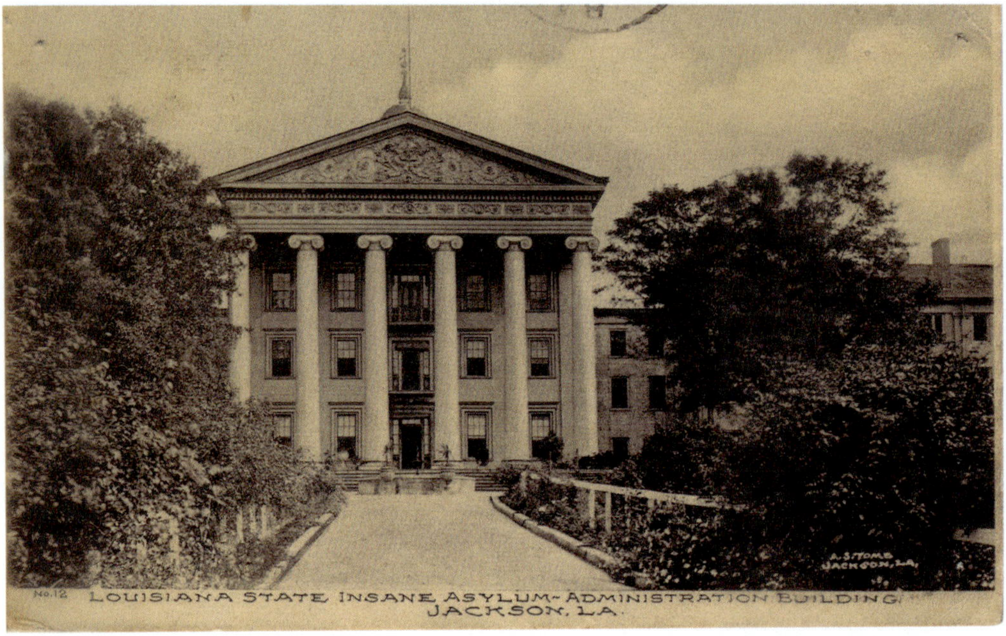

Figure 45

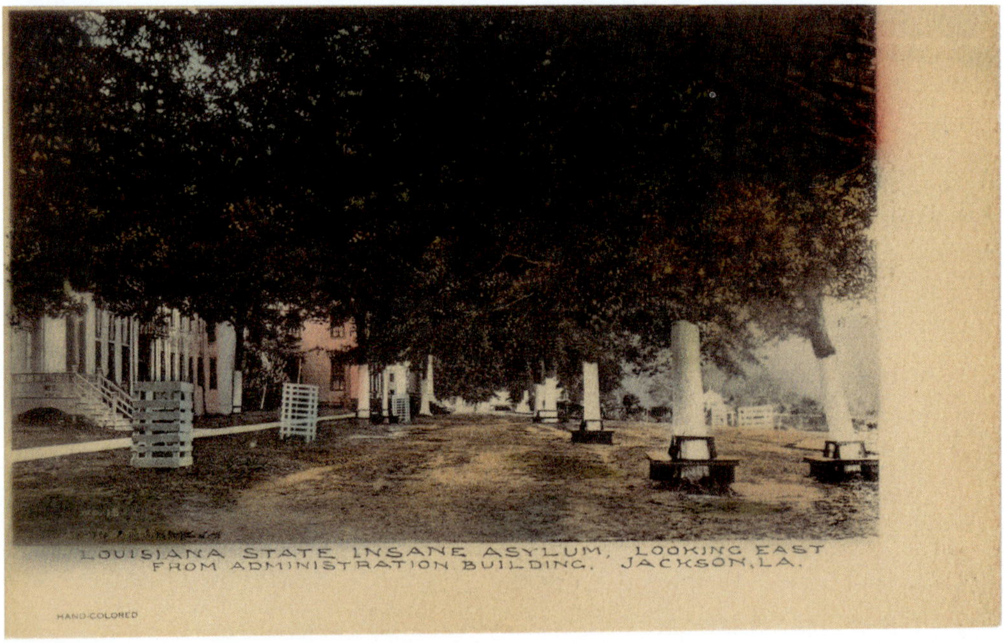

Figure 46

Pennsylvania State Lunatic Hospital and Union Asylum for the Insane
Harrisburg, Pennsylvania, 1851

Pennsylvania State Lunatic Hospital and Union Asylum for the Insane (figure 47) opened to patients in Harrisburg, Pennsylvania on October 6, 1851. In 1893, the original buildings were replaced with a series of buildings arranged on the cottage system with an administration building and about ten other buildings, all connected by corridors.

From the beginning of its history, Dorothea Dix showed an interest in the Harrisburg, Pennsylvania hospital. She had observed the "lunatics" in the area languishing in jails or wandering around without help or proper care. She visited the Pennsylvania and other state legislatures to urge the proper care and collected funds to provide a bowling alley, two buildings for reading, horses with a carriage, magic lanterns with slides, and musical instruments for this facility (figure 48).

Like other facilities, Harrisburg (figure 49) suffered early from overcrowding. By 1895, the Lunacy Committee recognized that larger buildings would not suffice. They adopted a county system plan, sending chronic patients to farm colonies. Caring for chronic patients became a source of revenue for the counties.

The backside of the postcard in figure 50, postmarked 1907, provides advertising about the facility, including its location, and boasts of it as "one of the best in the United States." This was a Tuck postcard published in England. They were considered one of the best publishers of postcards.

The postcard in figure 51 shows the entrance to the facility with an open driveway and a building that housed the guard.

In 2006, the Harrisburg State Hospital closed. Several of the buildings remain intact and have been repurposed, while others have been demolished over the years.

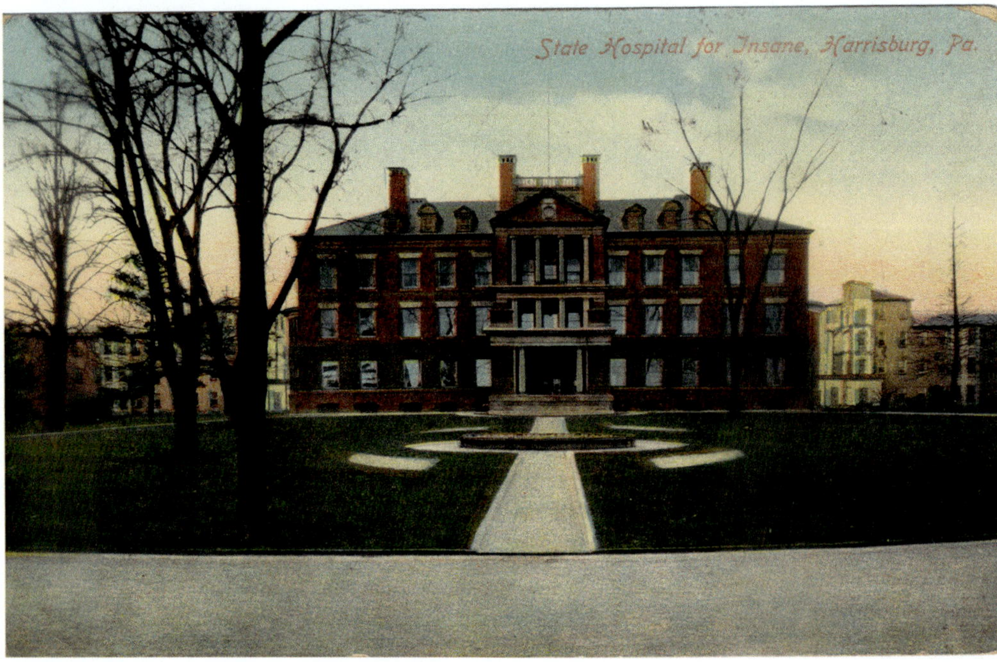
State Hospital for Insane, Harrisburg, Pa.

Figure 47

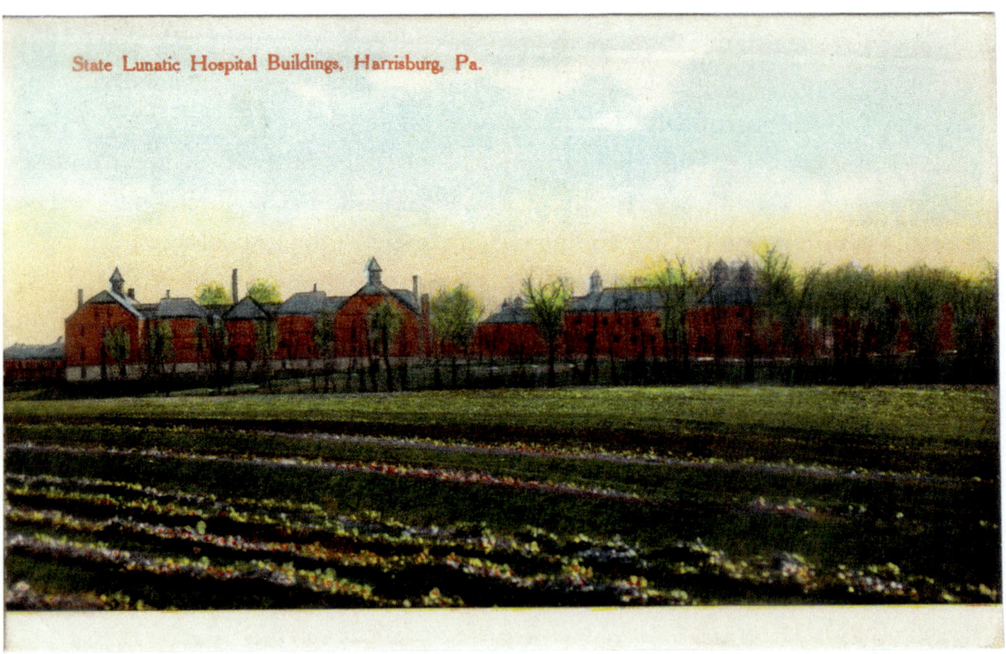
State Lunatic Hospital Buildings, Harrisburg, Pa.

Figure 48

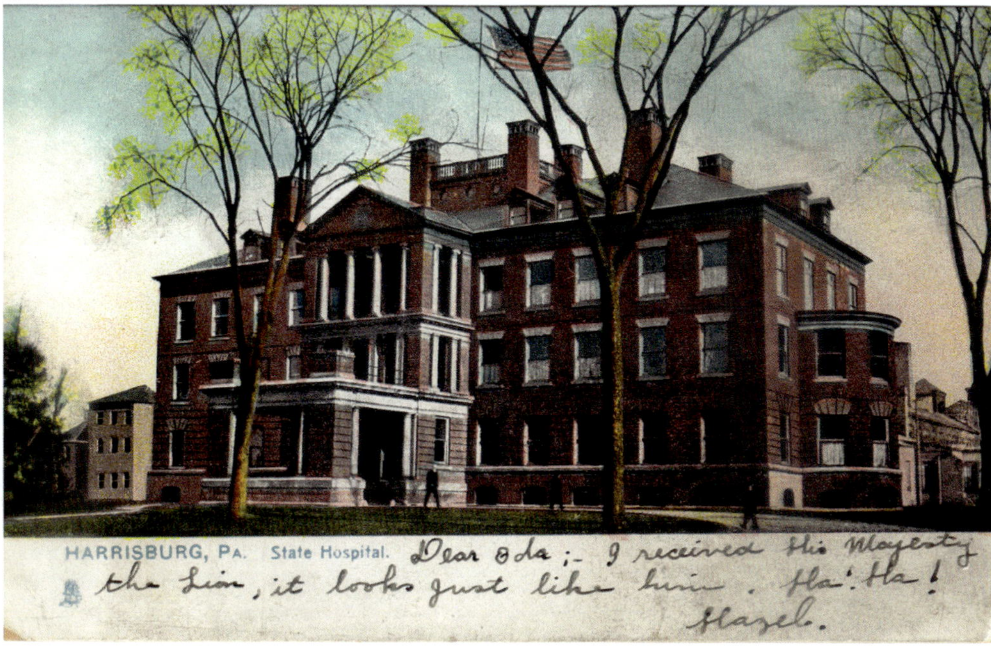
HARRISBURG, PA. State Hospital.
Dear Eda :- I received His Majesty the Lion, it looks just like him. Ha! Ha!
Hazel.

Figure 49

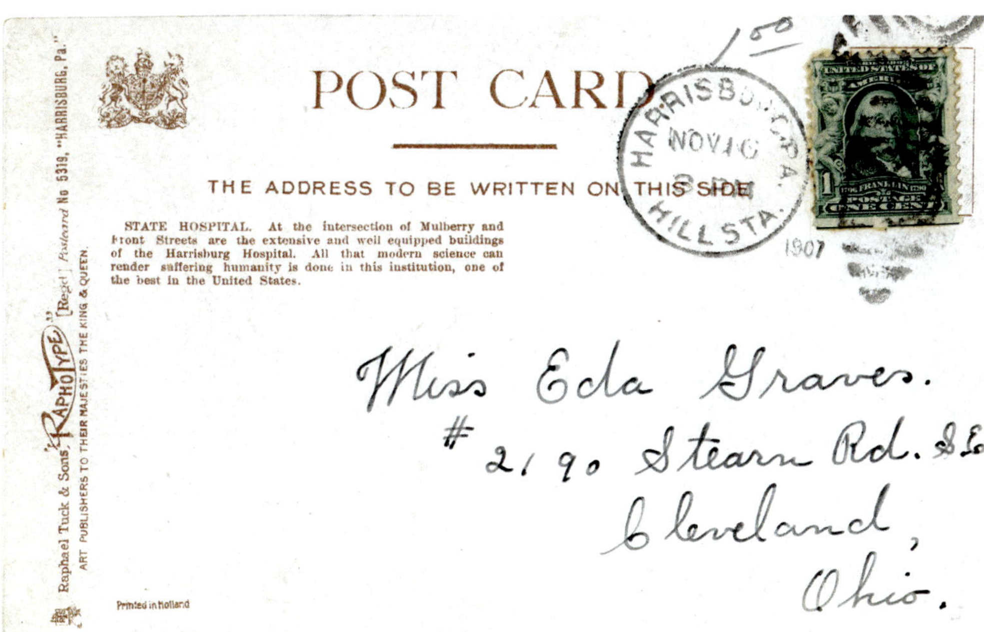

Figure 50

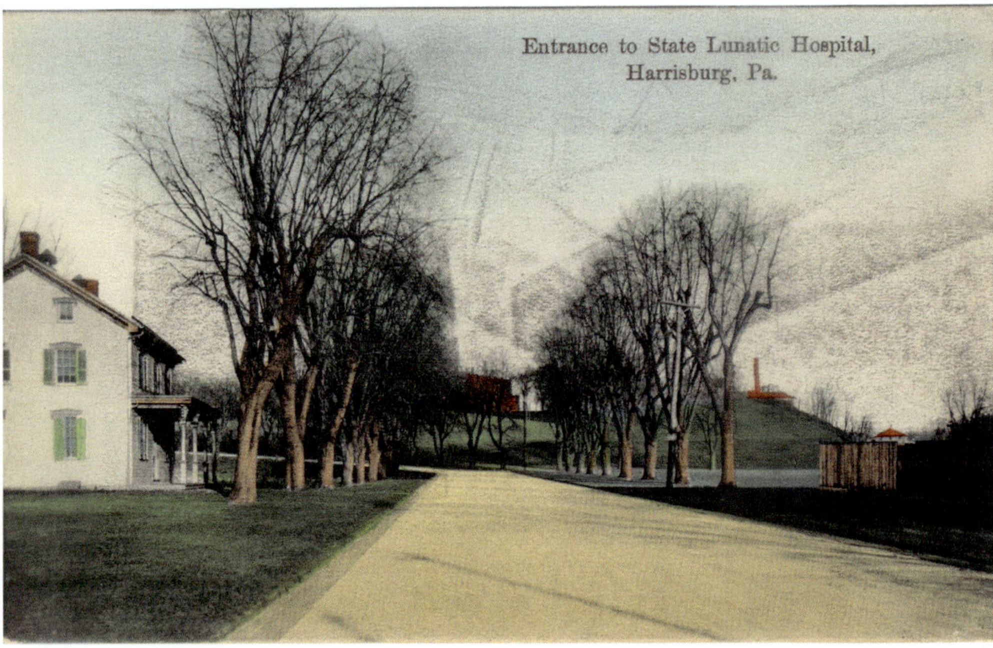
Entrance to State Lunatic Hospital,
Harrisburg, Pa.

Figure 51

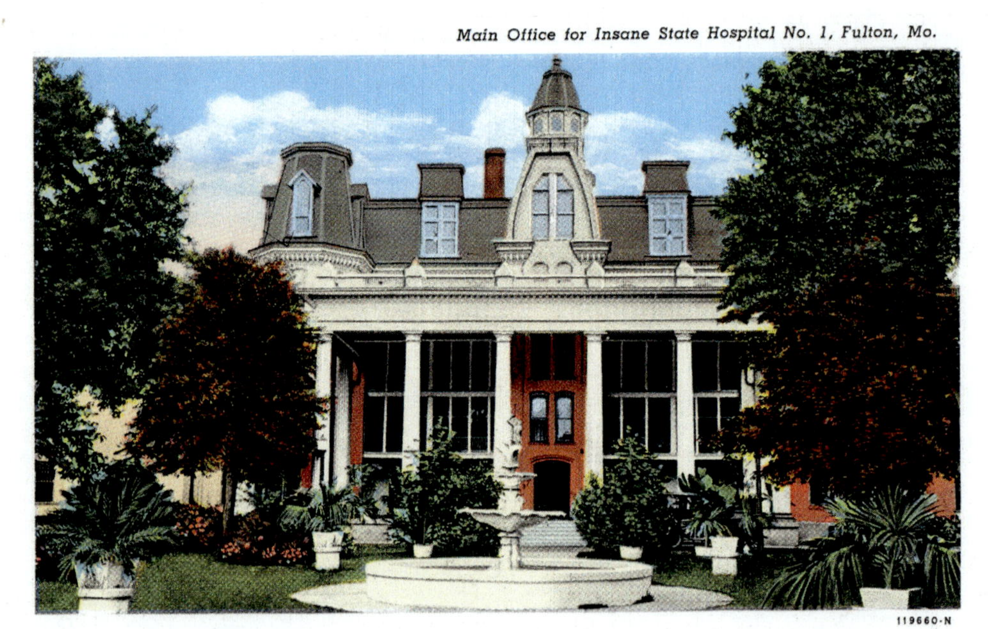
Main Office for Insane State Hospital No. 1, Fulton, Mo.
119660-N

Figure 52

Missouri State Lunatic Asylum,
Fulton, Missouri, 1851

Opened in 1851 as the Missouri State Lunatic Asylum, the original home of this facility consisted of a four-story brick structure with porticos in the front of the building supported by massive columns. The front portion was used by the officers of the institution while the rear of the administration building was used as the dining rooms for men and women. The sleeping rooms were in the wings on either side of the administration building.

By 1912, the census for the asylum had reached 1,027. A training school for nurses was established and a building for tubercular patients was completed. Movies were shown weekly and patients worked on the farm or on the grounds doing industrial work.

The original building was destroyed by fire in 1956. When a postcard of that building was found (figure 52), a copy was sent to that facility around 1990. It was their only picture of that building since all their early pictures had burned in the fire.

This facility (figure 53), later named the Fulton State Hospital, continued to grow throughout the twentieth century and continues to operate under this name today.

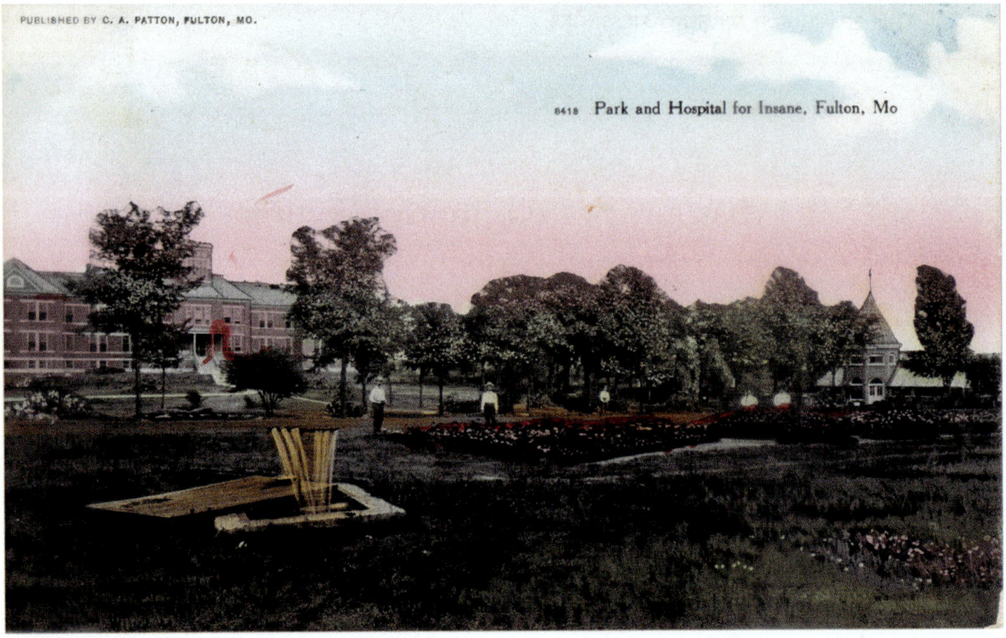
PUBLISHED BY C. A. PATTON, FULTON, MO.
8418 Park and Hospital for Insane, Fulton, Mo

Figure 53

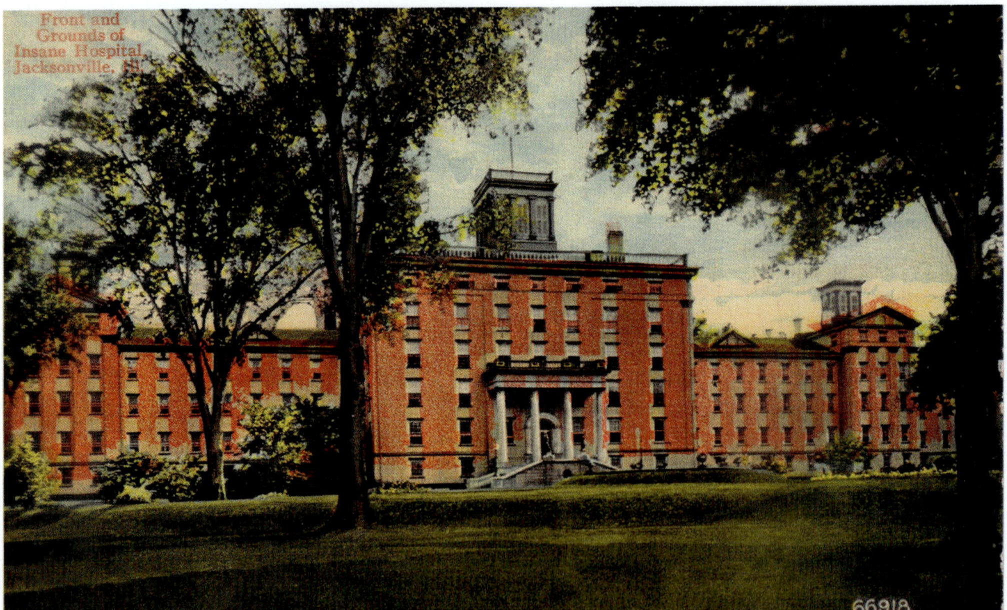
Front and
Grounds of
Insane Hospital,
Jacksonville, Ill.
66918

Figure 54

Illinois State Hospital for the Insane
Jacksonville, Illinois, 1851

The Illinois State Hospital for the Insane opened in 1851, after Dorothea Dix made a public appeal to the Illinois legislature. The facility (figure 54), located four miles from Jacksonville on 160 acres of land, was the first state-sponsored institution in Illinois.

When the facility opened, only two of the wards were completed for the 138 patients that were received. Seven years later, the population had risen to 229 cases. A new west wing was added in 1857. The east wing was completed in 1867, providing accommodations for 450 patients. By 1874, the hospital was crowded, housing 20 percent more patients than were permitted for by its allotted capacity. Two new wings for 75 patients each were completed in 1880 and the number of patients increased to 534. A one-story tubercular hospital was also added.

Efforts were made for the employment and amusement of patients. A paint shop and broom shop provided work for many of the patients.

The hospital underwent several name changes before finally closing as the Jacksonville Mental Health and Developmental Center in 2012. The majority of the original buildings, including the Kirkbride building pictured here, have been demolished.

Insane Asylum of California
Stockton, California, 1851

The Insane Asylum of California in Stockton (figure 55) opened in 1853, shortly after the gold rush created a significant rise in the state's population.

The original buildings consisted of a women's building, a men's building (figure 56), and an administration office, all within one-third of a mile of each other. A receiving building accepted all new patients and also housed a space for hydrotherapy treatment. By 1915, the population of the hospital consisted of 1,256 males and 799 females for a total of 2,155 patients. There were 262 officers and employees.

In the fall and winter months, dances were held weekly and were accompanied by moving pictures. Patients participated in many industrial activities, including working in the shoe shop where all shoes and slippers for the hospital were made. Other industries included mattress-making and broom-making. The hospital also included a herd of 118 cows, producing an average of 7,500 gallons of milk per month.

The hospital grounds (figure 57) included lush lawns and gardens.

The medical superintendent and associate physicians were housed in dwellings (figure 58) situated on the main avenue.

Stockton State Hospital closed in 1996. Nearly all of the original buildings have been demolished or destroyed by fire. The superintendent's home, built in 1900, still survives. The site is currently occupied by California State University.

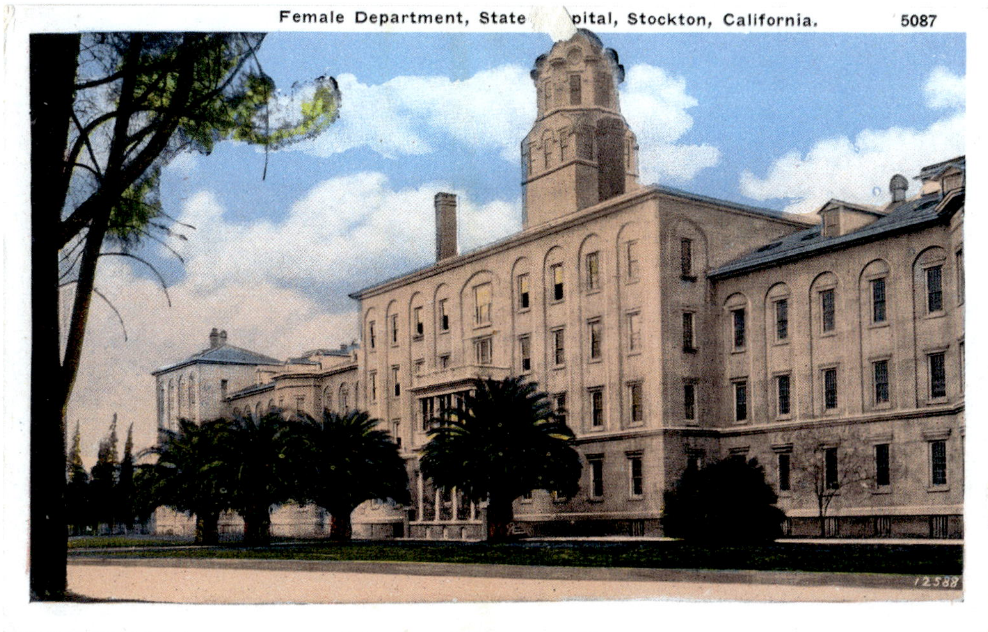
Female Department, State pital, Stockton, California.
5087
12588

Figure 55

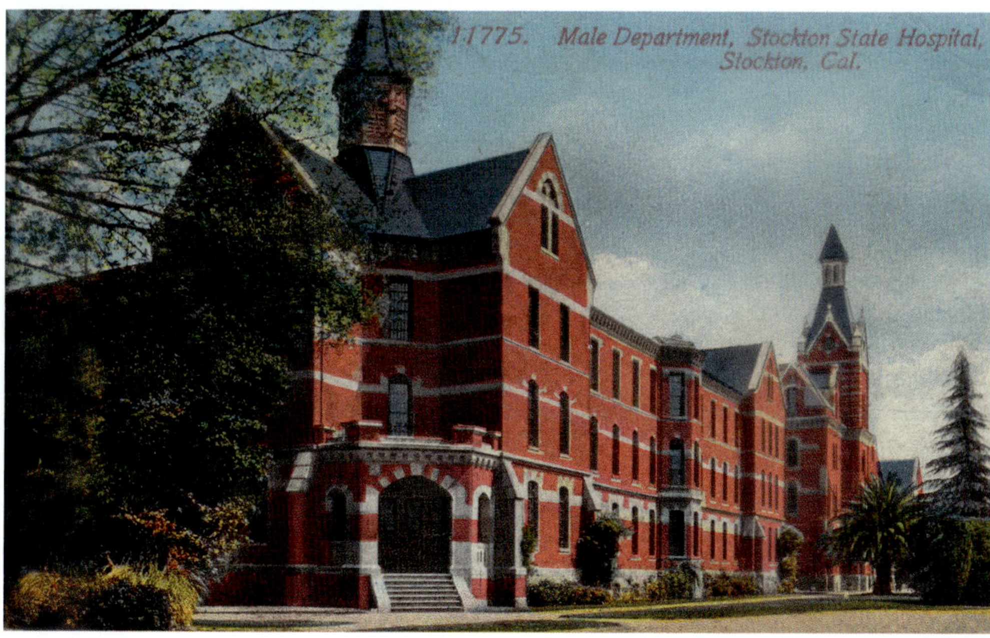
1775. Male Department, Stockton State Hospital, Stockton, Cal.

Figure 56

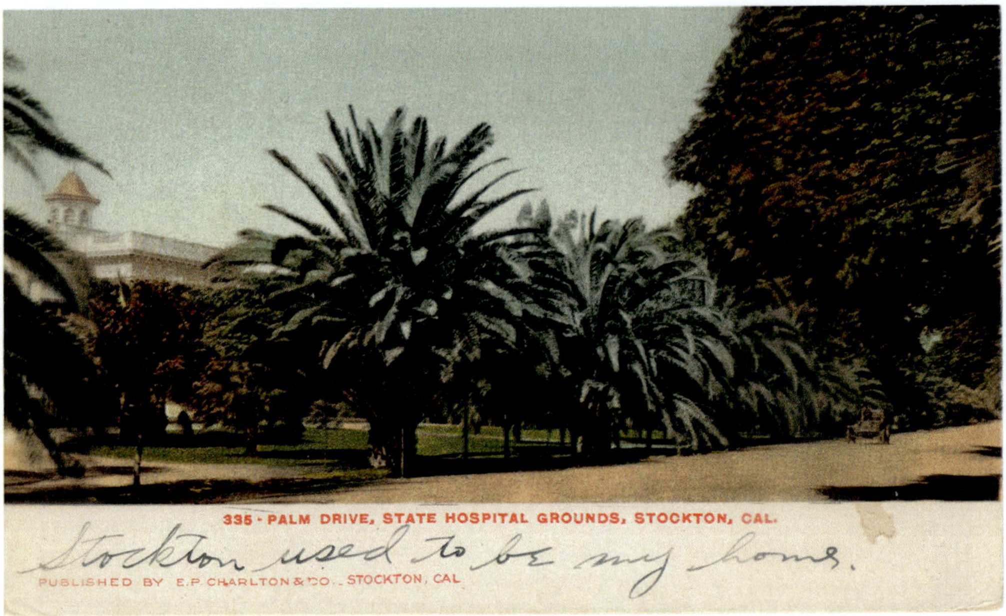
335 - PALM DRIVE, STATE HOSPITAL GROUNDS, STOCKTON, CAL.
Stockton used to be my home.
PUBLISHED BY E.P. CHARLTON & CO., STOCKTON, CAL

Figure 57

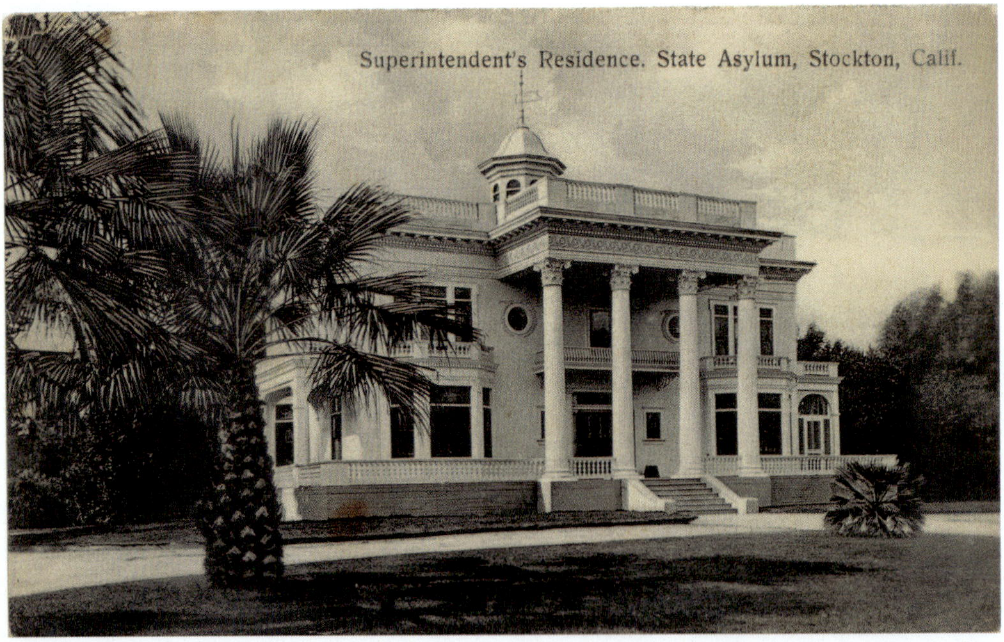
Superintendent's Residence. State Asylum, Stockton, Calif.

Figure 58

Taunton Insane Hospital
Taunton, Massachusetts, 1854

The Taunton Insane Hospital opened in 1854 as the second state-supported facility for the mentally ill in Massachusetts.

The original hospital (figure 59) was expected to accommodate 250 patients. The facility included 42 rooms designed to restrain violent patients. However, these rooms were never used because the first superintendent argued against them and argued in favor of the use of wards for these patients. In 1892, a male and female infirmary building was added and a training school for nurses was established in 1894. Furthermore, a farm colony was added in 1899.

A home for female nurses was built in 1902 and a home for male nurses was built in 1904. The building for male nurses included 12 rooms for married couples and is thought to be the building in figure 60.

The Taunton State Hospital remains open with new facilities, though there are plans to close the institution. All of the original buildings were demolished, destroyed by fire, or decayed over the years.

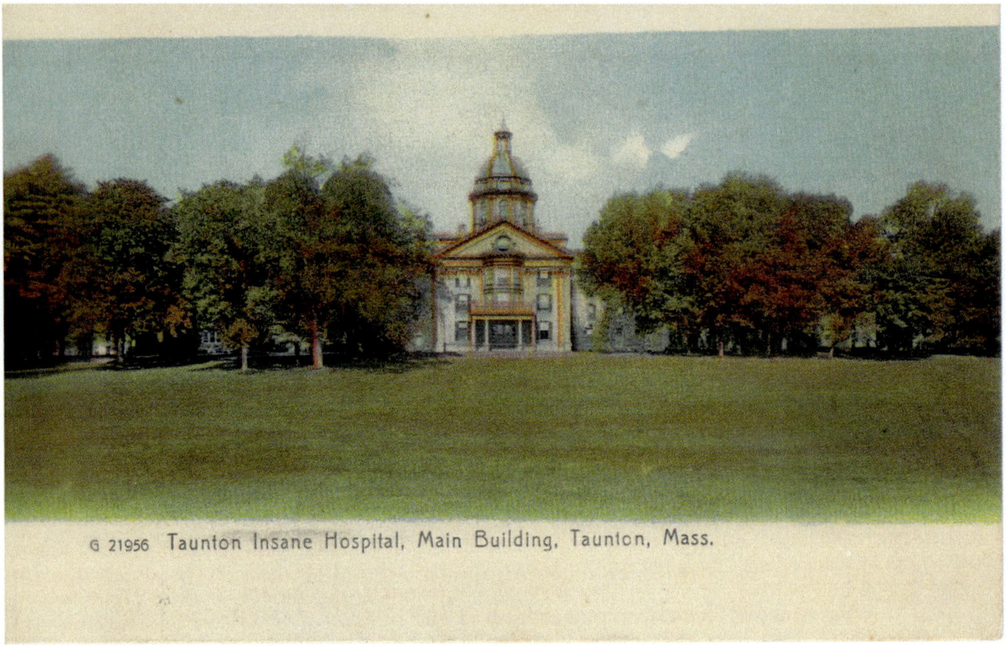

Figure 59

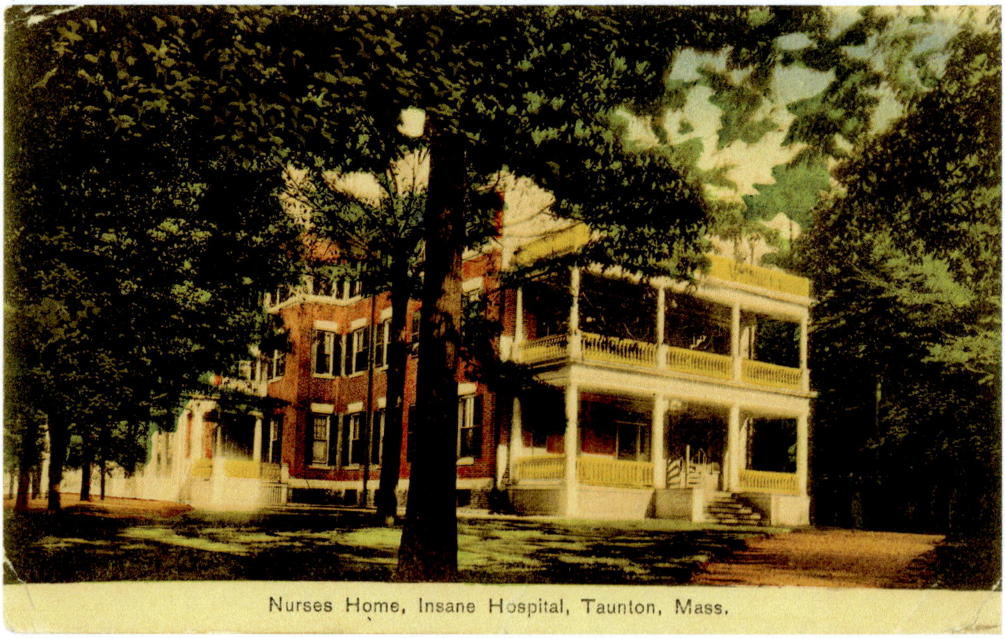

Figure 60

Western Lunatic Asylum
Hopkinsville, Kentucky, 1854

The Western Lunatic Asylum opened in 1854 two miles east of Hopkinsville, admitting 113 patients in the first year. This institution was the second to be erected in the state of Kentucky. It was situated in the western part of the state to reduce overcrowding at other state hospitals and to accommodate the counties of that district. The original 370-acre site was expanded to 727 acres by the purchase of two adjoining farms.

The facility (figure 61) accommodated all classes of insane, including "criminal," "epileptic," and "dangerous idiots" (Report, 1873). Wards were arranged as large hallways with individual rooms on the sides, along with two small dormitories. Each ward had its own dining room, supplied from a central kitchen. The original buildings accommodated 350 patients. After a fire in 1860, the main building had to be completely rebuilt.

By 1912, the arrangement of the buildings consisted of a main building with two wings, comprising four extensions at right angles to each other, four stories high to accommodate 800 patients. Six additional cottages and a colony accommodated 400 more patients. The main building (figure 62) was equipped with a hydrotherapeutic apparatus, shower, tub, and continuous baths.

This facility continues to exist as Western State Hospital and much of the campus is comprised of many of the original buildings.

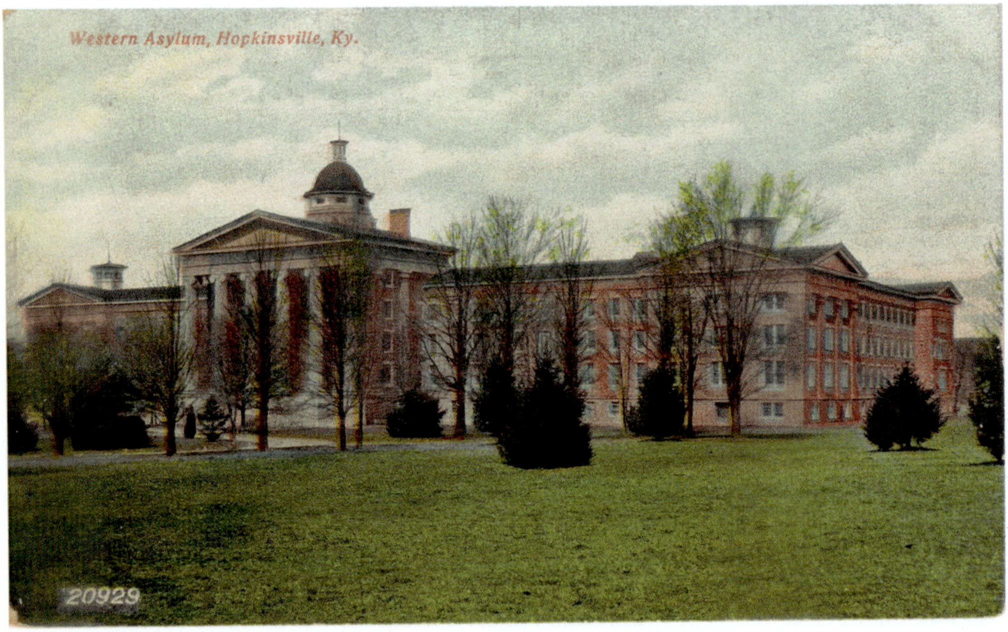

Figure 61

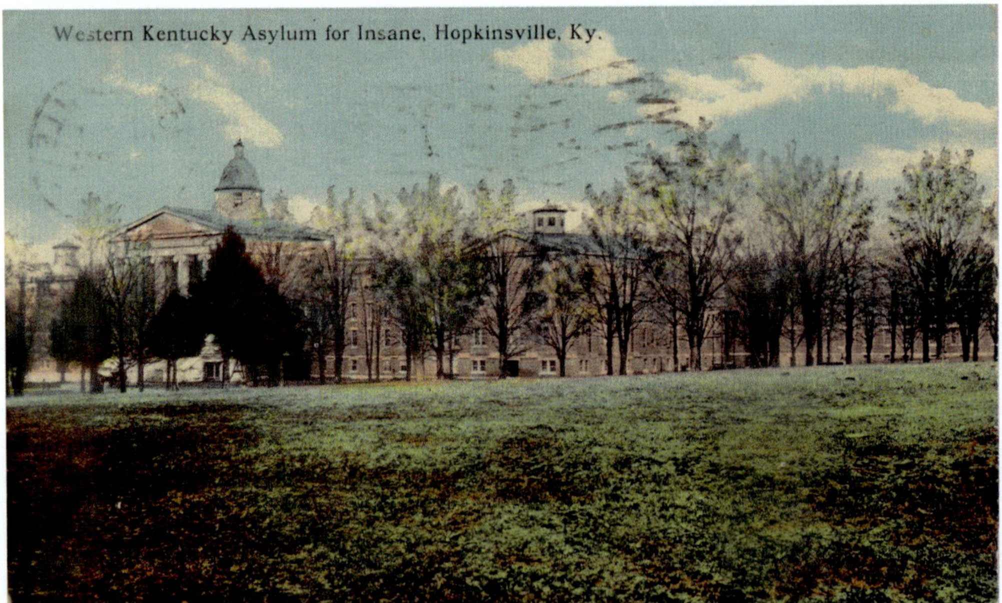

Figure 62

Northern Ohio Lunatic Asylum
Cleveland, Ohio, 1855

This Northern Ohio Lunatic Asylum, later named the Cleveland State Hospital, was opened in 1855 with a capacity of 100 beds. It had increased to 300 when it was almost destroyed by fire in 1872. The facility was rebuilt by 1875. By 1893, two cottages for convalescent patients were added, with each cottage housing 80 patients. By 1912, the hospital had a capacity of 1,300, but cared for over 1,600 patients.

In 1897, the amusement hall was remodeled and converted into a dining hall with a capacity of 600. This same year, a chapel and amusement hall were constructed with a capacity of 800. A training school was established for nurses in 1891 and in 1907, an industrial building was erected with a machine shop in the basement and a carpenter's shop on the first floor. The second floor housed 14 double rooms for outside help. The grounds consisted of 83 acres that included a baseball field, lily ponds, and flowering plants grown in the hospital greenhouse.

The postcard in figure 63 is the only postcard that was identified as part of the Cleveland State Hospital.

Cleveland State Hospital became the Cleveland Developmental Center in 1975. The Center closed in 1987 and none of the original structures have survived.

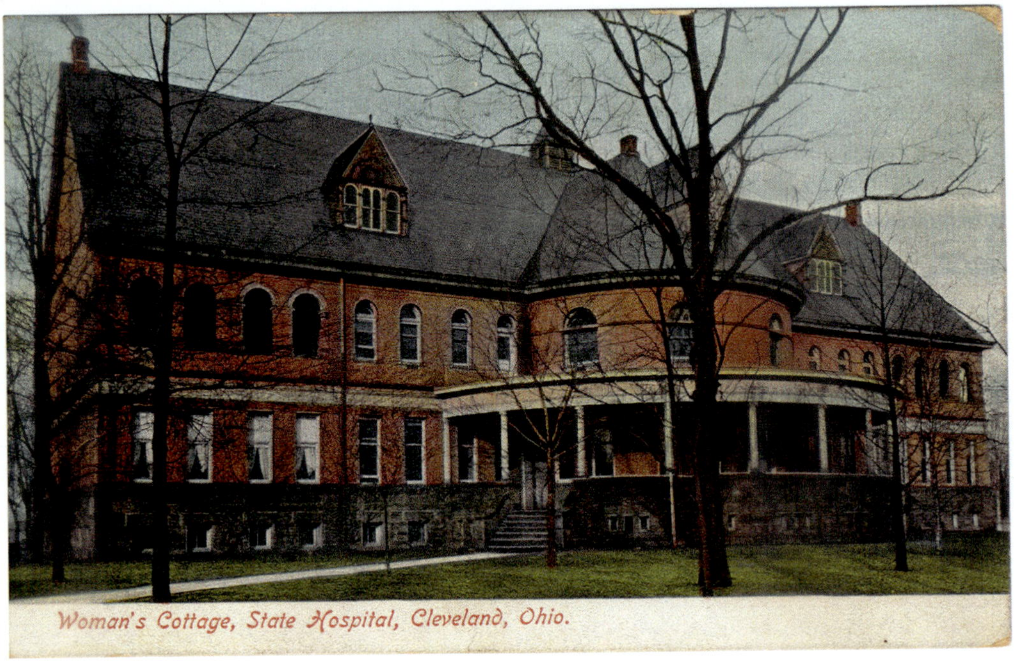
Woman's Cottage, State Hospital, Cleveland, Ohio.

Figure 63

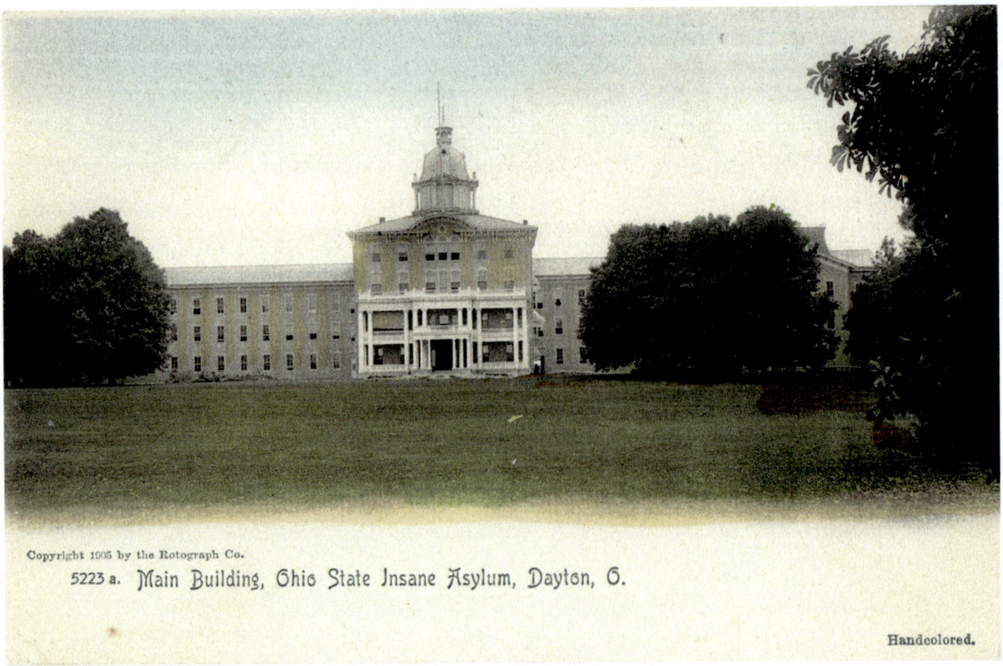
Copyright 1905 by the Rotograph Co.
5223 a. Main Building, Ohio State Insane Asylum, Dayton, O.
Handcolored.

Figure 64

Ohio State Insane Asylum
Dayton, Ohio, 1855

This Ohio State Insane Asylum in Dayton, Ohio was opened in 1855 under the name of the Southern Ohio Lunatic Asylum. It was one of two asylums (the other located in Cleveland) opened in Ohio after the first asylum in Columbus became overcrowded. The name was later changed to the Dayton State Hospital.

The 1910 picture on the bottom of the previous page (figure 64) shows the administrative building, one of the Kirkbride buildings that underwent a variety of additions and renovations over time.

By 1914, there were 20 wards for patients, an amusement hall and chapel, and four detached cottages.

The facility was a small city of about 1,400 patients and staff. It conducted its own farming operation that provided congenial and healthful labor for the patients.

This hospital was located in a beautiful park containing 50 acres of lawn, ornamental trees, and artificial lakes (figure 65).

The facility, which later became known as the Dayton Mental Health Center, is now closed. Most of the original buildings of this facility were demolished, but the main building has been preserved and currently serves as a retirement home.

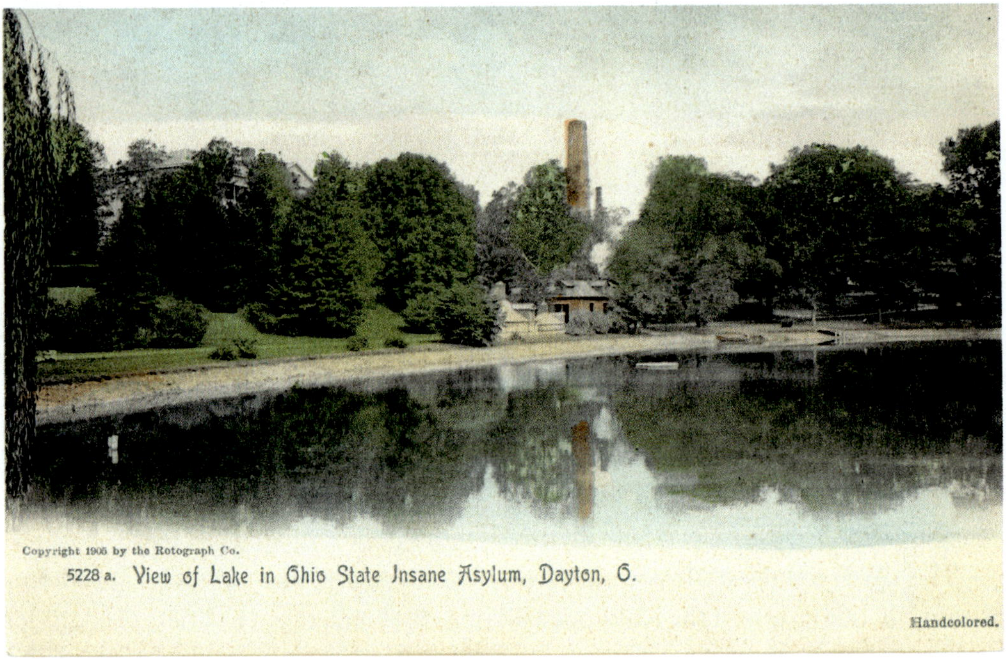
Copyright 1905 by the Rotograph Co.
5228 a. View of Lake in Ohio State Insane Asylum, Dayton, O.
Handcolored.

Figure 65

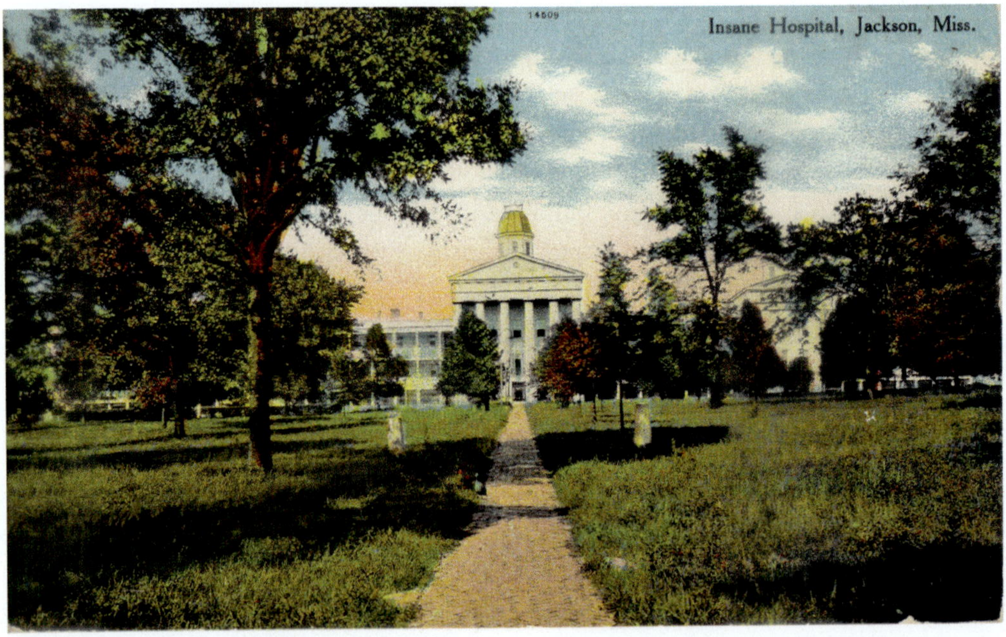
14809
Insane Hospital, Jackson, Miss.

Figure 66

Mississippi State Lunatic Asylum
Jackson, Mississippi, 1856

The Mississippi State Lunatic Asylum, opened in 1855, was located on about 140 acres of land approximately two miles from Jackson, Mississippi. Dorothea Dix appeared before the legislature to secure funds for the facility (figure 66).

In 1892, the administration building was rebuilt due to a fire. The postcard pictured in figure 67 is thought to be of the second regeneration of the building.

It is important to note that this institution began admitting black patients during the reconstruction period. The capacity of the institution was 830 patients, and before 1900, nearly 400 of the institution's patients were black.

The rare postcard in figure 68, sent in 1909, shows a collage of images of buildings in Jackson, Mississippi, including the Mississippi Lunatic Asylum. This postcard illustrated the importance of each facility to the city, including the asylum.

In 1935, the institution moved to the southeast city of Whitfield, Mississippi and a new facility was established based on the cottage plan. The Kirkbride building at the original location was demolished and the site was developed for the University of Mississippi Medical Center. The hospital, with the cottage-style buildings, continues to operate at the Whitfield location.

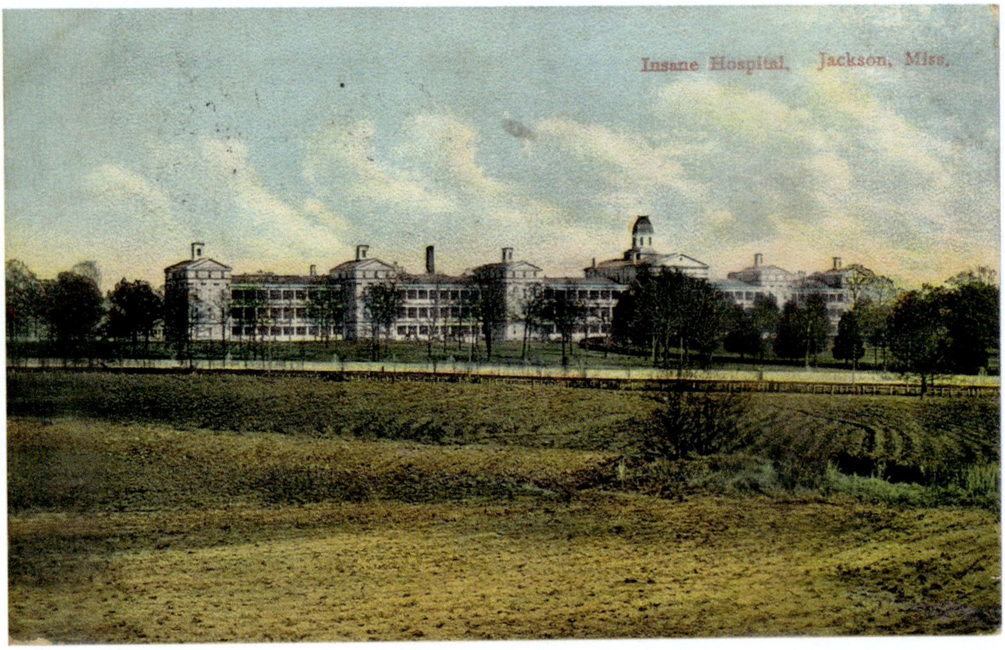

Figure 67

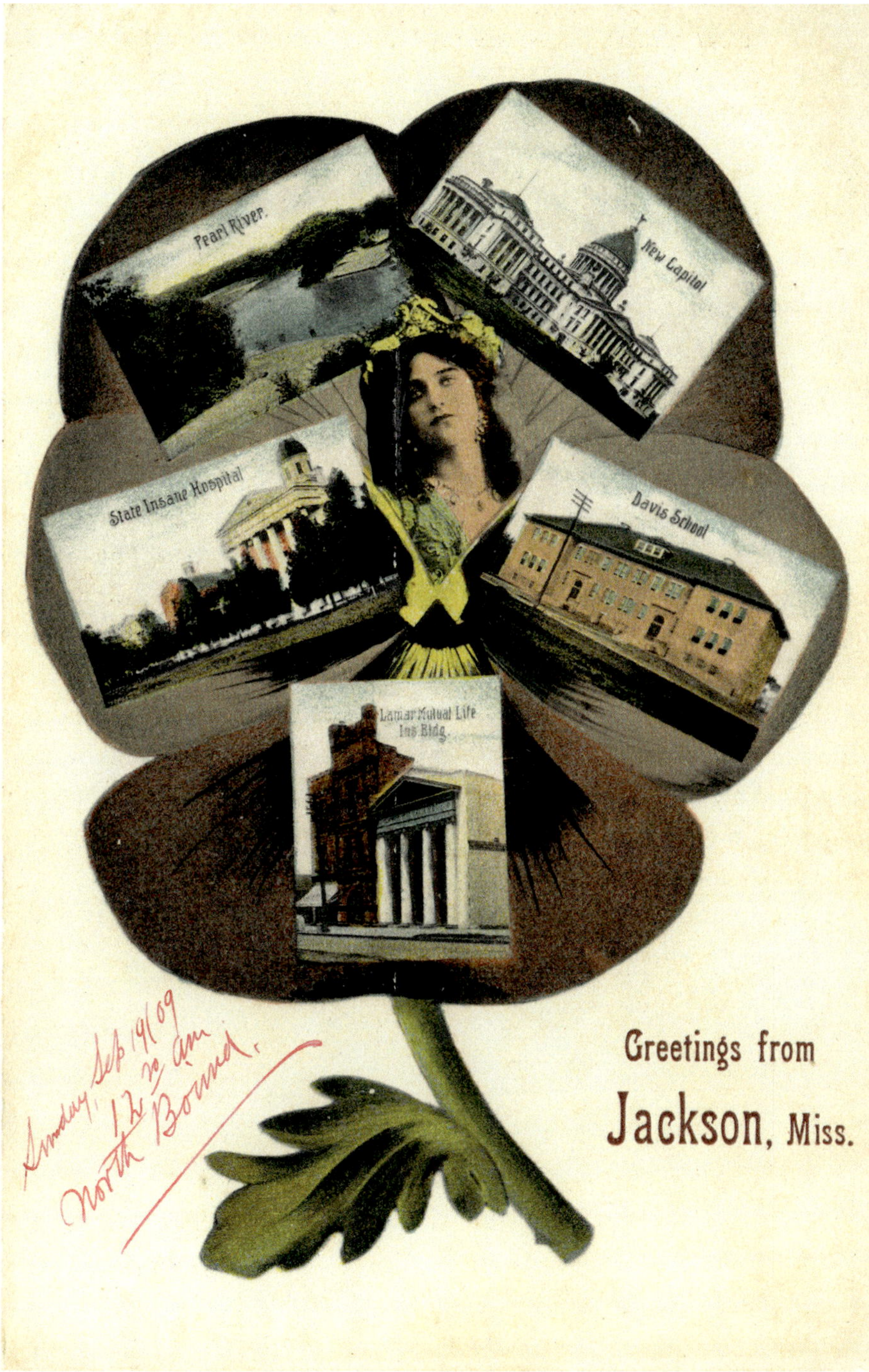
Pearl River.
New Capitol
State Insane Hospital
Davis School
Lamar Mutual Life Ins Bldg.
Greetings from
Jackson, Miss.
Sunday, Sep 19/09
12 20 am
North Bound.

Figure 68

Insane Hospital of North Carolina
Raleigh, North Carolina, 1856

The Insane Hospital of North Carolina accepted its first patient in 1856, after much lobbying by Dorothea Dix. The facility included a large central section with wings on either side. The central building (figure 69) included living spaces for the medical staff on the second floor and the wings served as patient wards. The building consisted of three stories with the third floor being used as an amusement hall. The building was the first public building in Raleigh to use steam heating and gas lighting. Two other buildings on the grounds housed the laundry, a kitchen, a bakery, and staff apartments.

The postcard in figure 70 shows a side view of the buildings.

By 1912, there were 1,114 patients in the facility with 58 attendants and 15 buildings. Chronic and acute cases were housed together. The original building and wards were destroyed by fire in 1926. Patients were housed in the four undamaged wards, sent to nearby institutions, or temporarily returned to live with relatives or friends until the facility could be rebuilt.

The facility, later named Dorothea Dix Hospital, was closed in 2012 and sold to the city of Raleigh, where it is now used as a city park.

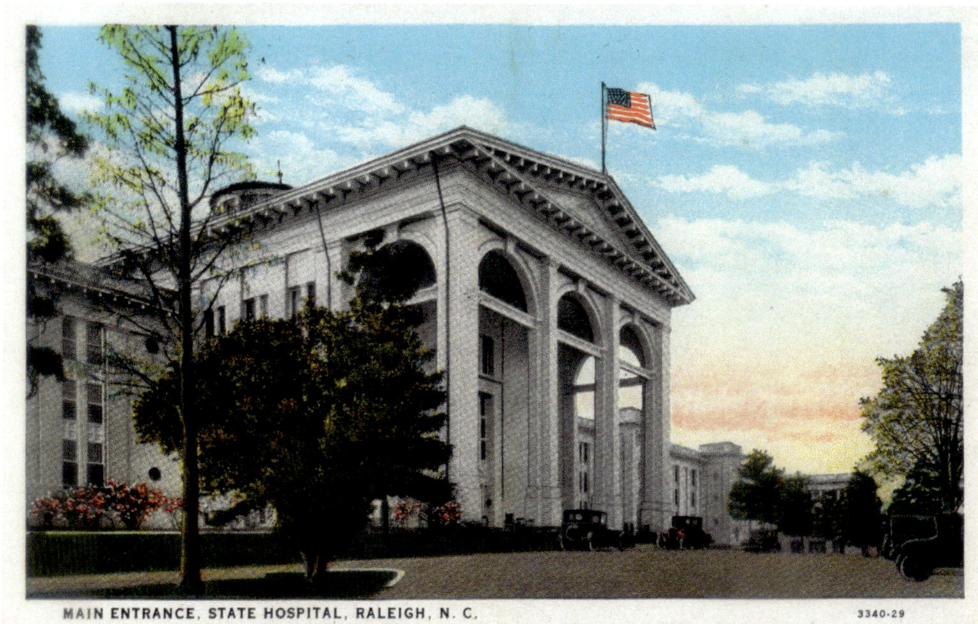
MAIN ENTRANCE, STATE HOSPITAL, RALEIGH, N. C.
3340-29

Figure 69

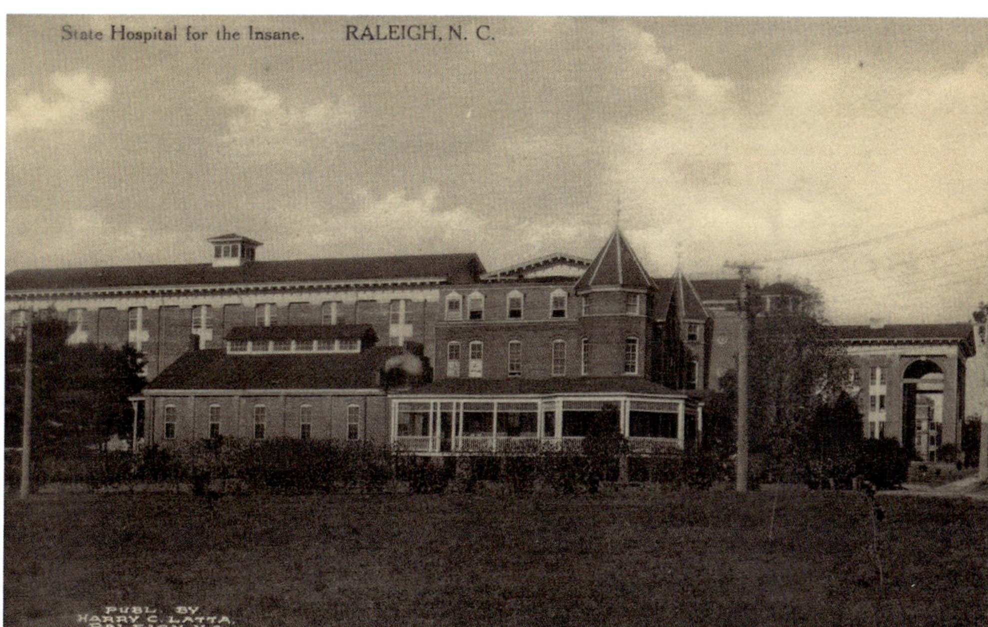
State Hospital for the Insane. RALEIGH, N. C.
PUBL. BY
HARRY C. LATTA,
RALEIGH, N.C.

Figure 70

State Lunatic Hospital
Northampton, Massachusetts, 1858

The State Lunatic Hospital in Northampton accepted its first patients in 1858. Prior to the opening of this facility, there were already three state facilities for the care of the insane in Massachusetts, but a survey indicated that there were still about 600 people in the state requiring care. After six weeks of operations, the hospital population had reached 220 and by 1935, it cared for more than 2,100 patients.

This Kirkbride institution (figure 71) consisted of a central building for administrative offices and had extended wings for patients. By 1905, the main building had been considerably enlarged and several buildings were added including a reception building and infirmary. A training school for nurses was established in 1892. In the early 1900s, a recreation pavilion was added for female patients and a clubhouse for male patients including a bowling alley, a billiard room, and a reading and smoking room. A greenhouse, added in 1870, can be seen in figure 72.

The renamed Northampton State Hospital was closed in 1993. The original main building of Northampton was abandoned in 1986 and demolished in 2006. All the buildings were torn down in 2007. There is now a residential development on the site of the original Kirkbride building.

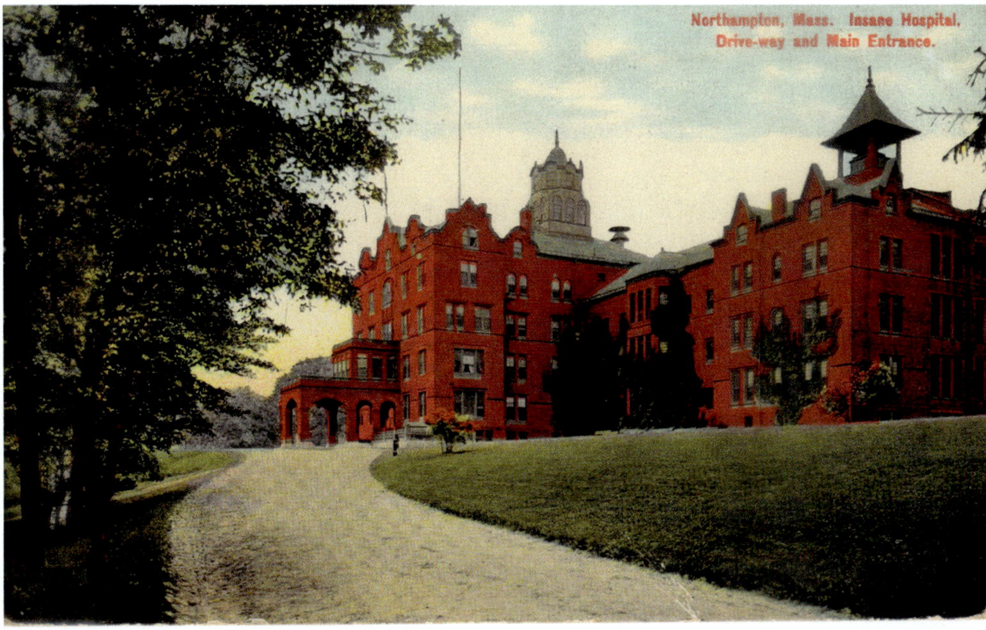
Northampton, Mass. Insane Hospital.
Drive-way and Main Entrance.

Figure 71

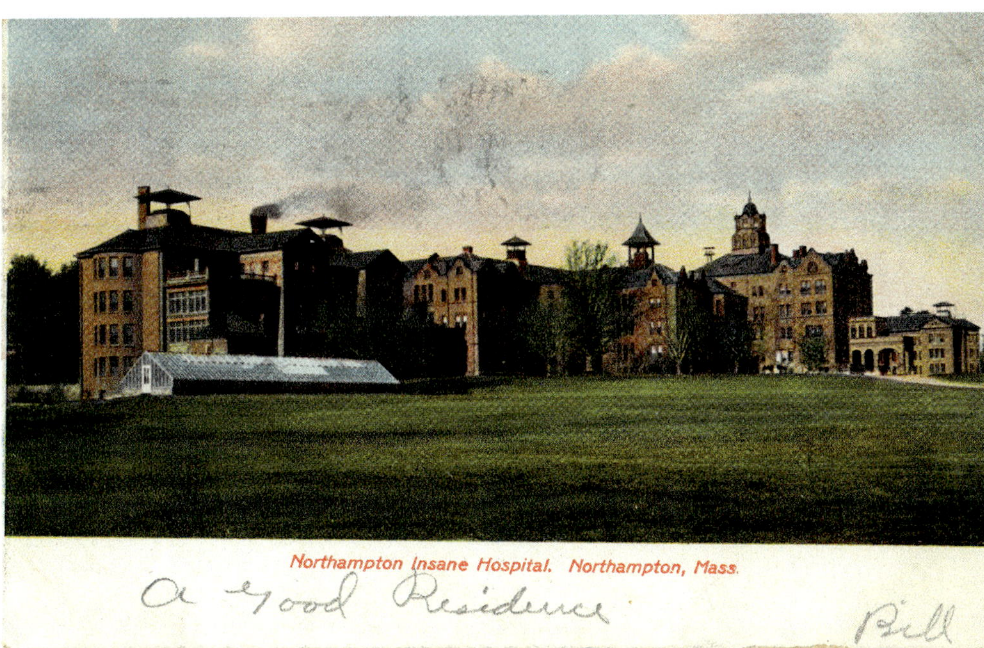
Northampton Insane Hospital. Northampton, Mass.
a Good Residence
Bill

Figure 72

Michigan Asylum for the Insane
Kalamazoo, Michigan, 1859

The Michigan Asylum for the Insane opened in 1859 to provide services for the more than 300 people who had been deemed insane but were still living in county houses and jails. A board of trustees was given the authority to purchase 160 acres to build a facility capable of accommodating 200 patients near the village of Kalamazoo. This Kirkbride asylum (figure 73) included six wings that could accommodate 300 patients.

By 1885, the trustees purchased a tract of 250 acres and erected a two-story farm house with room for 40 male patients and a barn for 60 cows. This was the first experiment in distant segregation of patients, since it was located about 3 miles from the central buildings. Soon a colony plan with four houses built on 320 acres of land was completed.

By 1910, a three-story brick structure centrally located to the cottages was added and increased the capacity of the cottages to 50 beds and two new wards for the male patients (figure 74) were added. Four years later, the whole facility was comprised of 73 buildings on a tract of 1,053 acres with 141 patients. By 1914, there were 2,111 patients at Kalamazoo.

The postcard in figure 75, postmarked 1907, shows several of the buildings as they appeared at that time.

In 2000, the Kalamazoo Psychiatric Hospital closed. All of the original buildings had been destroyed, aside from the 175-foot water tower that had been built in 1895.

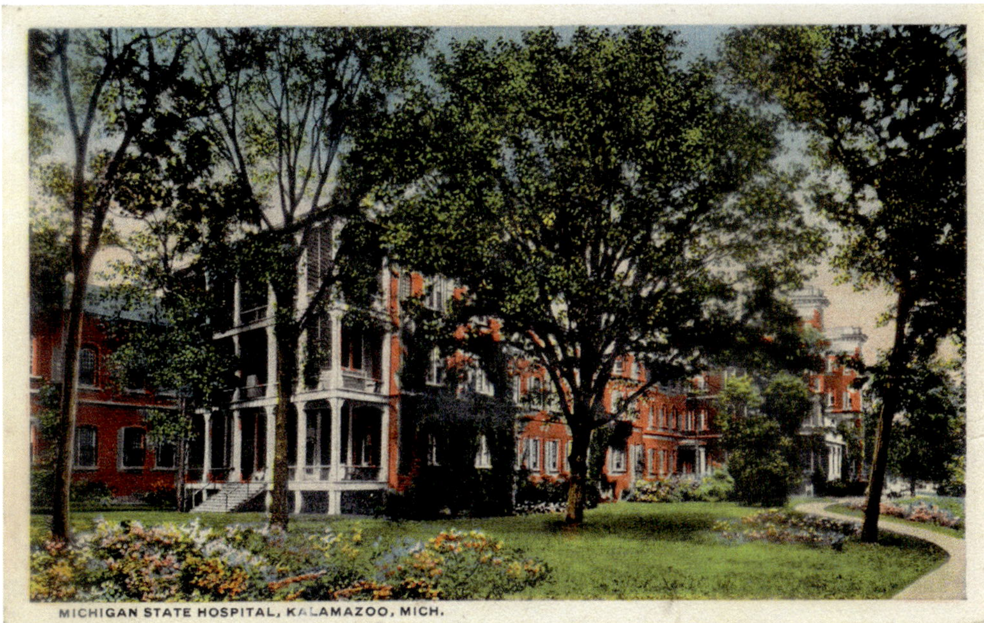
MICHIGAN STATE HOSPITAL, KALAMAZOO, MICH.

Figure 73

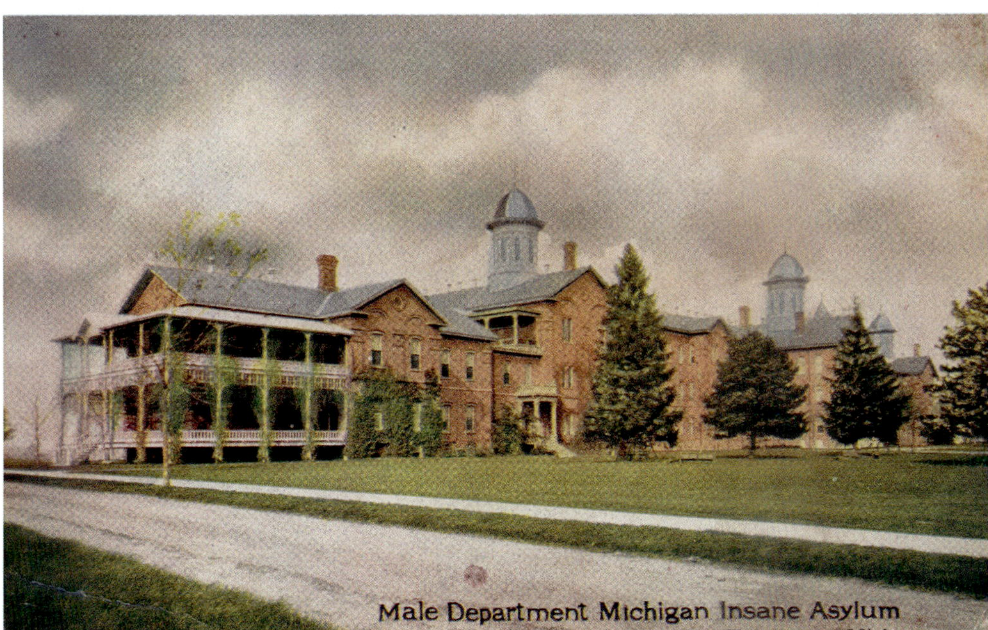
Male Department Michigan Insane Asylum
Kalamazoo, Mich.

Figure 74

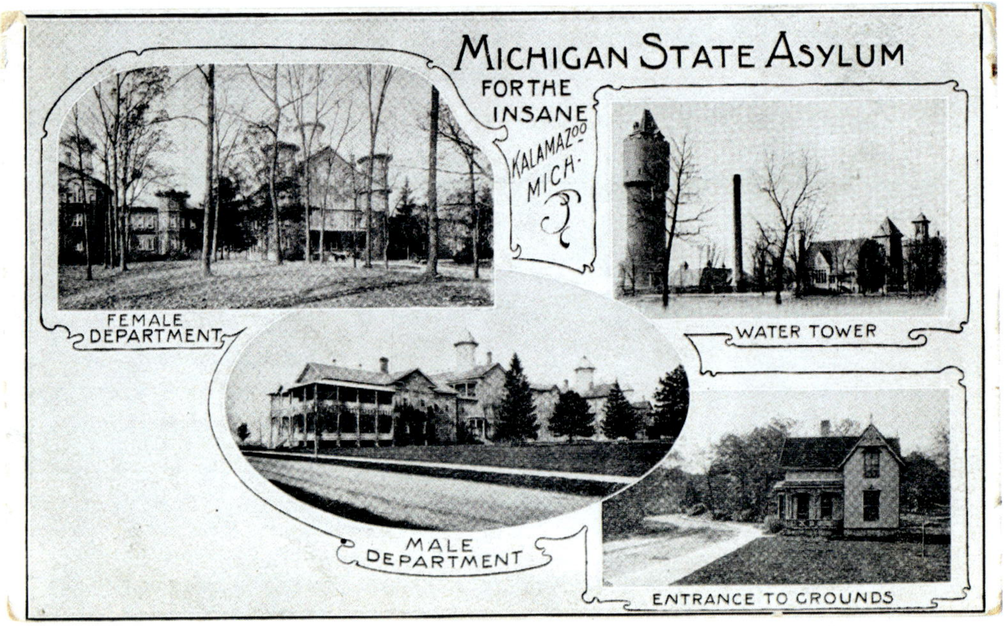

Figure 75

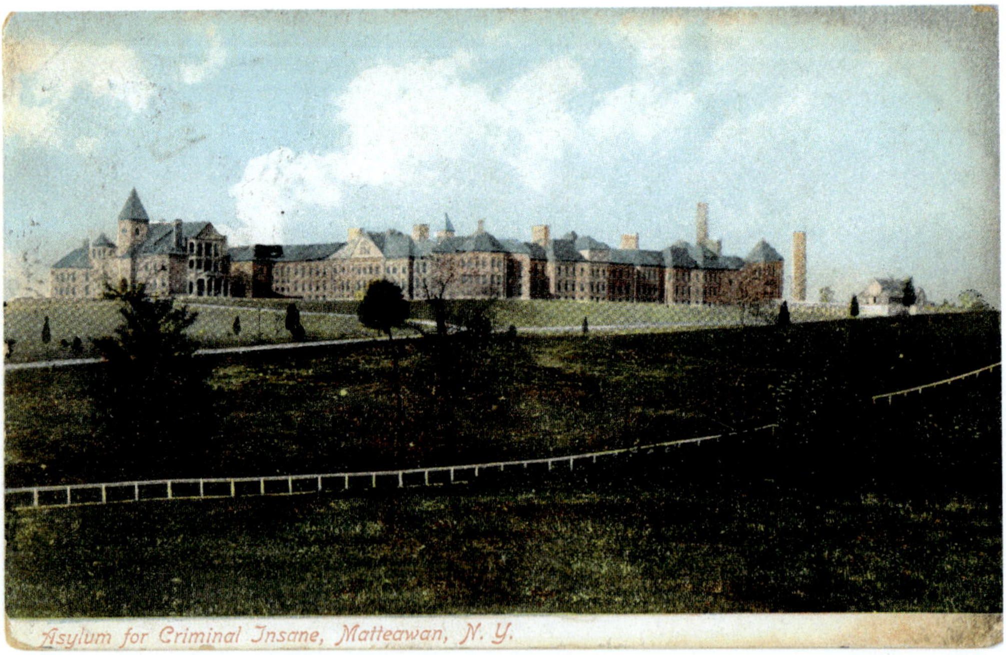

Figure 76

State Lunatic Asylum for Insane Convicts
Beacon, New York, 1859

The State Lunatic Asylum for Insane Convicts opened in 1859 on the grounds of Auburn prison. It was established to care for convicts that had been deemed "insane." Over the years, the facility (figure 76) would change its name multiple times, becoming the State Lunatic Asylum at Auburn in 1874. In 1892, the asylum was moved to the village of Matteawan and the name was changed to the Matteawan State Hospital (figure 77).

The facility not only cared for convicted criminals who were mentally ill, but also those deemed unfit to stand trial and those acquitted by reason of insanity. By 1916, there were 804 patients and the facility was severely overcrowded.

The postcard in figure 78 shows the dining room, which was located on the first floor of the building between two wards, and was connected to the kitchen, scullery, bakery, and storehouse. This postcard also illustrates the chapel which provided services delivered by priests and rabbis from the surrounding communities. The chapel was also used as an amusement hall.

As prison hospitals were slowly phased out, the Matteawan site underwent various changes until the late 1970s, when it was absorbed by new facilities providing psychiatric services. The Fishkill Correctional Facility, a medium-security prison, continues to occupy the site. Several of the original buildings have survived.

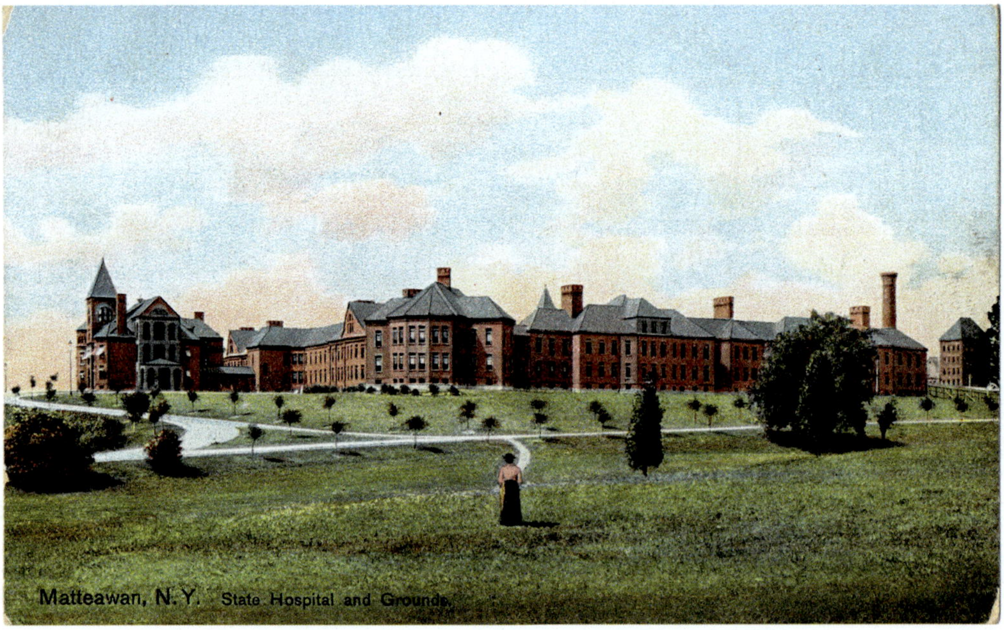

Figure 77

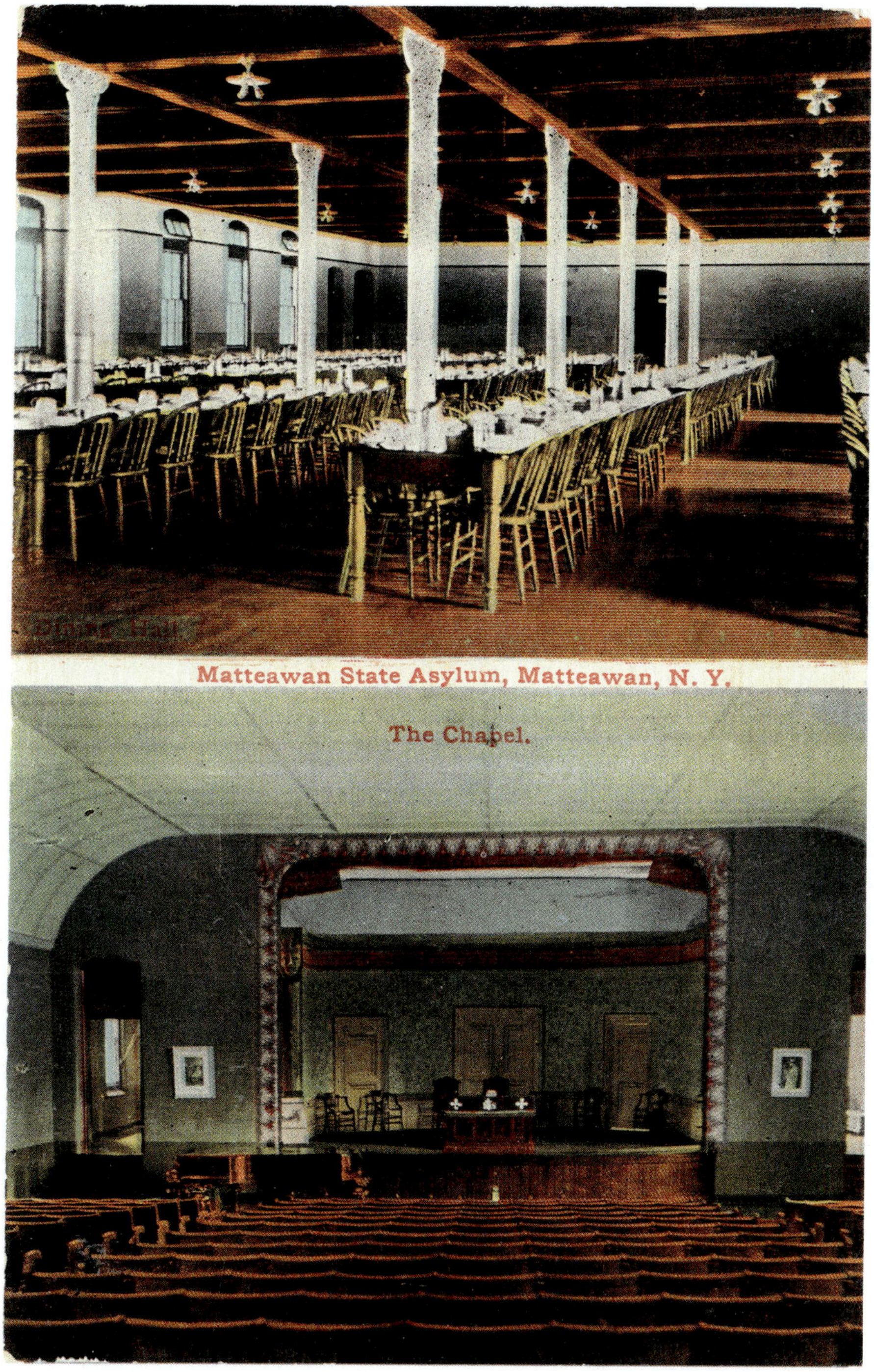
Dining Hall
Matteawan State Asylum, Matteawan, N. Y.
The Chapel.

Figure 78

Trans-Allegheny Lunatic Asylum
Weston, West Virginia, 1859

The Trans-Allegheny Lunatic Asylum was authorized in 1850 and opened in 1863 as the West Virginia Hospital for the Insane. It was the first publicly funded building in the state of West Virginia, which was established as a state the same year. Construction of the sprawling facility was interrupted by the Civil War in 1861, but was eventually completed in 1880. It is claimed to be the largest hand-cut stone building in the United States. At the end of the Civil War, the facility had a capacity for 250 patients, which increased as buildings were added over the years. By 1917, the patient population reached 1,023 and in 1950, the patient population peaked at 2,400.

The 1908 postcard (figure 79) shows the Kirkbride building, with wings extending to the north and south. Corridors connected all the wards to each other and to the central building. Two additional three-story buildings provided rooms for patients.

The grounds of the hospital (figure 80) consisted of approximately 335 acres fronting on the West Fork River, opposite the town of Weston.

The 1928 postmarked image in figure 81 provides a view from the front of asylum.

The facility, renamed Weston State Hospital in 1913, was closed in 1994. The original buildings have survived and are currently open for tours.

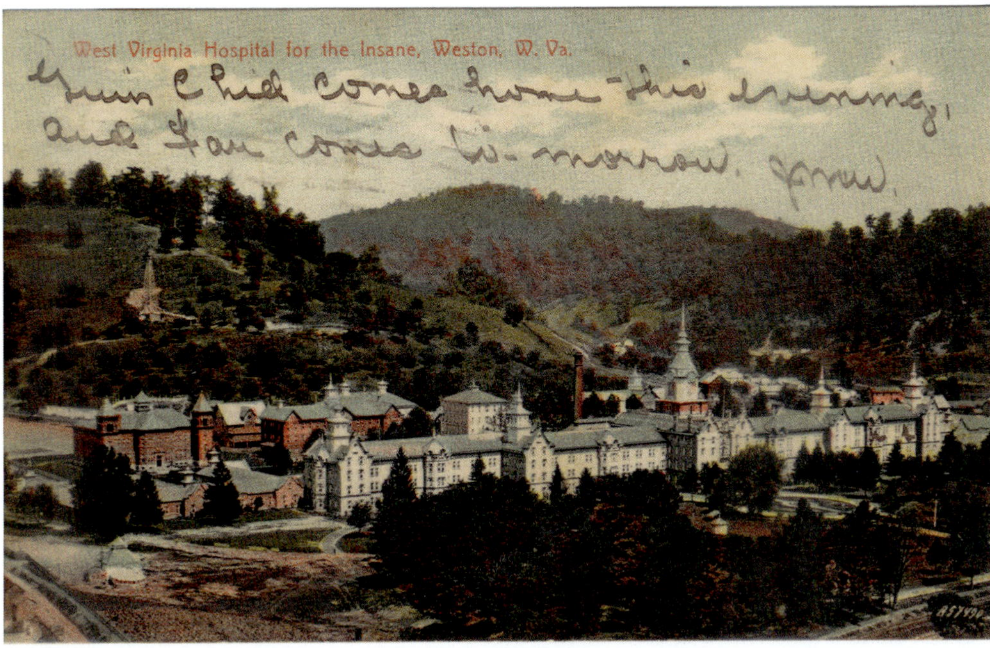

Figure 79

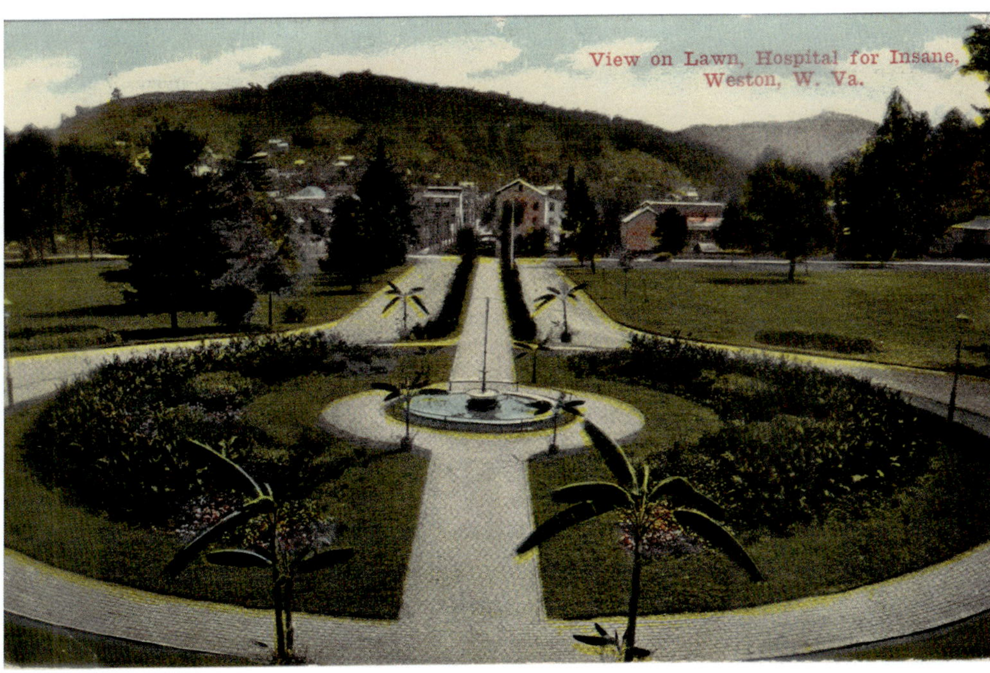

Figure 80

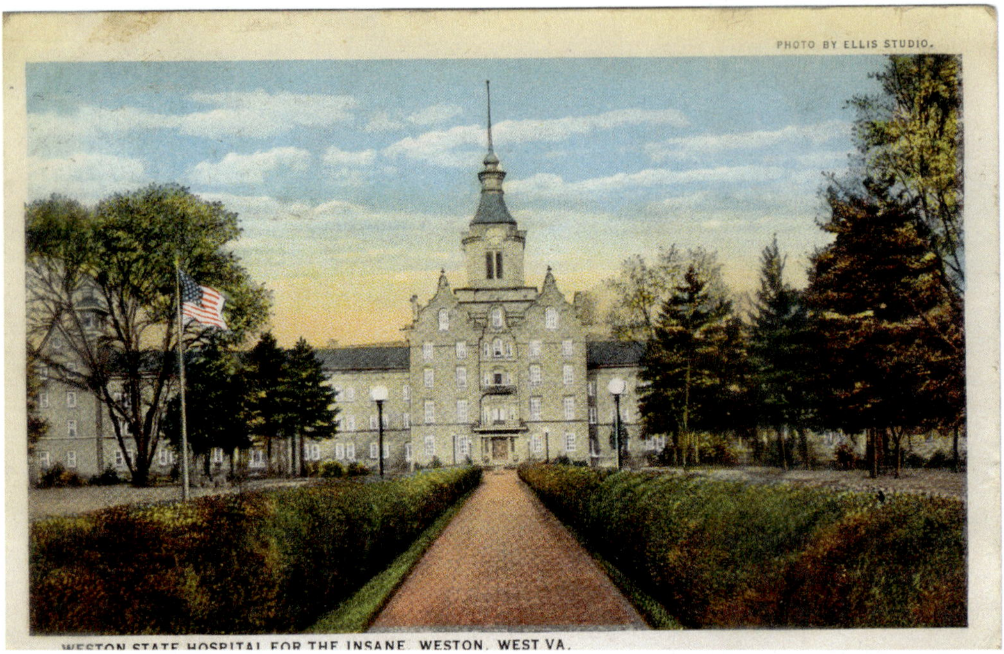
PHOTO BY ELLIS STUDIO.
WESTON STATE HOSPITAL FOR THE INSANE, WESTON, WEST VA.

Figure 81

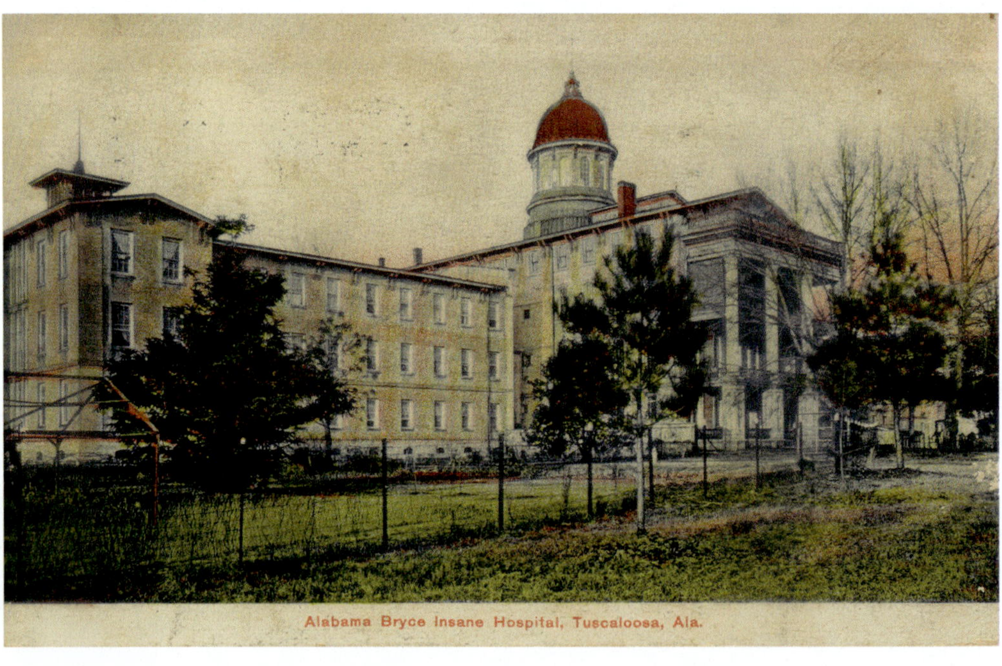
Alabama Bryce Insane Hospital, Tuscaloosa, Ala.

Figure 82

Alabama Insane Asylum
Tuscaloosa, Alabama, 1861

Bryce Hospital in Tuscaloosa was the first state facility for the care of the mentally ill, with a second facility located in Mt. Vernon for the care of black individuals suffering from mental illness. The Tuscaloosa facility was established on the Kirkbride plan. Originally named Alabama Insane Asylum, the facility was renamed to honor its first superintendent, Peter Bryce, who had been recommended by Dorothea Dix.

The postcard on the opposite page (figure 82), postmarked 1908, reflects the early structure of this facility.

The postcard at the top of the next page (figure 83), postmarked 1934, shows a different view of the main entrance to the facility.

A colony consisting of 75 white males was established 2 miles from the main buildings. These patients were responsible for all of the farm work and seldom returned to the main hospital.

There was a separate psychopathic ward for new patients and separate wards for violent, "demented," and medical patients. Out of the 1,500 acres, about 500 were used for field crops and gardens.

The postcard on the bottom of the next page (figure 84) is a linen era (1930–1945) postcard depicting the vast size of the facility and grounds.

In 1912, the hospital census reached 1,441 patients, including 1,377 white patients and just 64 black patients.

By 1970, there were a total of 5,200 patients. In 2009, the facility was relocated and the University of Alabama took over the old campus. The original buildings are expected to be restored. The relocated facilities consist of 268 beds for acute care with treatment and rehabilitation for addictions and include a 100-bed geriatric care facility.

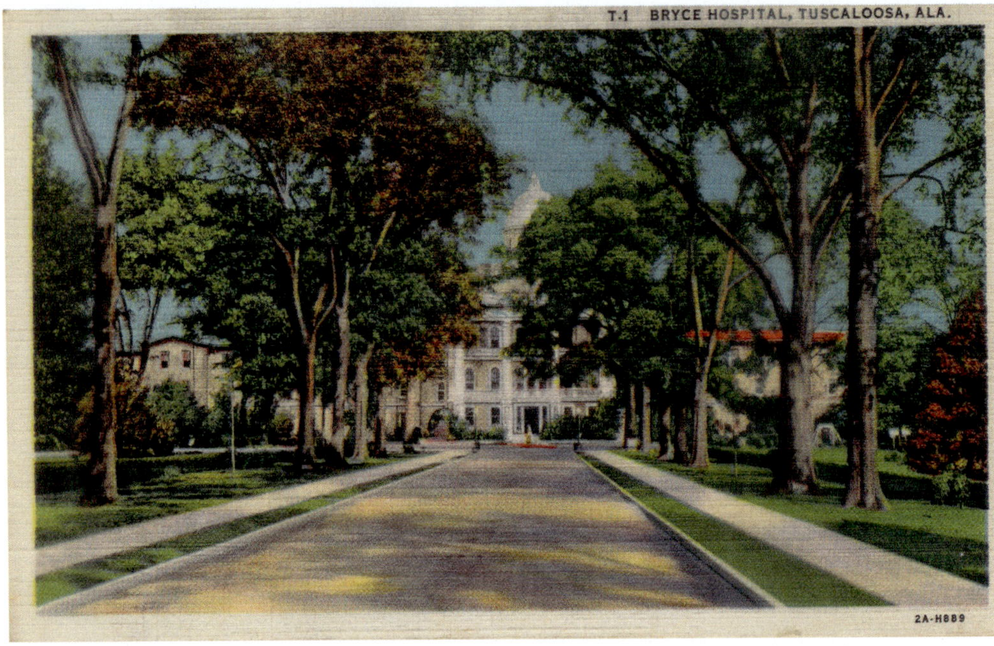

Figure 83

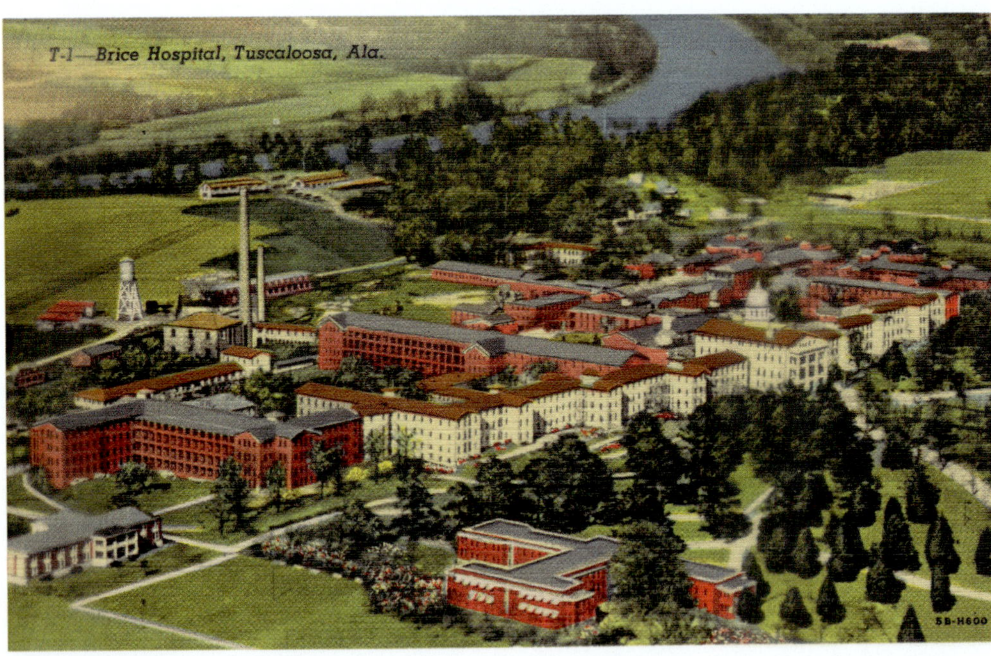

Figure 84

Wisconsin Hospital for the Insane
Mendota, Wisconsin, 1860

The facility opened as the Wisconsin Hospital for the Insane and the first patient was admitted on July 14, 1860. It had an expected population of 45, but by 1870, there were 362 patients.

This building originally followed the Kirkbride plan with a center building, one longitudinal wing, and one transverse wing. The center building was four stories high and three-story wings were later added.

The early postcard on the next page (figure 85) shows a horse and carriage in front of the administration building.

In 1910, a training school for nurses was opened in the facility that included clinical and pathological laboratories. Another view of the administrative building is shown from a postcard postmarked 1909 (figure 86).

Another view of the administrative building and its grounds is depicted on the postcard in figure 87, postmarked 1914.

By 1916, an orchard of 1,200 trees and flowers were planted along the paved walkways throughout the grounds.

Male patients were employed to work on the farm, in the gardens or tending the lawn while women were employed in the dining rooms, in the kitchen, or in the sewing area. A hydrotherapeutic apparatus consisting of seven continuous bathtubs was used in treatment of patients. Hospital entertainment included musical concerts by the hospital orchestra and regular Friday night dances. Religious services were conducted by the pastors of various churches in the city.

By 1974, the hospital was renamed the Mendota Mental Health Institute at Madison, Wisconsin (figure 88), located on the same grounds of the original facility. By 1997, there were fewer than 300 patients.

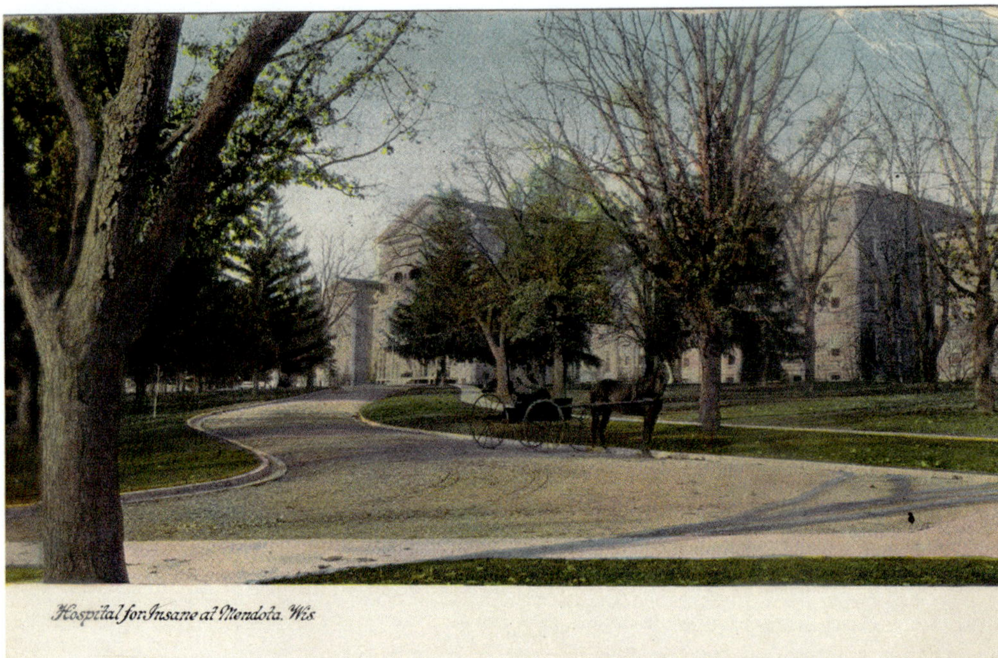
Hospital for Insane at Mendota, Wis.

Figure 85

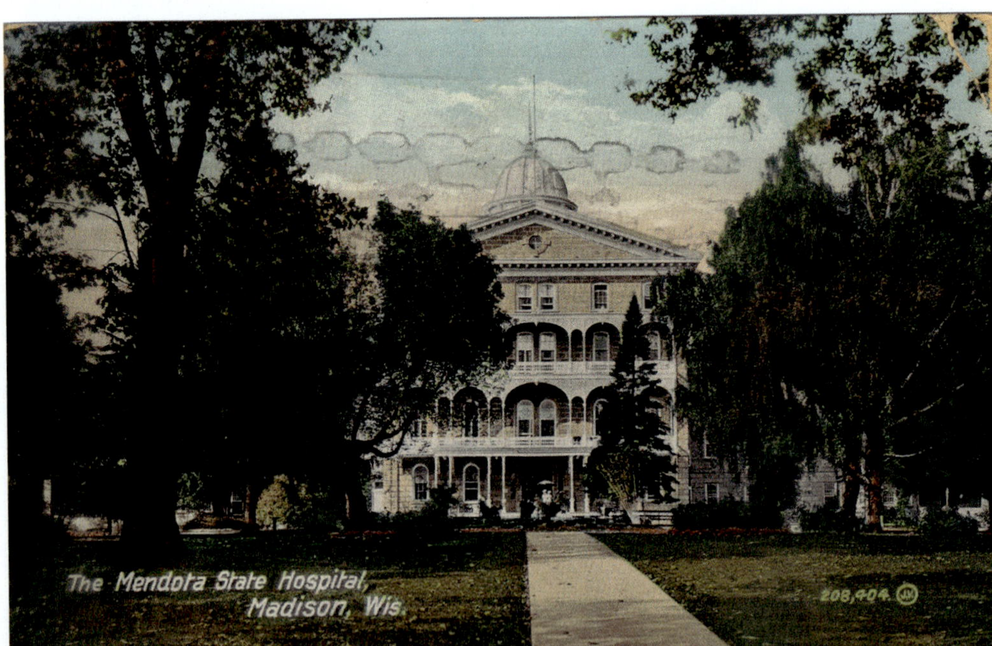
The Mendota State Hospital,
Madison, Wis.
208,404.

Figure 86

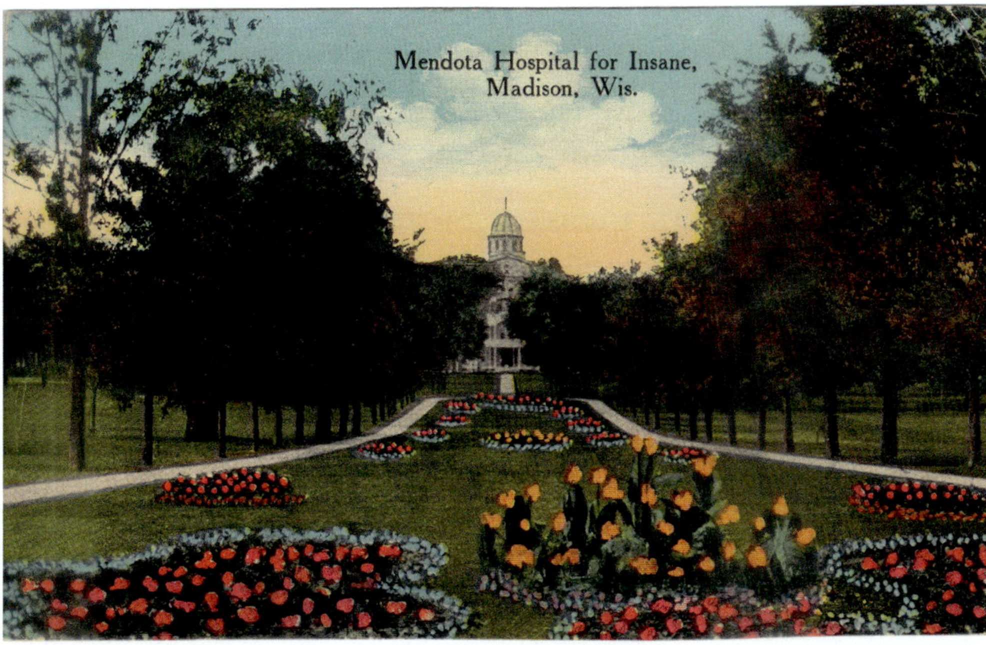
Mendota Hospital for Insane,
Madison, Wis.

Figure 87

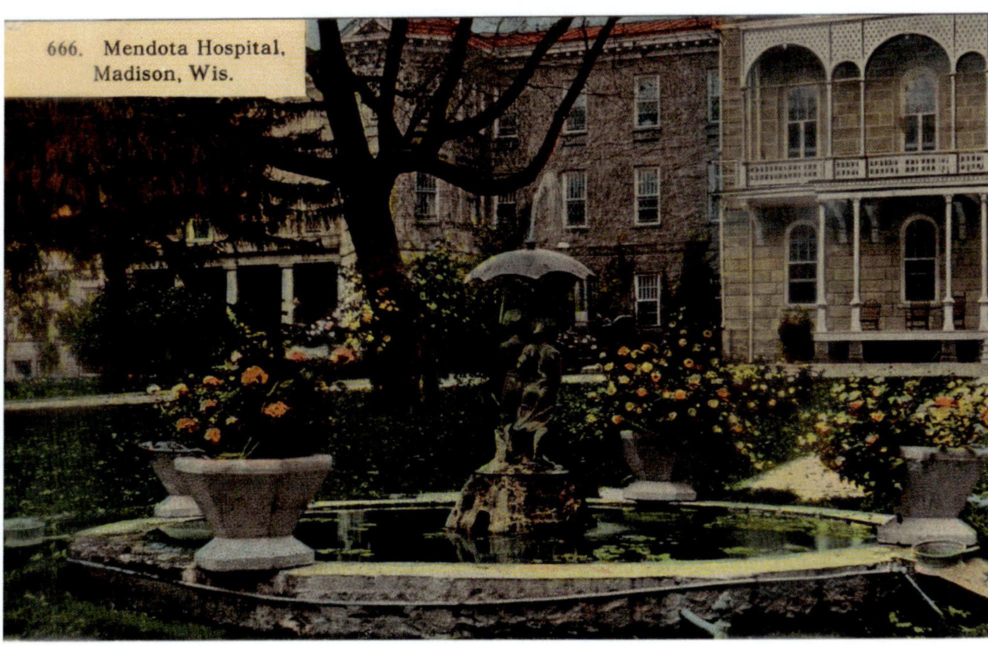
666. Mendota Hospital,
Madison, Wis.

Figure 88

Mount Pleasant State Hospital
Mount Pleasant, Iowa, 1861

Mount Pleasant State Hospital was opened in 1861 on 173 acres of land adjoining the city of Mount Pleasant with a capacity to care for 300 patients. However, by 1865, the facility became overcrowded with approximately 400 patients. As a result, patients who were deemed harmless or incurable were ordered back to their respective counties of origin without considering the counties' capacity to accommodate or provide care for these patients.

A county infirmary was located on the grounds adjacent to the hospital and that facility drained their sewage on to the hospital's farm, polluting all water in both facilities. As a consequence, typhoid fever and other diseases were prevalent until an extensive filtration system was constructed at the hospital. Problems with the water supply continued until the city of Mount Pleasant improved the water supply.

The image in figure 89 shows the administrative building.

By 1883, a wing on the east side of the main building added rooms for 200 male patients and two years later a west side was added for 200 female patients. These two wings doubled the capacity of the institution.

The farm was enlarged by 1901. A new psychopathic hospital for women was in use and a tuberculosis hospital was completed and occupied. The farm had been enlarged to 1,000 acres of adjoining land and the garden was increased to 60 acres.

Figure 90 shows the expanded facility around 1920.

Mount Pleasant State Hospital was the second oldest state institution in Iowa. A prison at Fort Madison was the oldest.

Currently, the facility is called the Mount Pleasant Mental Health Institute and is located on the same campus as the Mount Pleasant Correctional Facility. The previous facility closed in 1936 after a massive fire destroyed most of the buildings and left the rest of the complex beyond repair.

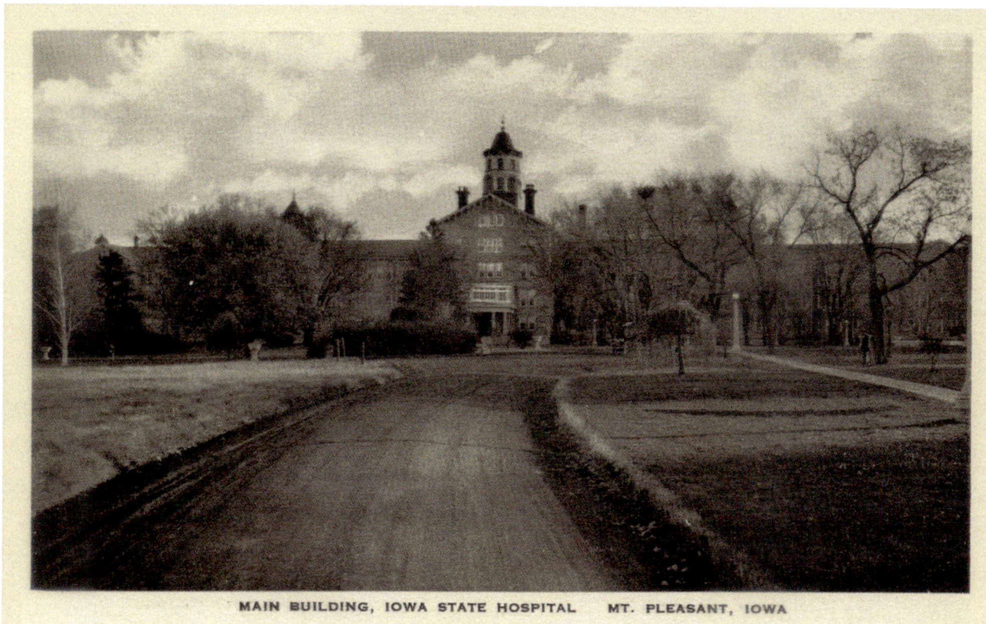

Figure 89

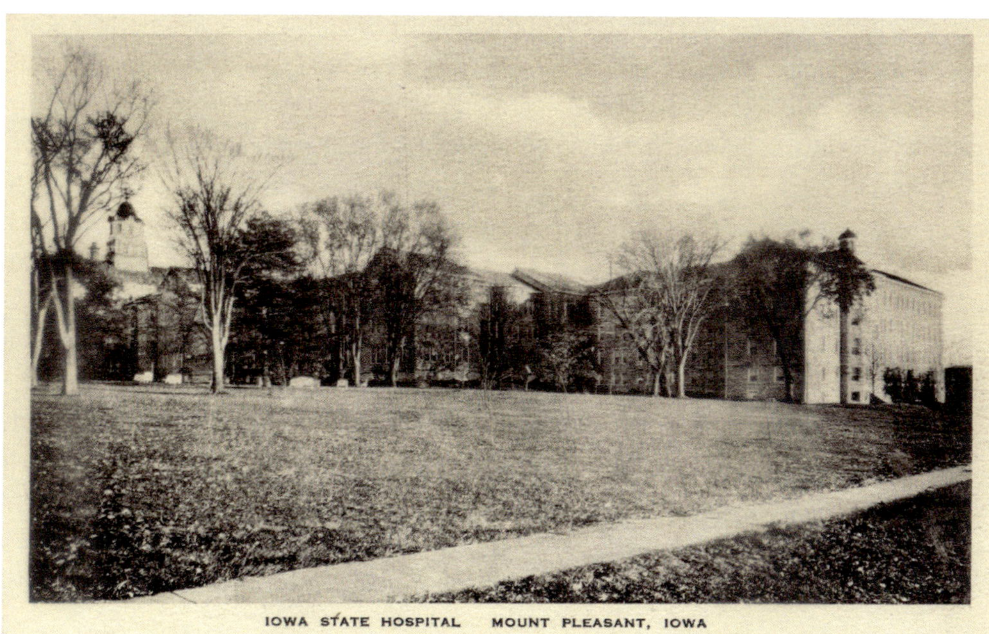

Figure 90

Texas State Lunatic Asylum
Austin, Texas, 1861

Upon this facility's opening in 1861, the structure consisted of a main building and three wards with capacity for approximately a dozen patients. The institution was originally called the Texas State Lunatic Asylum. The casebooks of the early period of the asylum describe some of the causes of illness as "war," "fright from soldiers," and "soldiers' marauding."

The early buildings were eventually expanded to accommodate 60 or 70 patients. Airing courts or enclosed yards were built for the patients' exercise. However, by 1883, the airing courts were discouraged and long walks were encouraged by the attendants. An infirmary was also built at this time.

By 1896, the census had jumped to 696 as improvements were made to the original buildings. The grounds were improved with the planting of many trees and a brass band of patients and employees was organized.

The postcards in figures 91 and 92 show the administration and other buildings.

By 1909, two cottages for tuberculosis patients were added, with a separate ward to accommodate 150 black patients. Patients continued to have weekly dances, as well as picture shows and band concerts on the lawn. Farming became part of the institution as the population reached 1,575 patients and 175 employees.

A final postcard in figure 93 shows what appears to be a water fountain in front of the buildings.

In 1968, the patient census reached 3,318 patients with an additional 900 elderly patients. In 1990, the original building was renovated and the facility is still currently operational.

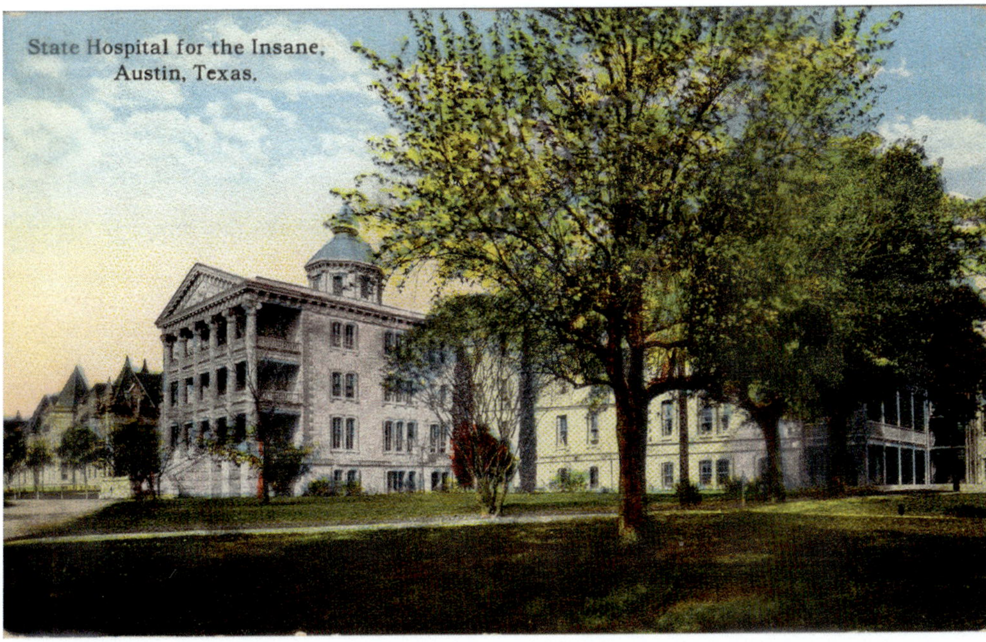
State Hospital for the Insane,
Austin, Texas.

Figure 91

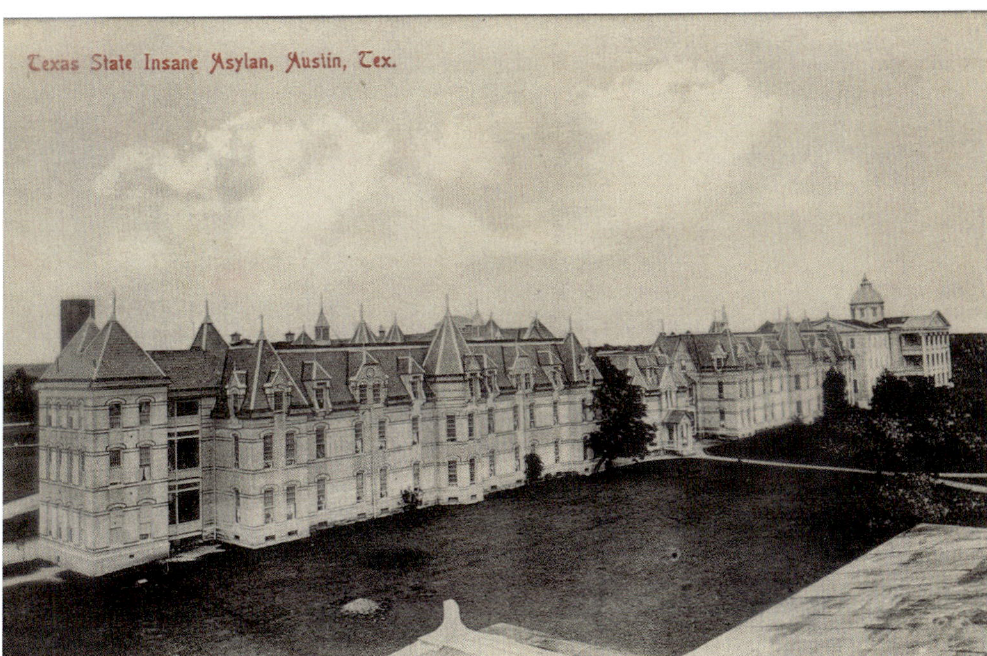
Texas State Insane Asylan, Austin, Tex.

Figure 92

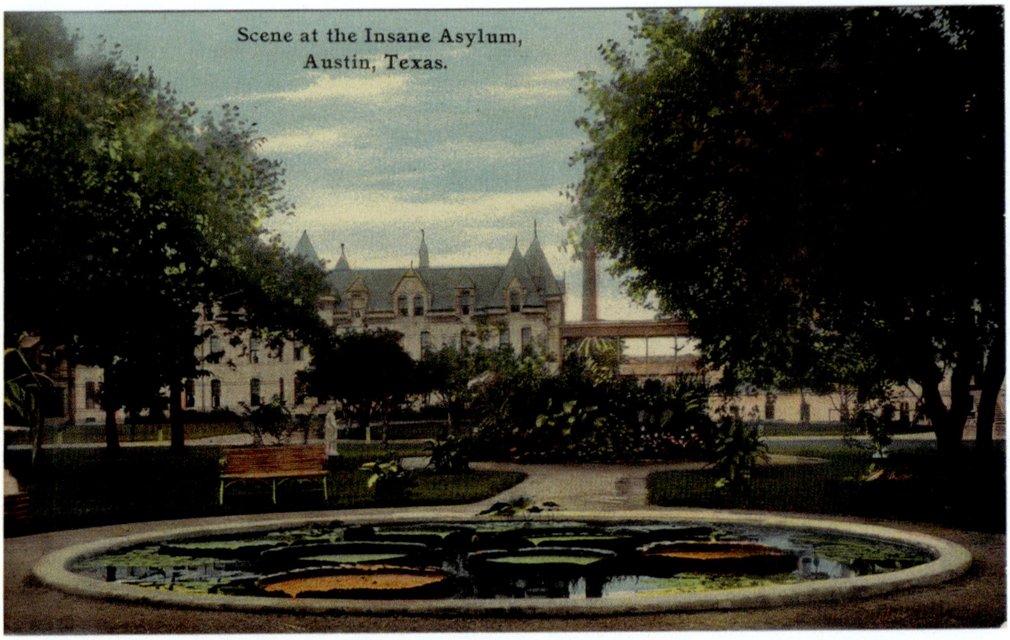
Scene at the Insane Asylum,
Austin, Texas.

Figure 93

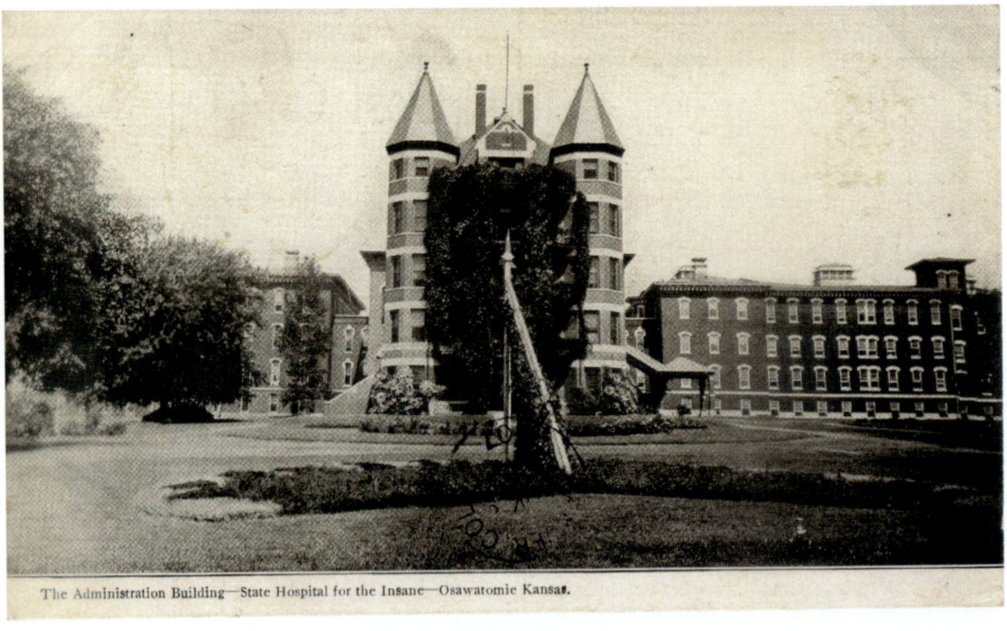
The Administration Building—State Hospital for the Insane—Osawatomie Kansas.

Figure 94

Kansas Insane Asylum
Osawatomie, Kansas, 1866

Prior to the establishment of this facility, there had been no provision for the care and treatment of the mentally ill in Kansas. Originally called the Kansas Insane Asylum, the hospital consisted of a central administrative building with side buildings for male and female patients. Shops and a power plant were located in the rear of the facility. Two detached buildings for chronic cases, a detached infirmary accommodating 100 patients, and two tuberculosis pavilions were also added. There were also separate cottages for female nurses and a commissary building for food storage and handling.

Figure 94 is an early postmarked postcard of 1907.

The lands and buildings of the facility were expanded by 1911, with 1,300 patients in residence.

Both of the postcards in figures 95 and 96 were sent after 1920.

The Asylum's name changed in 1901 to Osawatomie State Hospital and still serves the state of Kansas for the mentally ill. The original buildings were abandoned in 1986 and torn down in 2002.

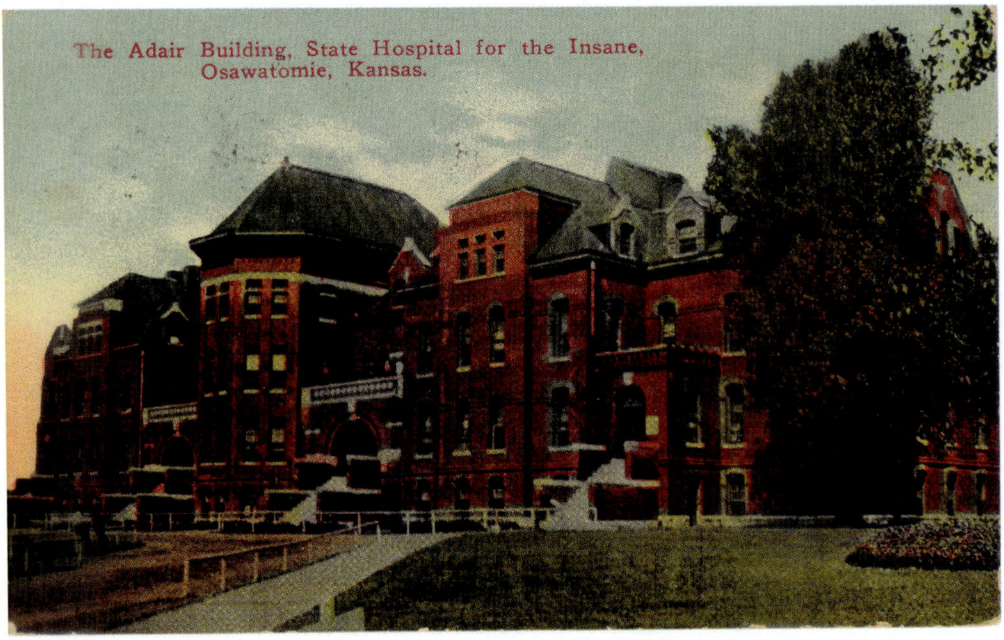

Figure 95

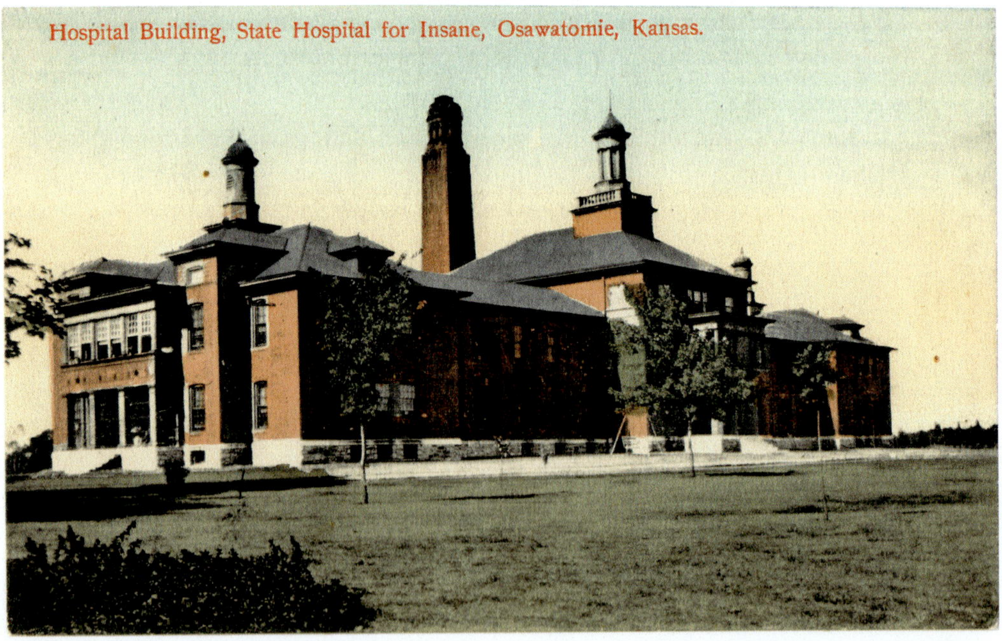

Figure 96

St. Peter Asylum for the Insane
St. Peter, Minnesota, 1866

Originally called St. Peter Asylum for the Insane, this facility opened in 1866 to temporarily care for Minnesota residents who were previously cared for in facilities located in Iowa and St. Louis. Shortly afterwards, the hospital buildings were made permanent, following the Kirkbride plan with a central administration building and diverging wings. The top postcard on the next page (figure 97) shows the administration building and wings.

The bottom postcard on the next page (figure 98) depicts the entrance to the facility.

By 1915, a detention hospital and a hospital for the criminally insane were opened. The detention hospital housed voluntary patients and the criminal building housed patients who were sent from the state prison, either under indictment or acquitted on the grounds of insanity.

The training school for nurses was created in 1912 since the superintendent insisted on only hiring graduate nurses at this facility. Postcards on page 95 (figures 99 and 100) provide images of the nurses' building and other employee facilities.

From 1906 to 1908, the central portion of the facility was rebuilt to include a laboratory, a larger operating room, and kitchens.

The oldest building was demolished in 1968 but one building was saved as a museum. By 1990, this facility was organized into two inpatient psychiatric hospitals: the Minnesota Security Hospital and the St. Peter Regional Treatment Center.

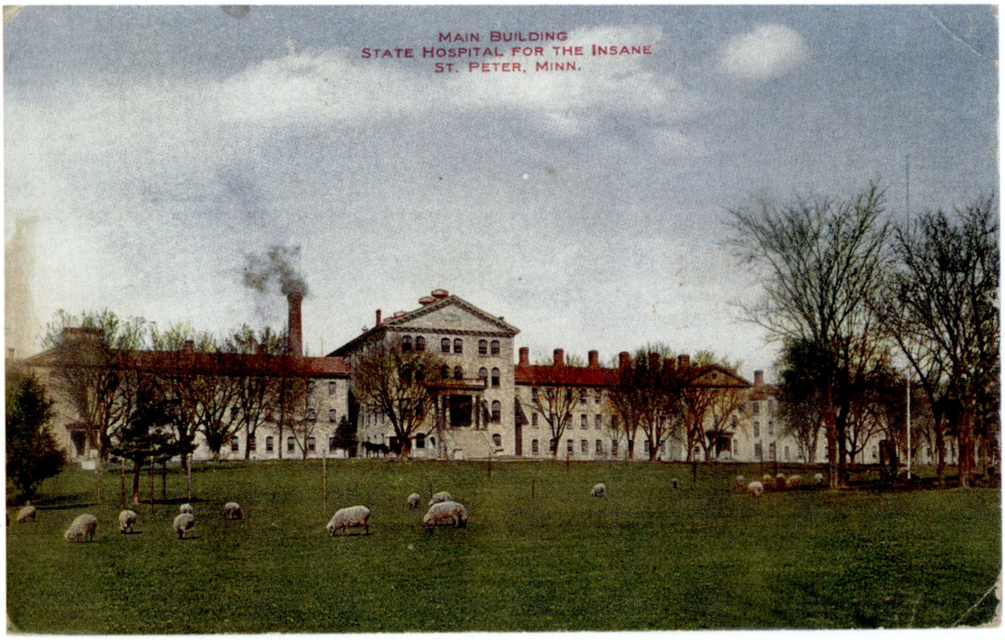

Figure 97

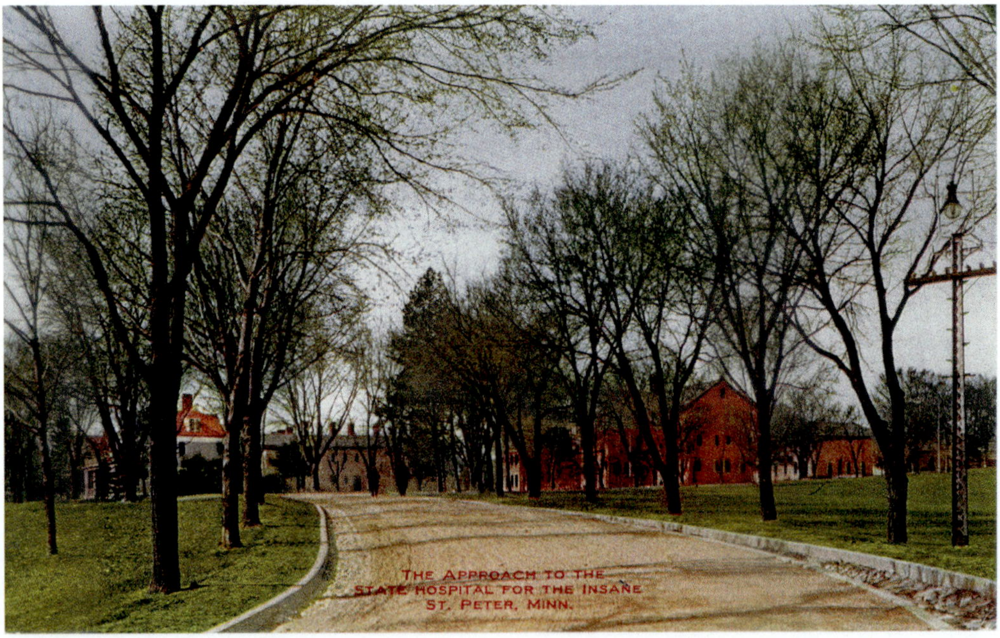

Figure 98

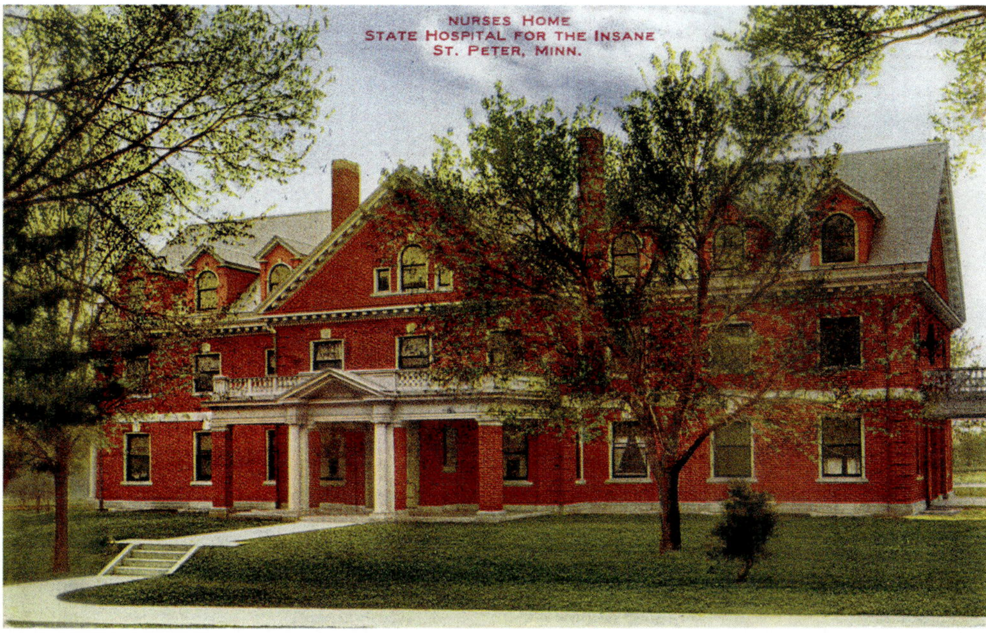

Figure 99

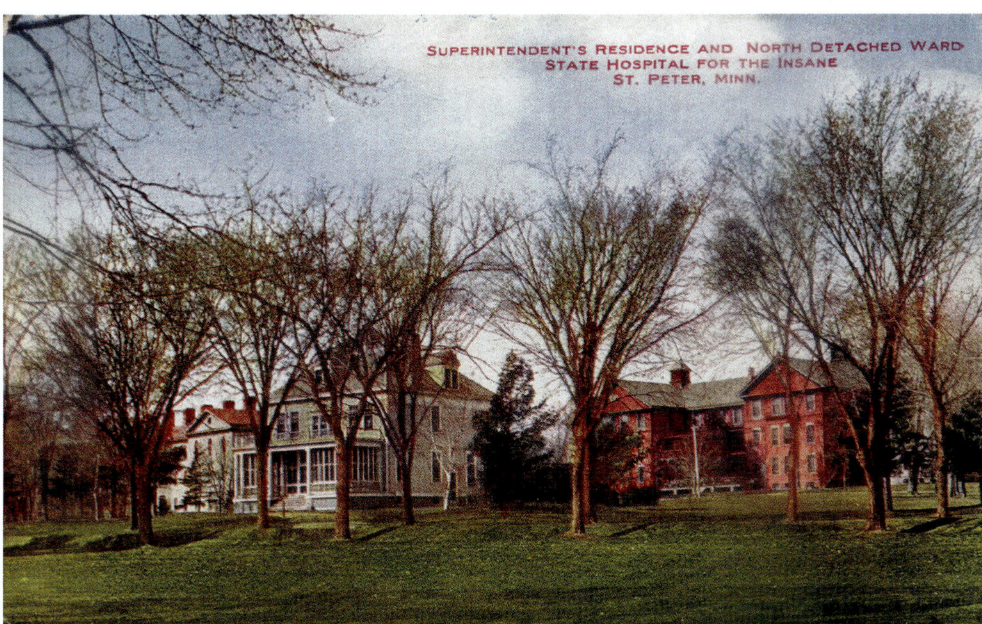

Figure 100

Tewksbury Almshouse
Tewksbury, Massachusetts, 1866

The Tewksbury Almshouse in Tewksbury, Massachusetts was opened on May 1, 1854, to care and provide for the poor. In the first year of operations, 2,193 individuals were admitted. In 1866, the institution also began accepting the "pauper insane," those individuals who were both poor and had received a diagnosis of chronic insanity. The almshouse officially became the Tewksbury State Hospital in 1900 (figure 101).

In the early decades of the 1900s, the facility (figure 102) was renovated and enlarged, eventually serving as a home for the "insane" and the sick, as well as the poor.

The facility reported having various kinds of entertainment and social gatherings for patients who were from different countries. The pictures in figures 103–105 illustrate the activities of the facility. These postcards were not commercially made; rather they were photos taken at an event where patients dressed to represent their country of origin.

Figure 106 shows the asylum #4 building.

The department for the mentally ill housed patients thought to be incurable but harmless. It included 3 farms, one wholly operated by male patients. The patients contributed significantly to the operation and economy of the whole institution by performing general housekeeping, laundry, and kitchen duties, and also working on the farm and grounds.

By 1914, Tewksbury consisted of 75 buildings, including four buildings for employees, one building for children, two large hospitals for tuberculosis, five isolation wards for those with infectious diseases, an observation building, a surgical building, a laboratory building, an administrative building, and a house for the superintendent of the whole facility.

The Tewksbury facility (figure 107) underwent several name changes over the years and now operates as the Tewksbury Hospital. The original administration building still stands and houses a public health museum.

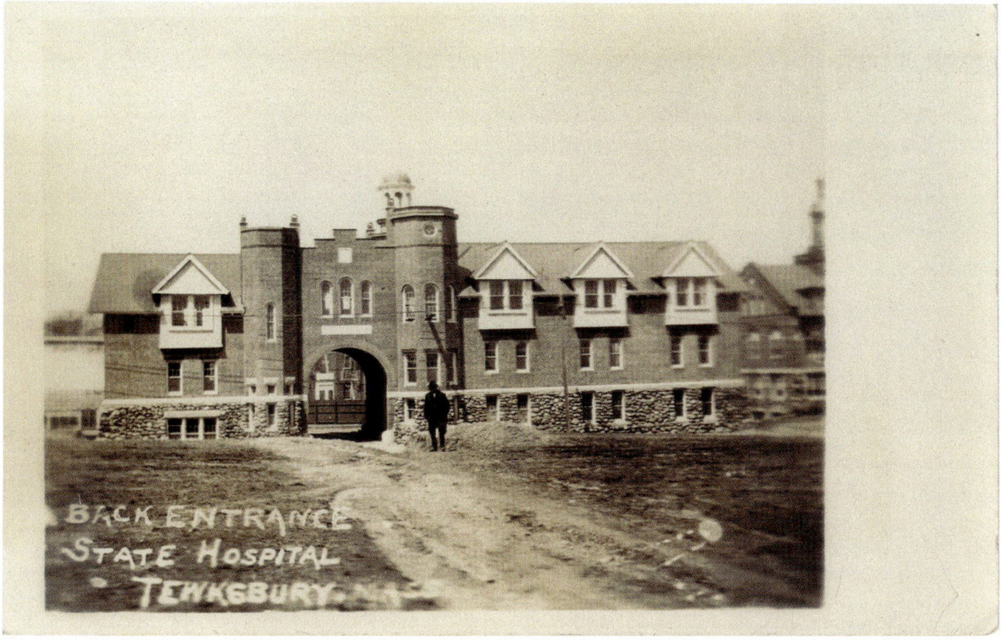
BACK ENTRANCE
STATE HOSPITAL
TEWKSBURY

Figure 101

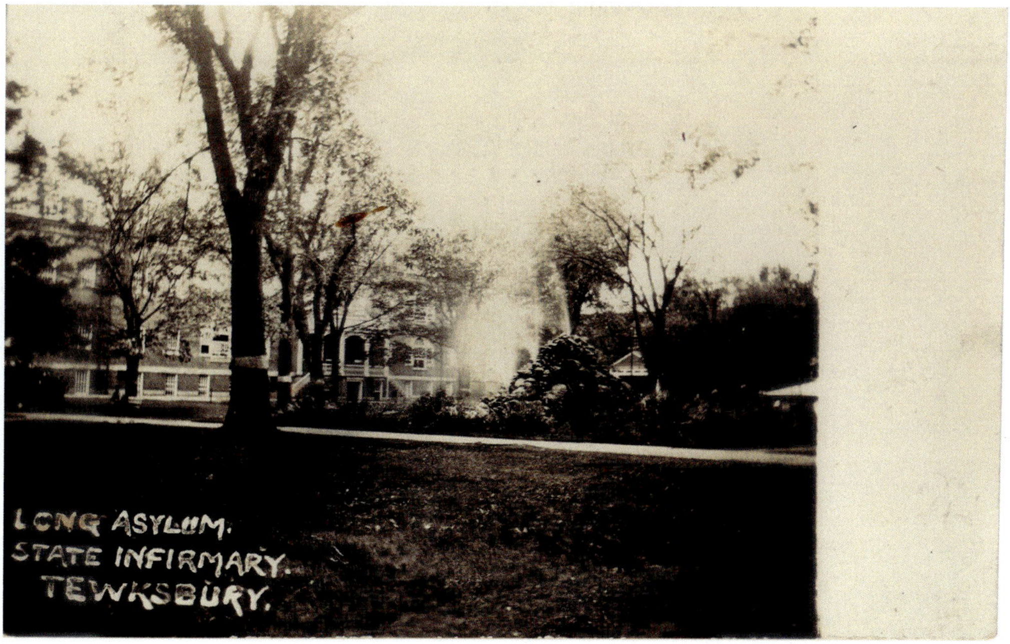
LONG ASYLUM.
STATE INFIRMARY.
TEWKSBURY.

Figure 102

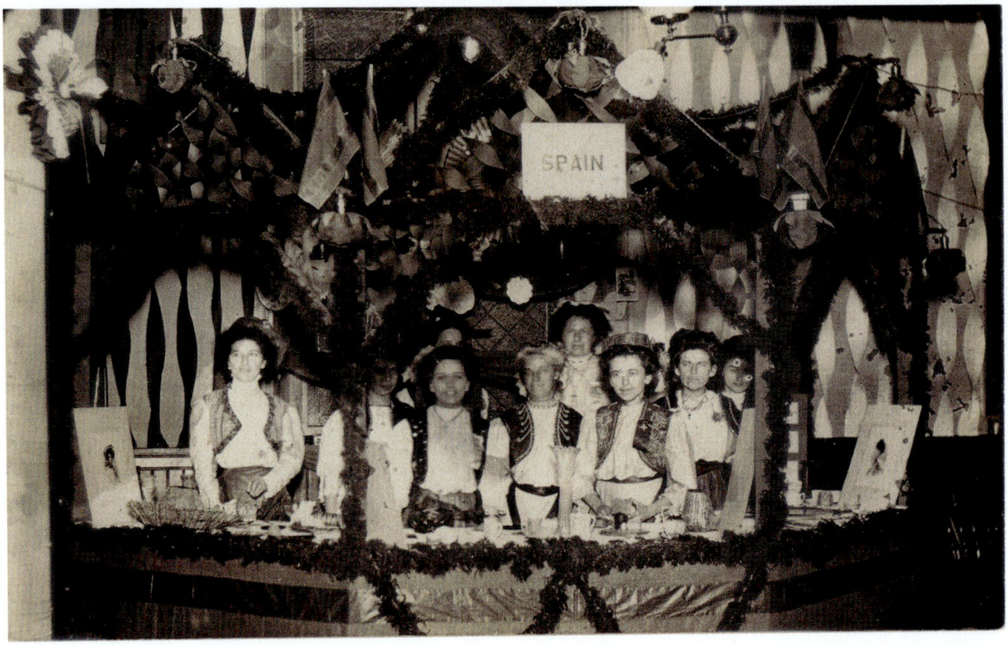

Figure 103

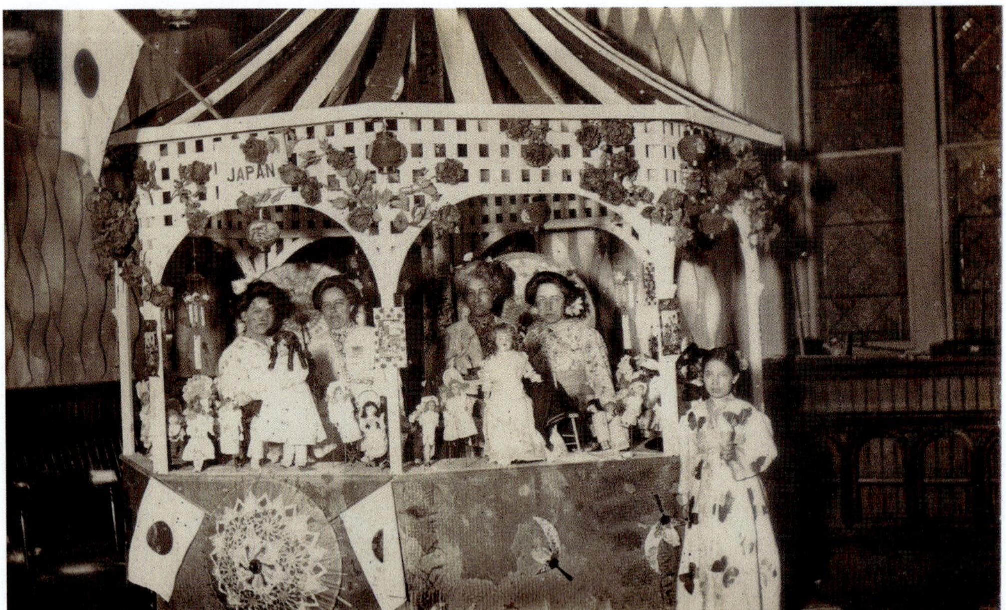

Figure 104

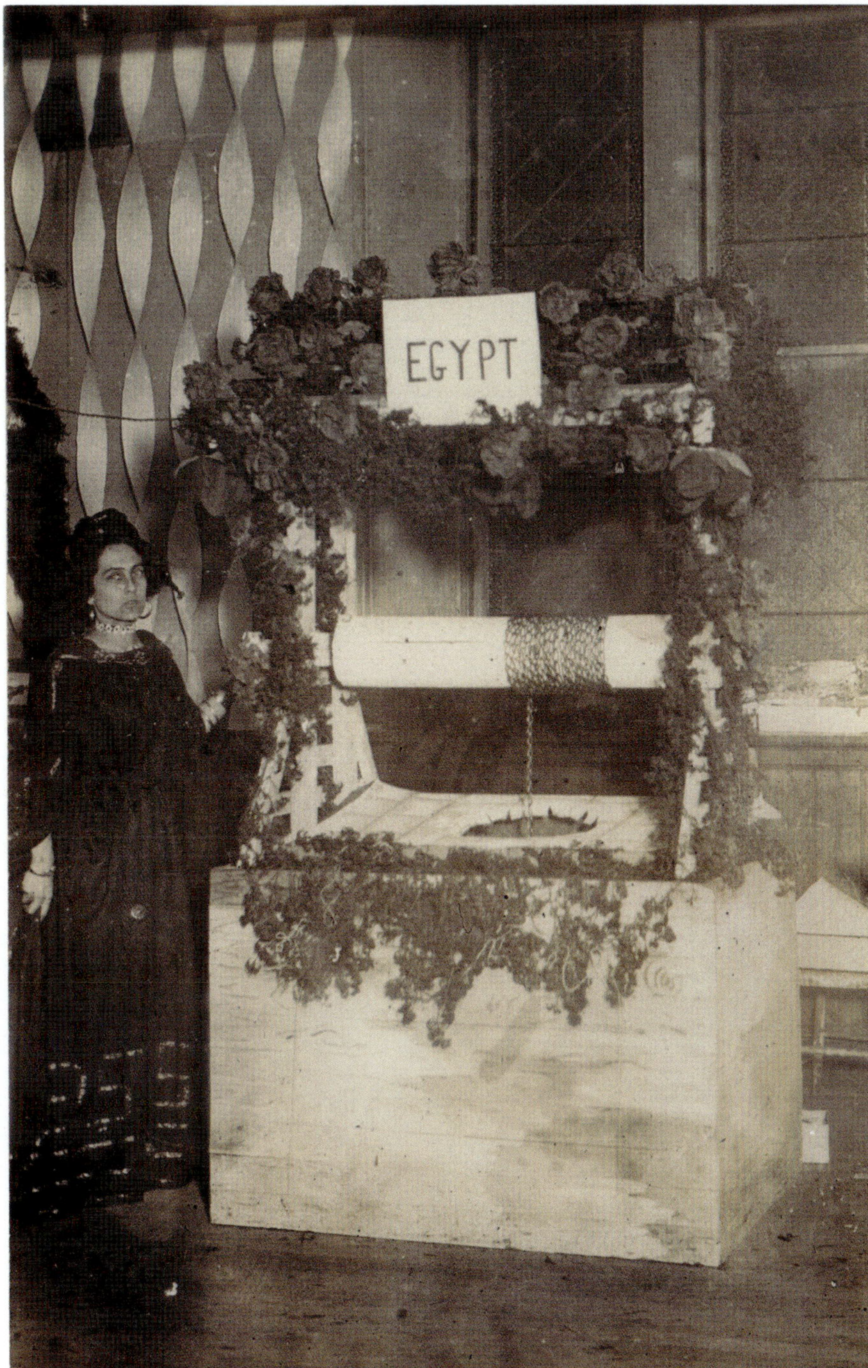

Figure 105

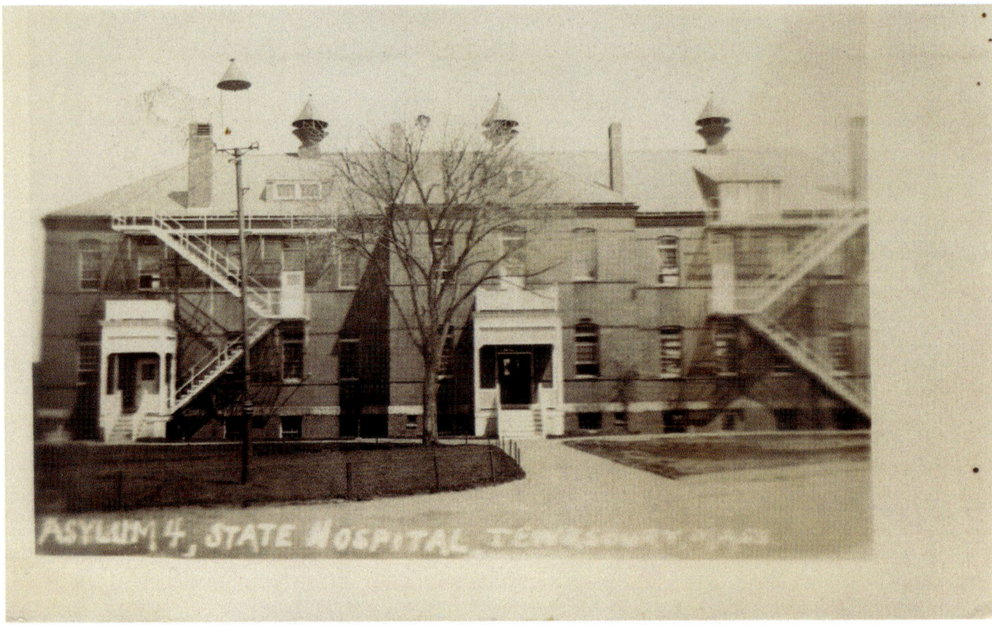
ASYLUM 4, STATE HOSPITAL

Figure 106

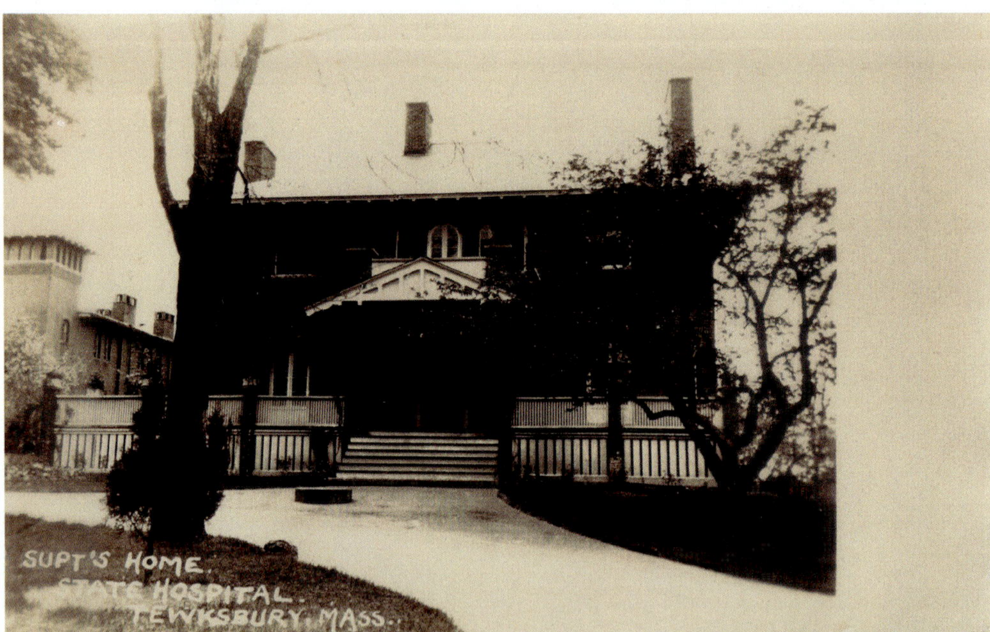
SUPT'S HOME.
STATE HOSPITAL.
TEWKSBURY, MASS.

Figure 107

Connecticut General Hospital for the Insane
Middletown, Connecticut, 1868

Opened in 1868 as the Connecticut General Hospital for the Insane, this facility was established to care for the growing number of Connecticut citizens that had been deemed "insane." The town provided land for the asylum and an additional 80 acres of adjoining land was also purchased. By 1912, additional land purchases provided a total of 650 acres for the hospital. The name was changed in 1874 to Connecticut Hospital for the Insane (figure 108), commonly referred to as Connecticut State Hospital until the name changed again in 1961 to Connecticut Valley Hospital.

A center building and one wing were ready for accommodating patients when the facility was opened, and over the next three years, three other wings were added providing a total of 450 beds by 1874.

By 1898, a new ward and five additional hospital buildings had been added and the population had risen to 1,895 patients. In the early 1900s, several buildings were destroyed by fire, including the amusement hall, chapel, and engine and tool rooms. No one was injured and planning began immediately for new fireproof buildings. By 1912, the number of buildings had increased to 34 (figures 109–111) with 2,535 patients in residence.

This facility continues to operate as Connecticut Valley Hospital. Although most of the original structures have been demolished, the central building, erected in 1867, remains standing.

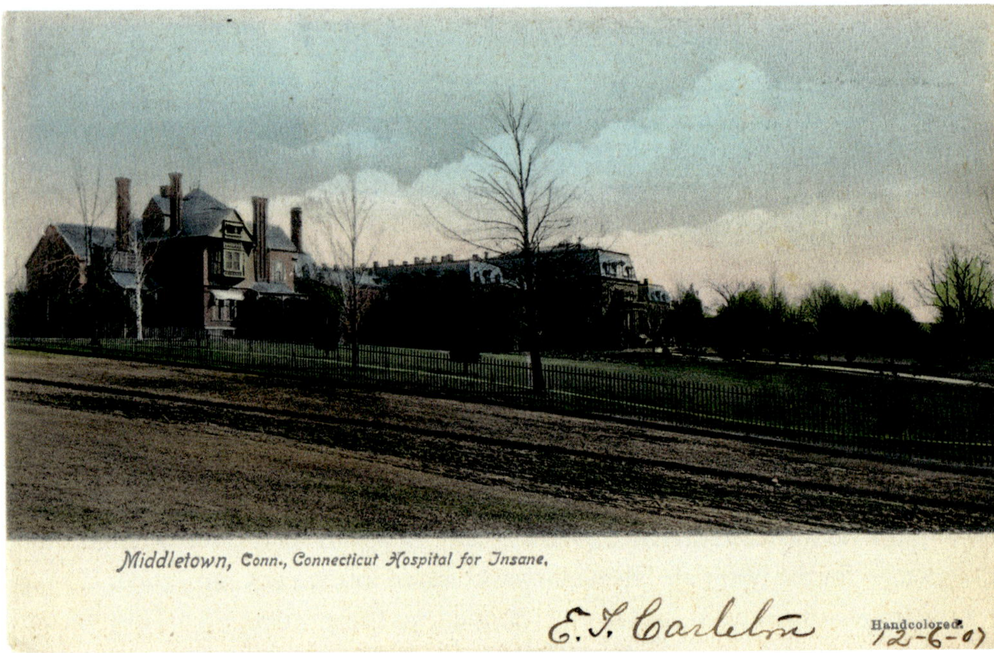
Middletown, Conn., Connecticut Hospital for Insane.
E. T. Carleton
Handcolored.
12-6-07

Figure 108

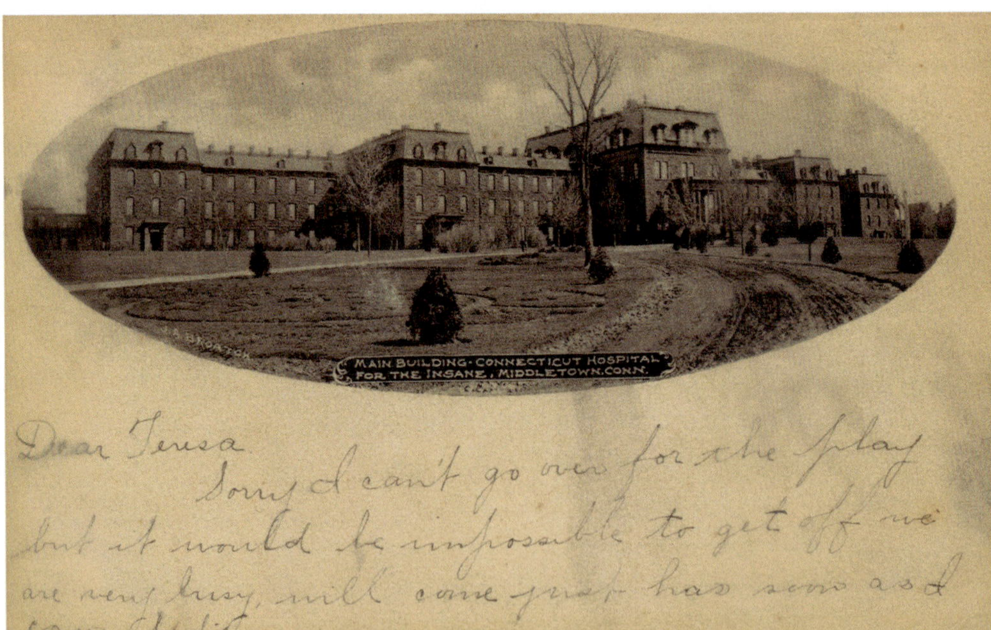
MAIN BUILDING - CONNECTICUT HOSPITAL FOR THE INSANE, MIDDLETOWN. CONN.
Dear Teresa
Sorry I can't go over for the play
but it would be impossible to get off we
are very busy, will come just as soon as I
can. Addie.

Figure 109

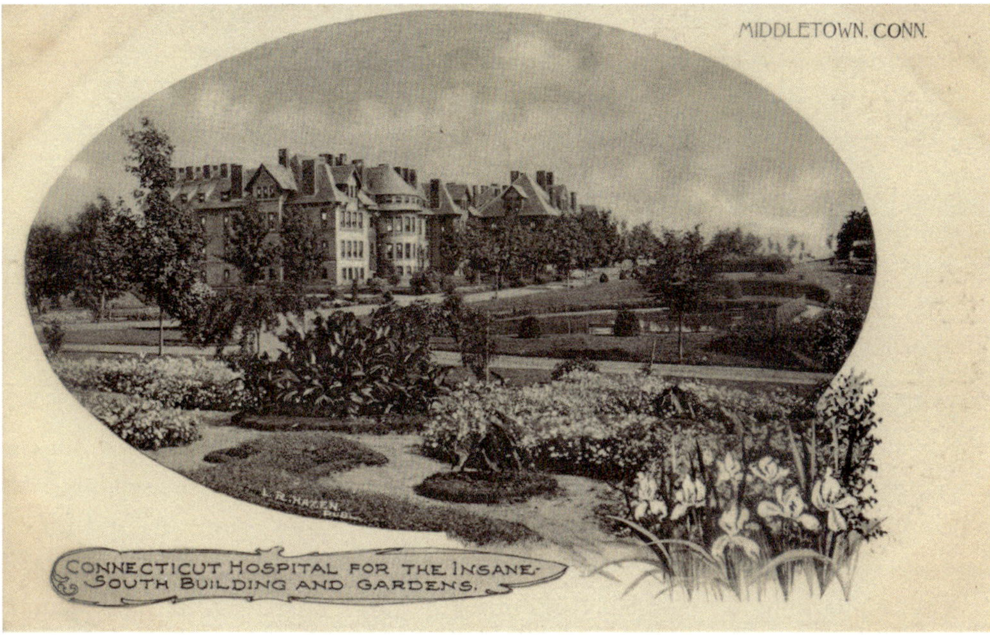
MIDDLETOWN, CONN.
CONNECTICUT HOSPITAL FOR THE INSANE-
SOUTH BUILDING AND GARDENS.

Figure 110

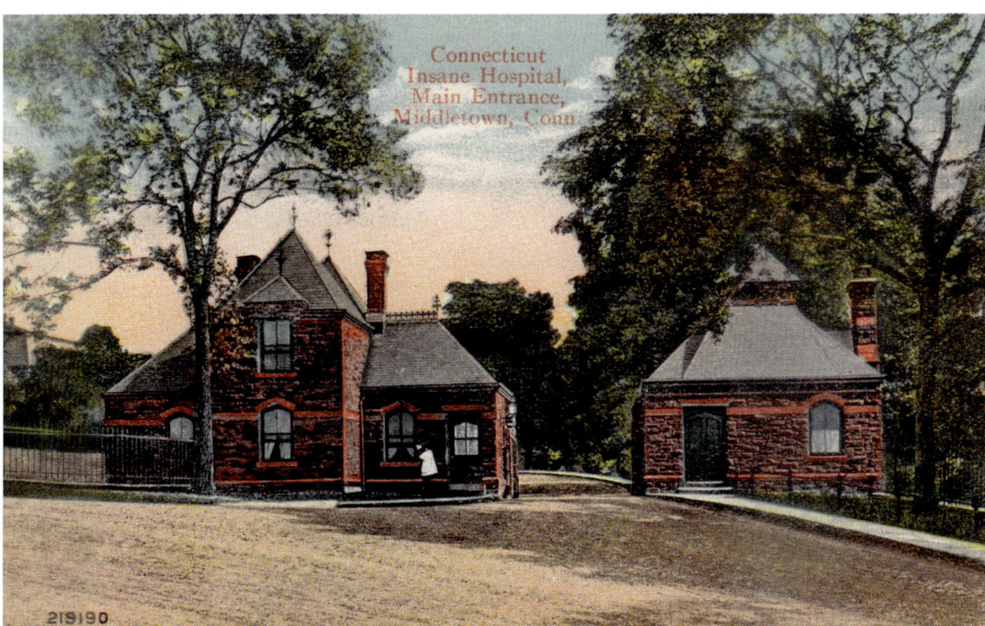
Connecticut
Insane Hospital,
Main Entrance,
Middletown, Conn.
219190

Figure 111

Willard State Hospital
Willard, New York, 1869

Willard State Hospital was opened in 1869 in Willard, New York to care for the chronically mentally ill. Willard was the first state asylum built to care only for the chronically ill as an experiment in relieving overcrowding at other asylums. This policy was discontinued in 1890 when patients with acute cases of mental illness were accepted.

The facility, built as a modified Kirkbride structure, included a three-story administration building with extended patient wards. Several detached cottage buildings were added over the years to accommodate patients and staff.

The Maples (figure 112), also known as "Detached Building #1," was opened in 1872. It was the first of five buildings opened by 1878.

The Hermitage building (figure 113), built in 1884, served as the male infirmary. In the early 1900s, its large enclosed porch was used to segregate tuberculosis patients.

The 1915 image in figure 114 shows field day, held every year in September. The annual field day included races, a parade, and booths displaying goods created at the hospital. These field days could attract up to 1,500 spectators.

In the early years of the hospital, patients frequently arrived by boat (figure 115).

The Grandview building (figure 116) was erected in 1860 as part of the New York State Agricultural College. It was repurposed as part of the asylum to house female patients.

The hospital closed in 1995, but the site is now home to the Willard Psychiatric Center. Most of the original buildings, including the original Kirkbride structure have been demolished, but some—including Grandview—have survived.

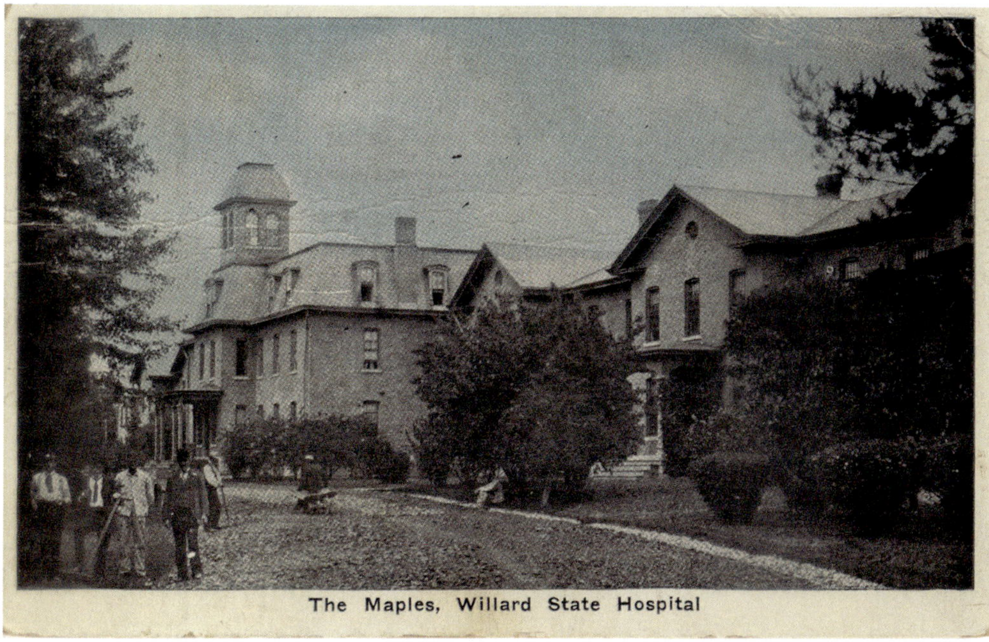

Figure 112

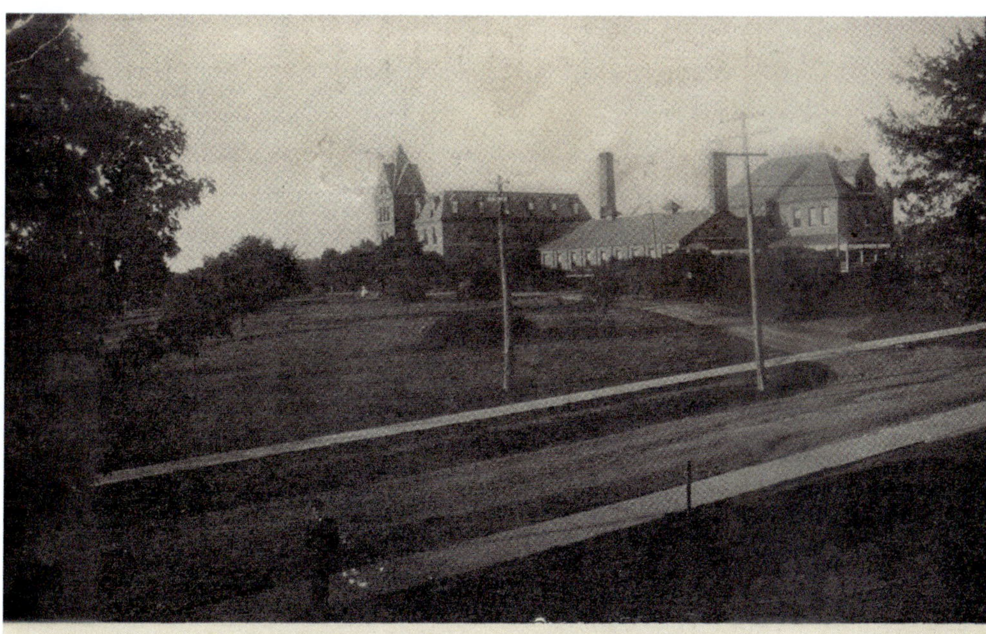

Figure 113

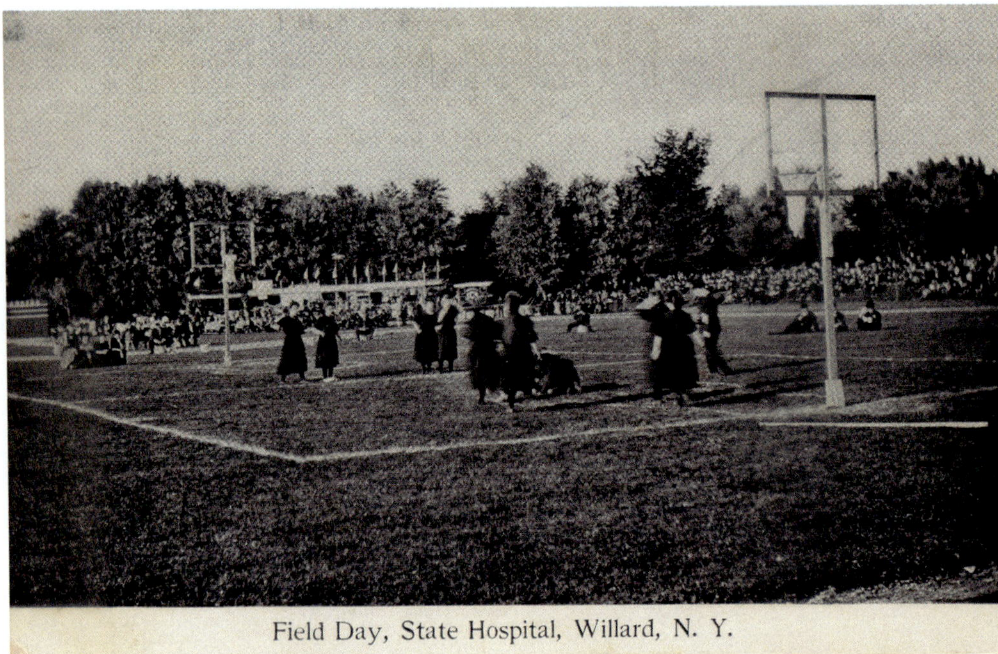
Field Day, State Hospital, Willard, N. Y.

Figure 114

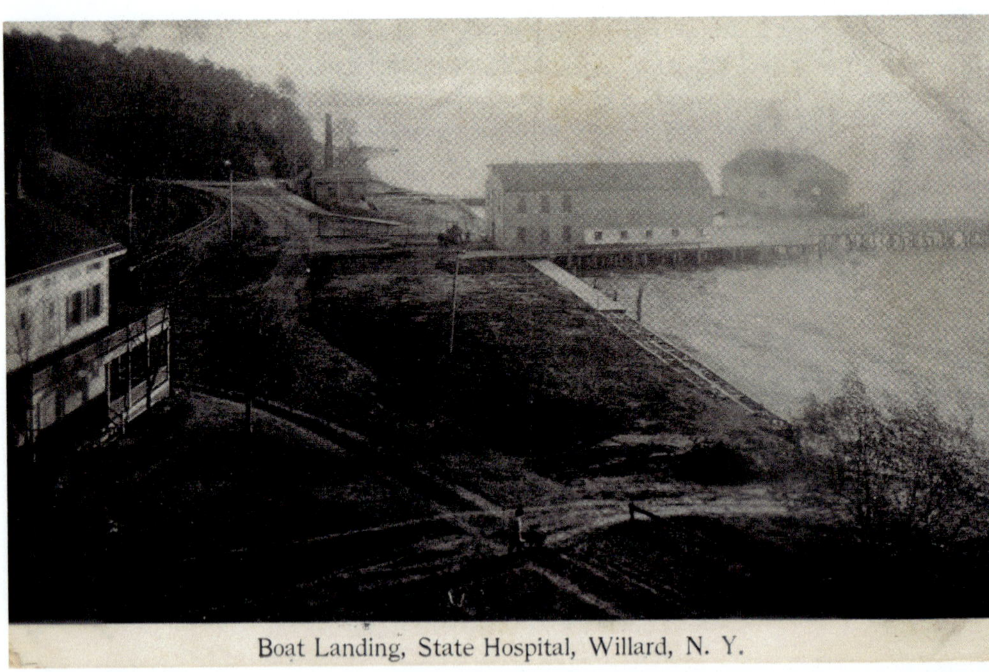
Boat Landing, State Hospital, Willard, N. Y.

Figure 115

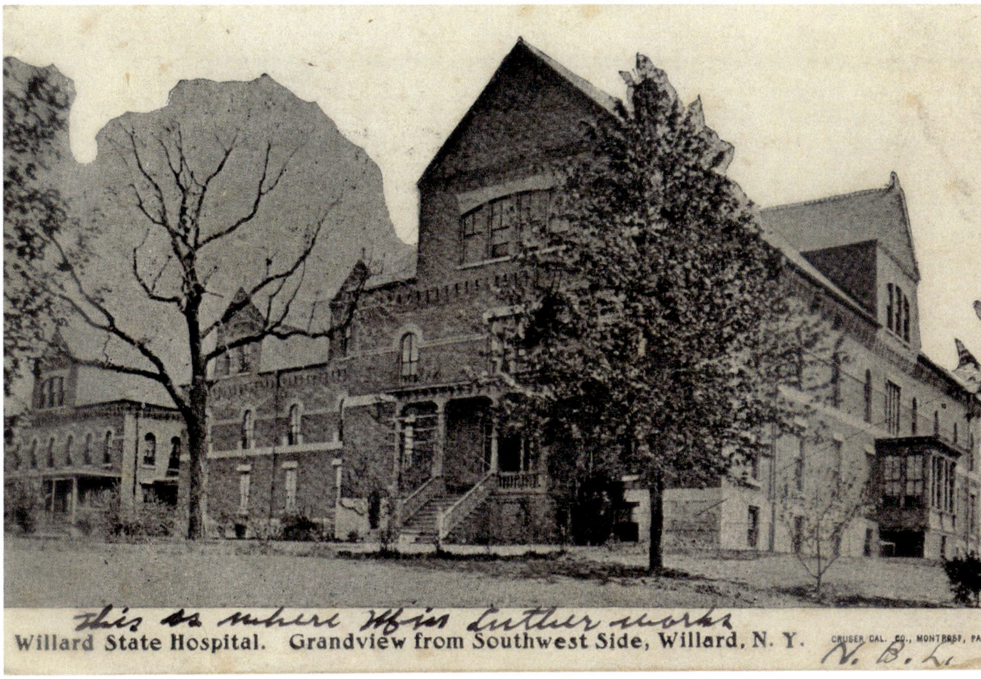
this is where Miss Luther works
Willard State Hospital. Grandview from Southwest Side, Willard, N. Y.
N. B. L.

Figure 116

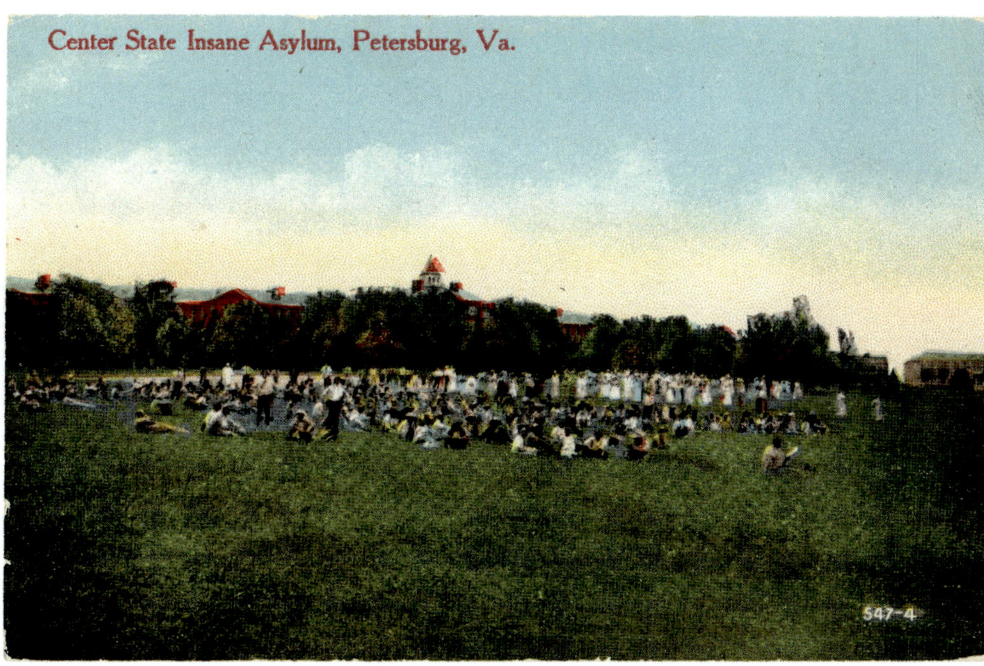
Center State Insane Asylum, Petersburg, Va.
547-4

Figure 117

Central Lunatic Asylum
Petersburg, Virginia, 1869

Originally called the Central Lunatic Asylum, the Central State Hospital began in 1869 as a hospital for mentally ill African American patients after the Civil War. Originally located in Howard Grover near Richmond, the hospital moved to St. Petersburg in 1885 and 373 patients from Howard Grover were transferred to the new facility. By September 1886, there were 436 patients in the asylum with 100 waiting for admission. By 1888, the patient census had risen to 576. In 1967, the facility began accepting people of all races.

The facility included a four-story administration building with three-story wings extending to each side. Construction continued and by 1914, there were 1,800 patients residing in 14 buildings.

Postcards of this facility are rare. This distant but significant image on the previous page (figure 117) shows the patients on the grounds.

Central State Hospital continues to occupy the same site in St. Petersburg. Mayfield Cottage, a building erected in 1750 and later used by the hospital for its headquarters, survives. It was sold privately and has been moved approximately one mile from its original location

Hudson River State Hospital for the Insane
Poughkeepsie, New York, 1871

Opened in 1871 as the Hudson River State Hospital for the Insane, this facility consisted of a beautiful Victorian-style Kirkbride which overlooked the Hudson River and the Shawangunk Mountains. This Kirkbride building was unique, in that one wing was slightly longer than the other, due to a lack of construction funds. The original plans specified a hospital capable of accommodating 500 patients. By 1872, there were 212 patients housed at the hospital. The capacity of this institution was increased from 800 beds in 1890 to 1,400 by 1893. By the early 1900s, the hospital staff included 20 physicians and 608 employees.

The postcard of this facility in figure 118 is postmarked 1908.

The main hospital buildings were located on a slope, which extended to the banks of the Hudson River (figure 119).

These facilities were closed in 2001, abandoned in 2003, and the property was sold. The original main building was destroyed by fire in 2007. Psychiatric services are presently provided by the Hudson River Psychiatric Center.

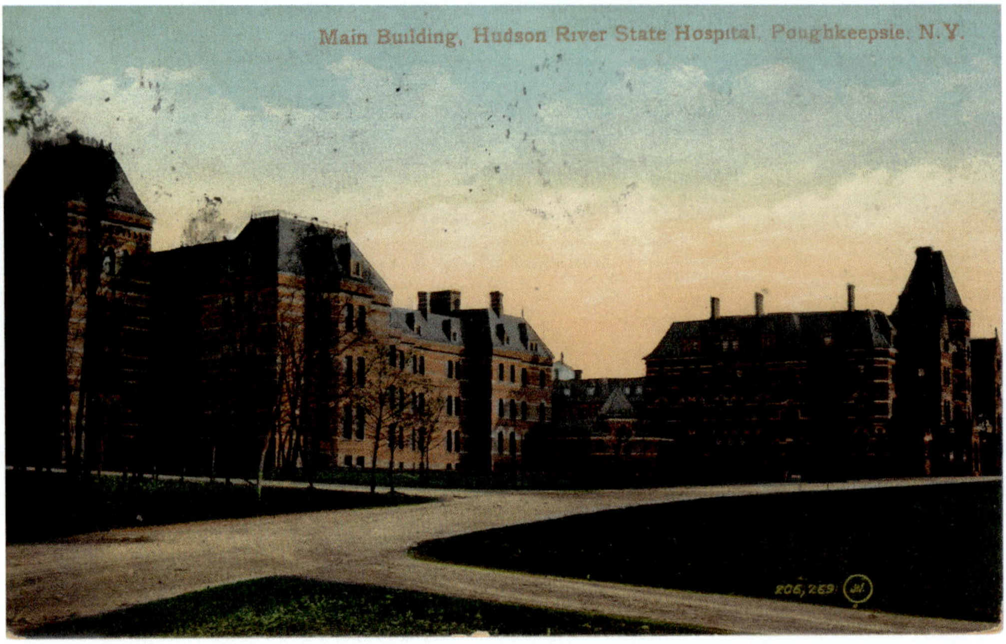

Figure 118

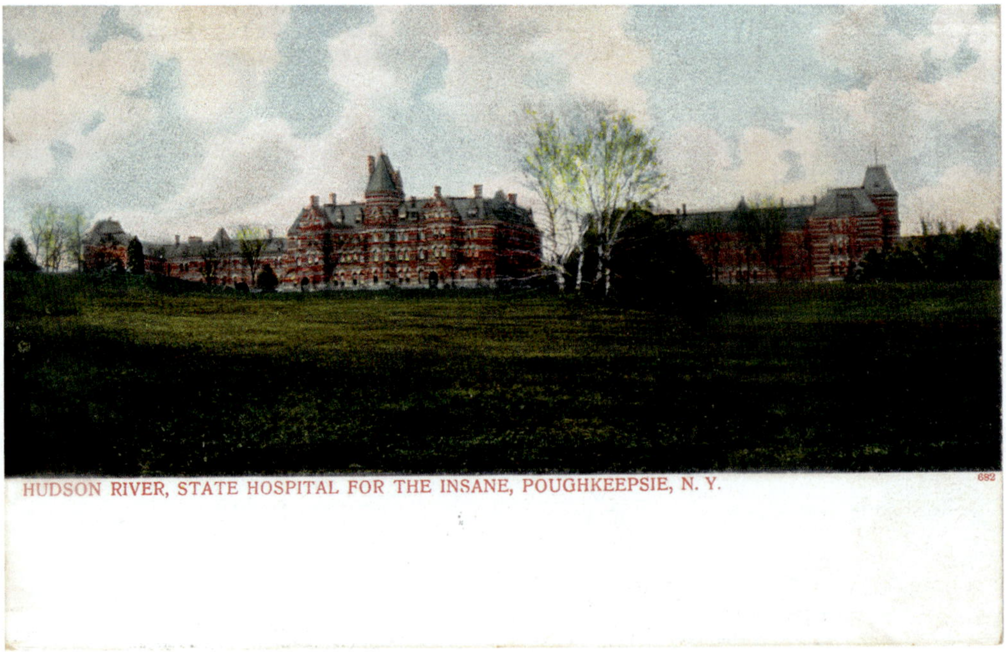

Figure 119

Insane Asylum of Washington Territory
Fort Steilacoom, Washington, 1871

The Insane Asylum of Washington Territory opened in 1871, making use of the buildings and grounds of a former US Army post at Fort Steilacoom. The total number of patients was 23 in October 1871.

Various improvements were made over the next few years, including the addition of an assembly room and chapel. The hospital also operated a 500-acre farm that included hogs, chickens, and cattle that supplied milk for the facility. Patients assisted in the farm and garden work and also worked in the kitchen, bakery, carpenter shop, and blacksmith's shop.

The original buildings were replaced by a new brick structure (figure 120) in 1887 and by 1900, the number of patients had risen to 694.

The facility was renamed Western State Hospital in 1915 and is still in operation. Some of the original officers' quarters that were part of Fort Steilacoom have survived, but the central asylum buildings have not.

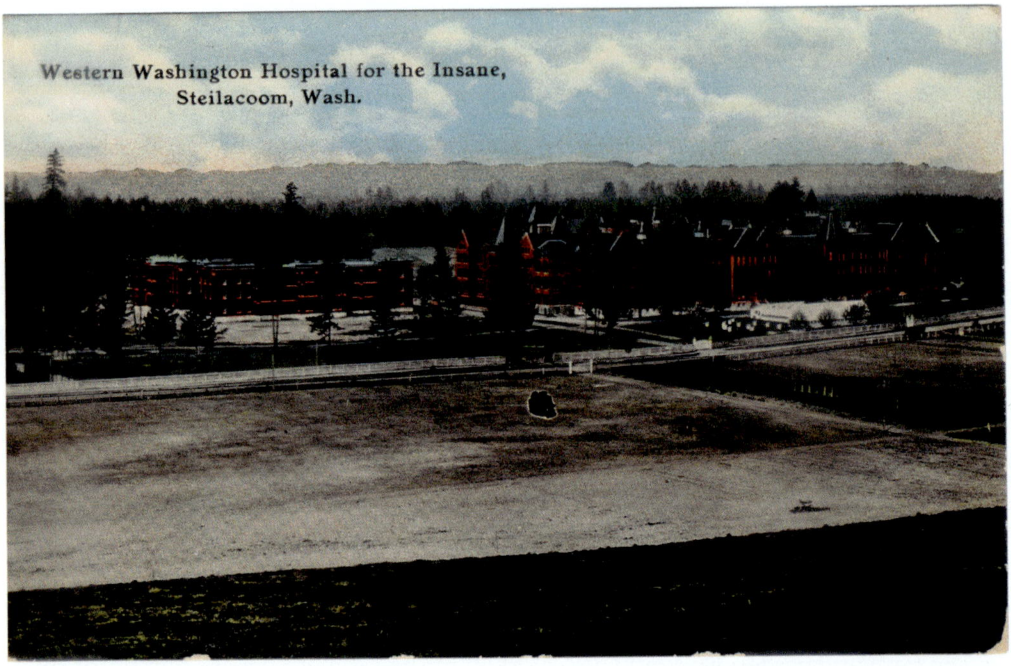

Figure 120

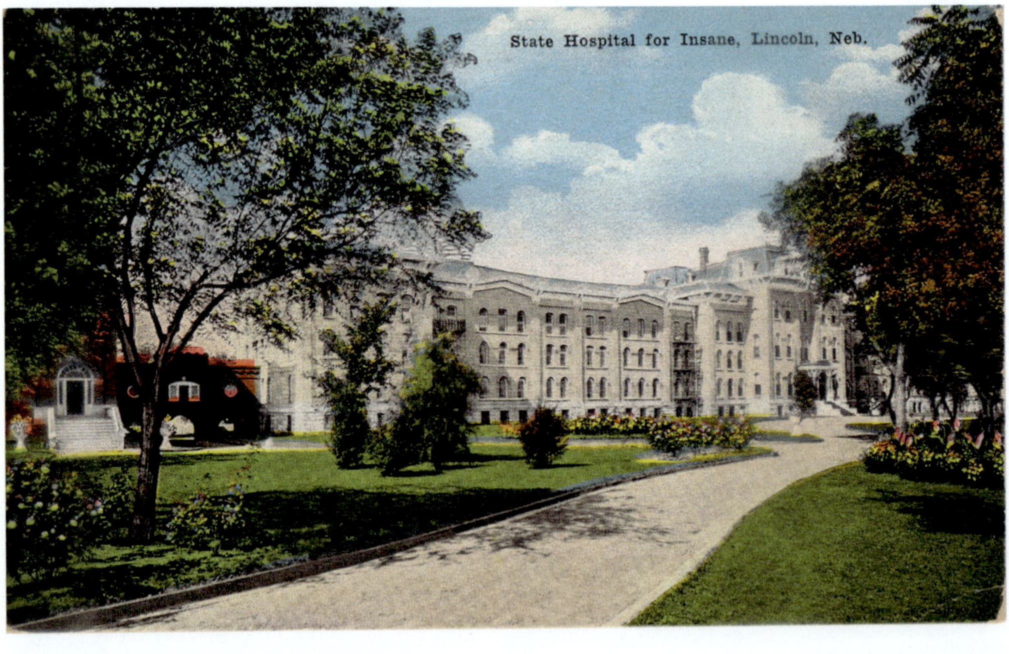

Figure 121

Lincoln State Hospital
Lincoln, Nebraska, 1871

Thirty-three people comprised the first group of patients admitted to this facility, with twenty-two of them coming from Iowa hospitals and eleven coming from prisons. The first building was destroyed by fire in April 1871 and a replacement building (figure 121) was enlarged and completed a year later. By 1900, the grounds spread over 800 acres, including the 20-acre campus (figure 122).

Thirteen years later, two buildings were added to accommodate 100 patients in each. Two complete hydrotherapy baths, one for males and one for females, were installed with a building for recreation. In 1913, the facility housed 800 people including patients and staff.

The facility was renamed the Lincoln Regional Center in 1969 and operates as a psychiatric hospital.

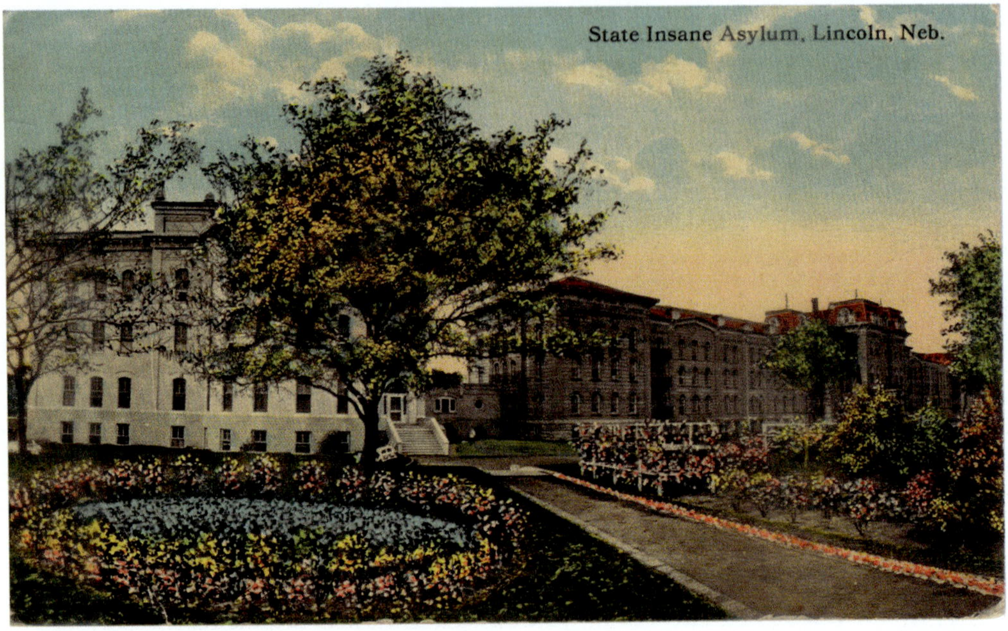
State Insane Asylum, Lincoln, Neb.

Figure 122

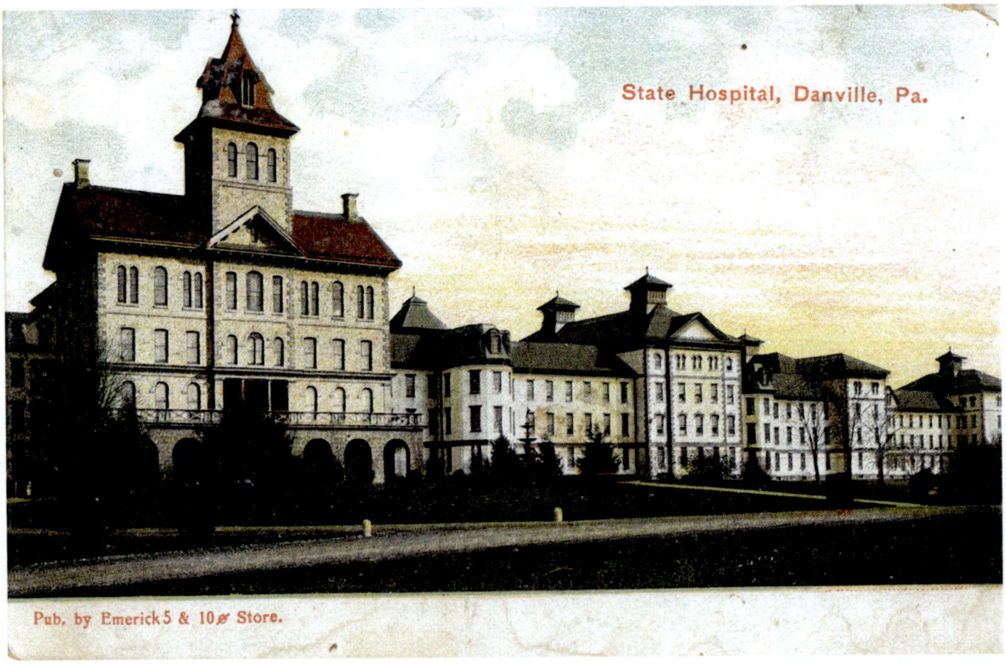
State Hospital, Danville, Pa.
Pub. by Emerick 5 & 10¢ Store.

Figure 123

Danville State Hospital
Danville, Pennsylvania, 1872

The Danville State Hospital (figure 124) opened in 1872 as the first state lunatic asylum in Pennsylvania. Previously, each county had been responsible for the care of the mentally ill. The opening of Danville provided relief from significant overcrowding at county institutions.

The original Kirkbride-style structure (figure 123) provided room for 200 patients. In 1881, fire destroyed the wing for female patients, the administration building, and one-third of the wing for male patients. By 1883, the wings were repaired to conform with the original design while the administration building was completely rebuilt.

A nurses' home was completed in 1900 and two buildings for the treatment of patients with acute cases of mental illness were completed in 1909. Five years later, the facility had a capacity for 1,450 patients.

The grounds and farm (figure 125) were repeatedly extended, growing from the original 250 acres to 663 in 1916. Thirty-five acres were occupied by gardens and 430 were used for the farm.

The postcard in figure 126 provides a rare inside look at the hospital from sometime around 1915.

Trains and carriages were the most common method of transporting patients to the hospitals in the early 1800s. The postcard in figure 127 shows the train going to the Danville Hospital.

The facility continues to operate as Danville State Hospital. The central Kirkbride building along with several detached buildings have survived.

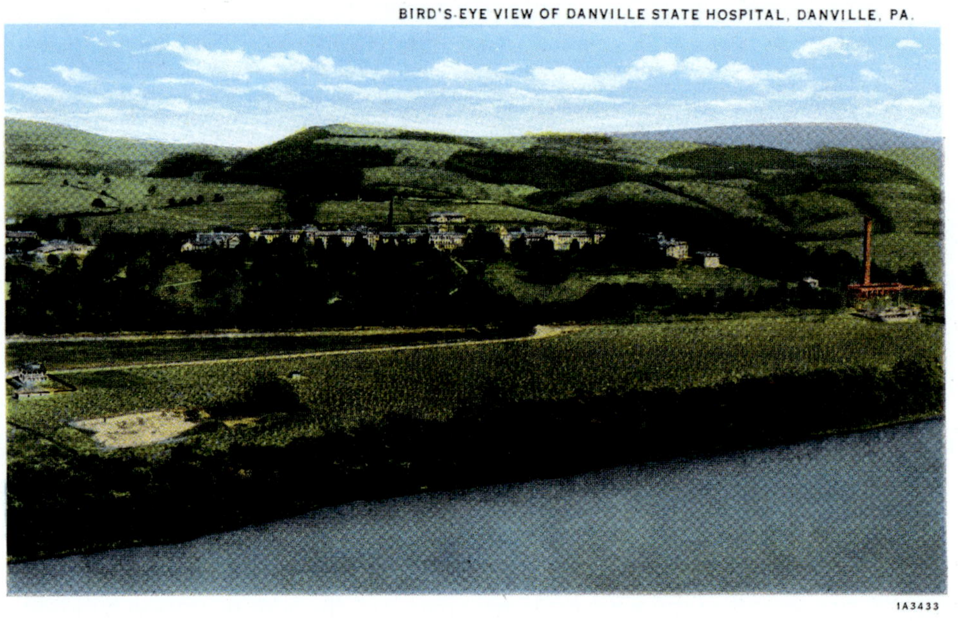

Figure 124

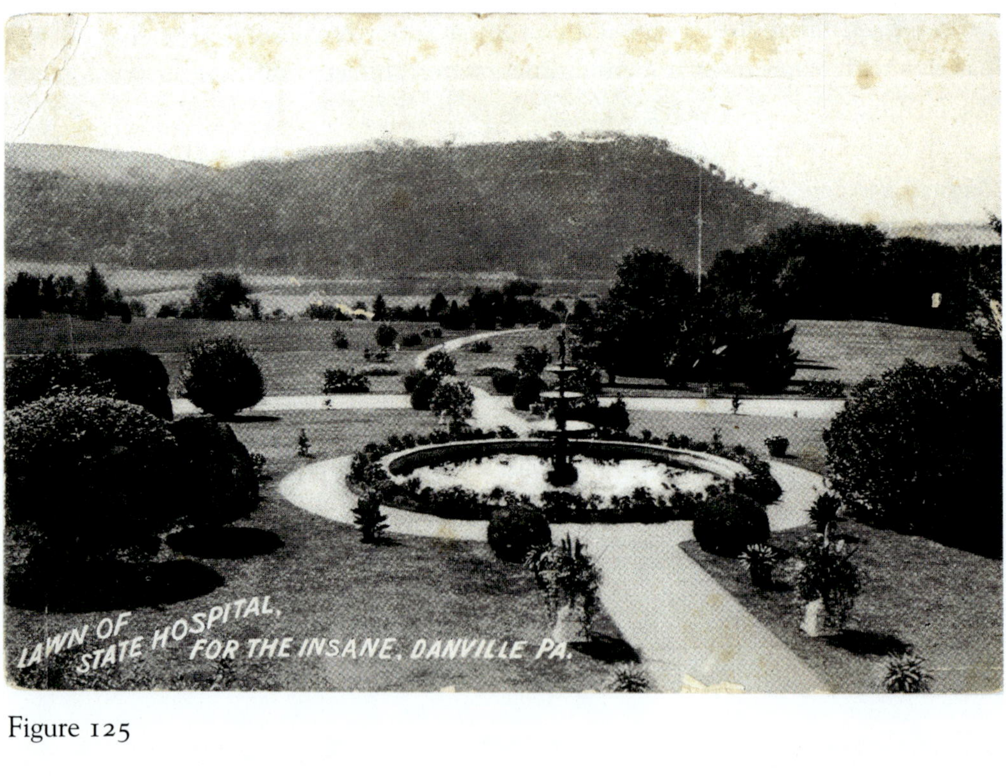

Figure 125

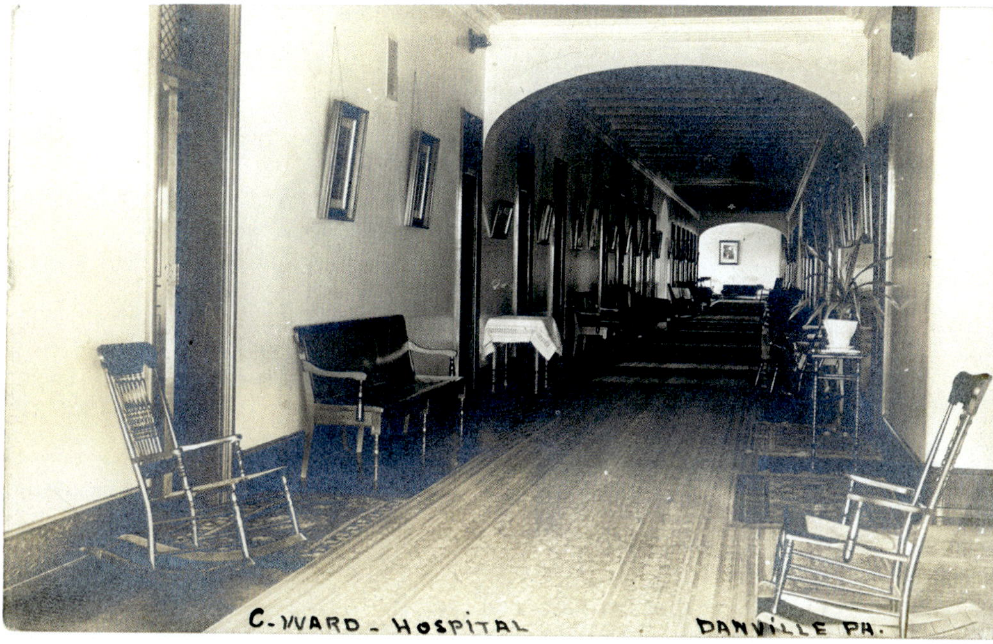

Figure 126

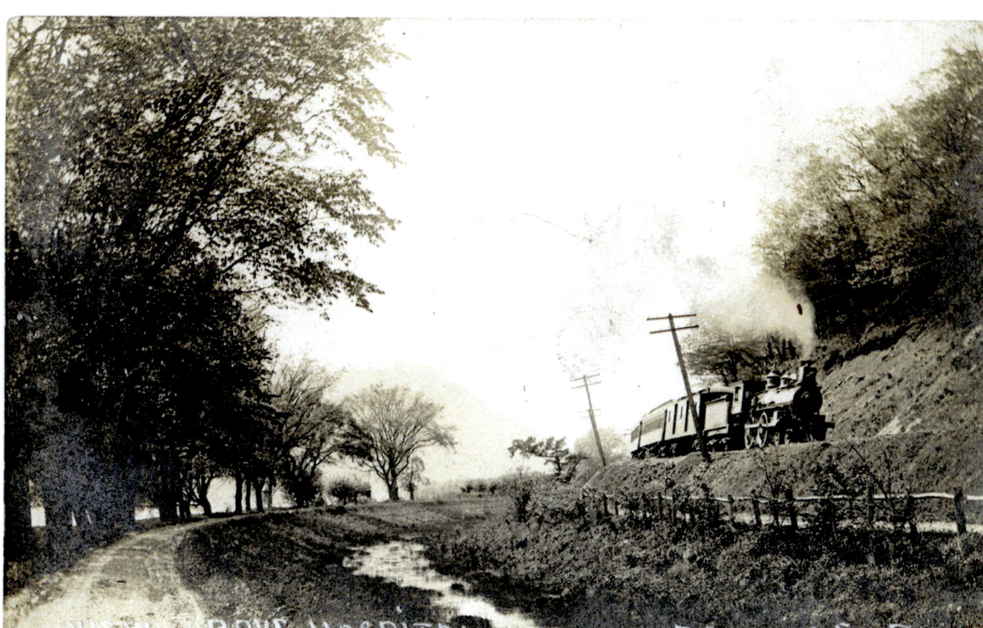

Figure 127

Northern Illinois Hospital and Asylum
Elgin, Illinois, 1872

This Northern Illinois Hospital and Asylum for the Insane (figures 128 and 131) opened in 1872 after a construction delay resulting from the Chicago Fire of 1871. Many of the first patients came from an overcrowded state hospital in Jacksonville, county poorhouses, and private homes. The three-story building (figure 129) housed male patients on the two lower floors and female patients on the third floor. The facility housed 183 patients by the end of the first year. By 1910, a new receiving ward was approved and later, a new building was added for tuberculosis patients. Additional buildings added housing for 170 more patients.

The patient census at Elgin was not published, so it is difficult to assess how many patients received care at any given time. As institutions became more overcrowded, the numbers of patients were often omitted from official institutional reports.

The facility, renamed the Elgin State Hospital in 1910, currently operates as the Elgin Mental Health Center. The Kirkbride building (figure 130) was demolished in 1993.

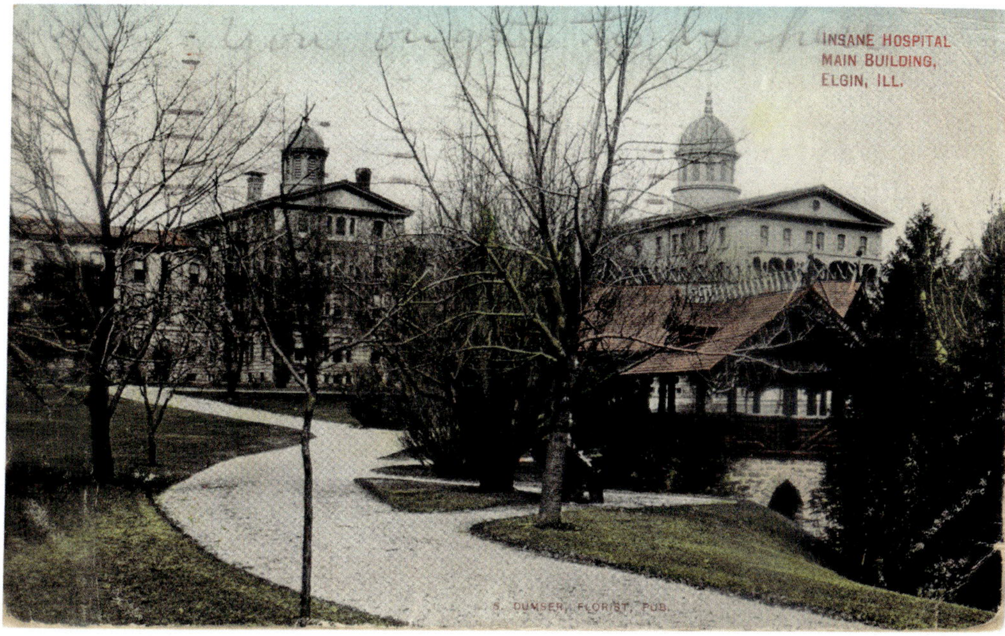
INSANE HOSPITAL
MAIN BUILDING,
ELGIN, ILL.
S. DUMSER, FLORIST, PUB.

Figure 128

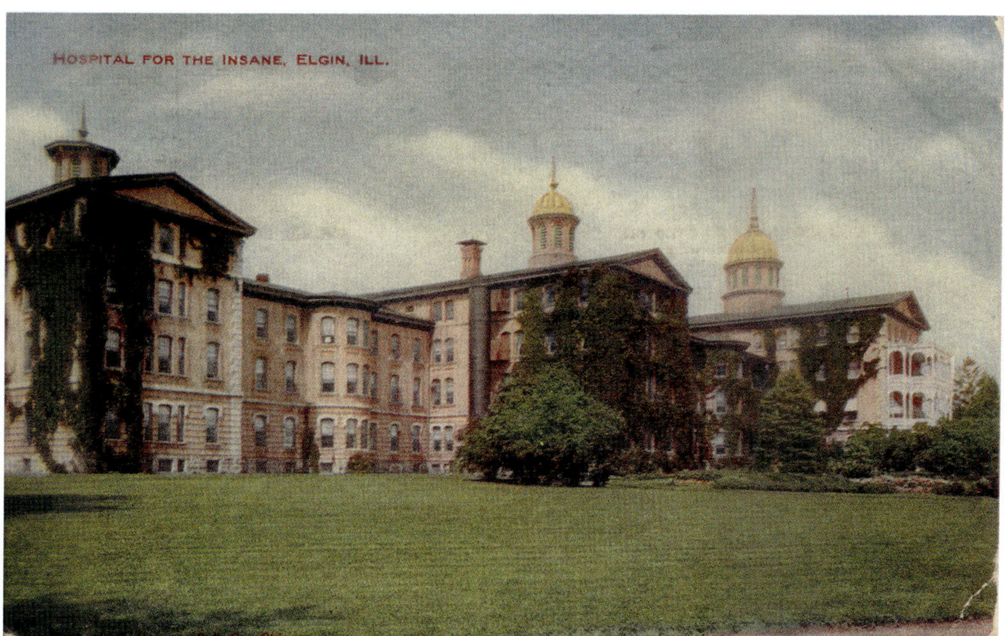
HOSPITAL FOR THE INSANE, ELGIN, ILL.

Figure 129

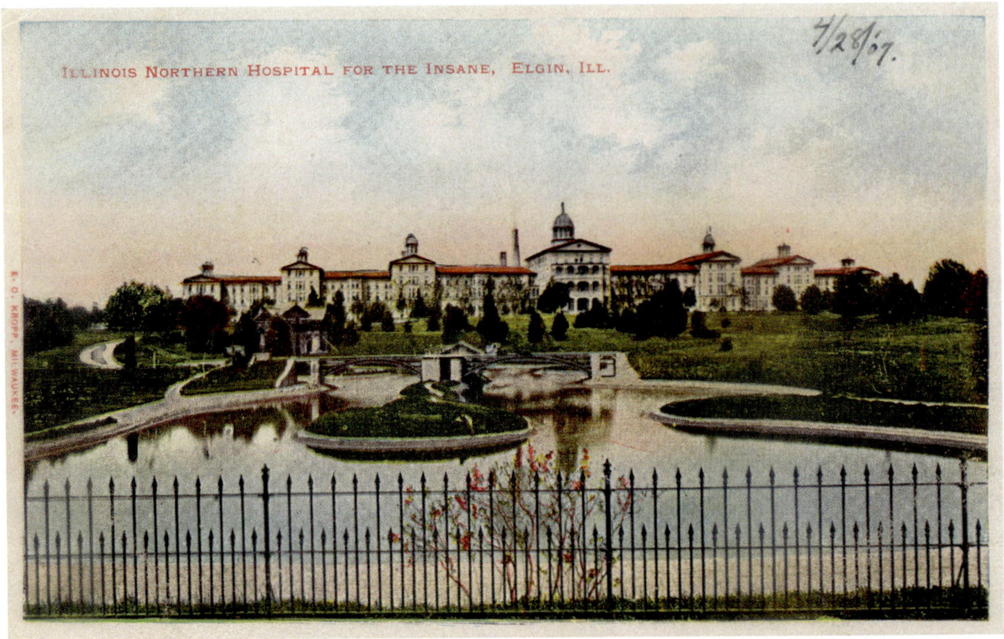
ILLINOIS NORTHERN HOSPITAL FOR THE INSANE, ELGIN, ILL.
4/28/07.
E. O. KROPP, MILWAUKEE.

Figure 130

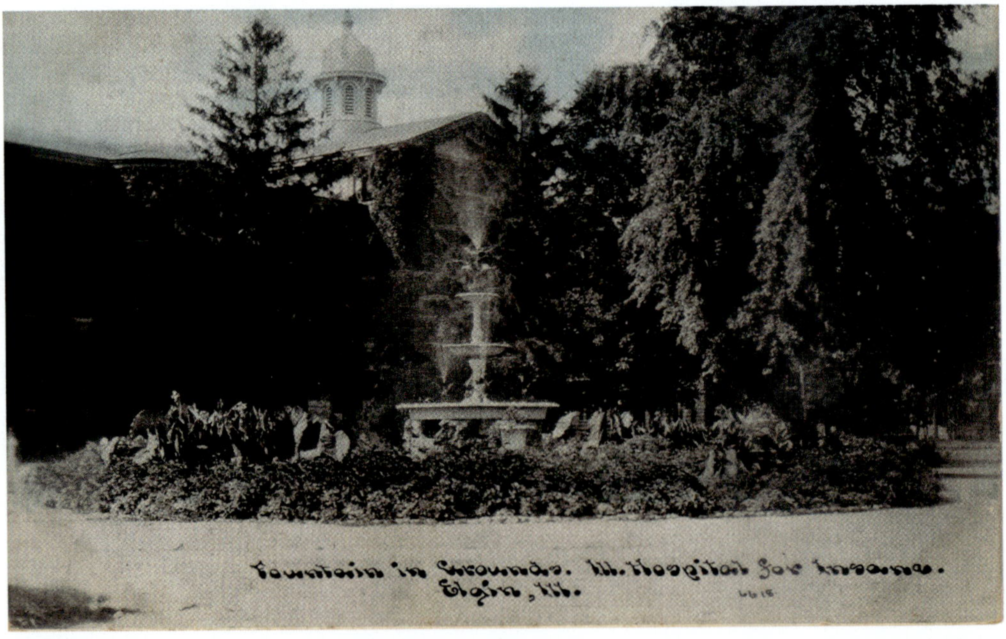
Fountain in Grounds. Ill. Hospital for Insane.
Elgin, Ill.

Figure 131

Iowa Hospital for the Insane
Independence, Iowa, 1873

This Iowa Hospital for the Insane opened in 1883 as the second state institution in Iowa, with the construction of the Kirkbride-style building beginning a decade earlier in 1873.

The original central building (figure 132) was five stories with attached three-story wings. The facility could house up to 600 patients when it was completed in 1883. Three detached cottages were later added to increase the capacity.

In 1907, a hospital intended for patients requiring acute care was added with a capacity of 134 beds. It included an operating room and hydrotherapy and electrotherapy equipment. By 1907, the patient census reached 1,200 with 200 employees. The farm consisted of 1,366 acres.

The green house, pictured in figure 133, was a common structure in asylums, providing work for patients.

The original Kirkbride building is still in use as part of the current facility now called the Independence Mental Health Institute.

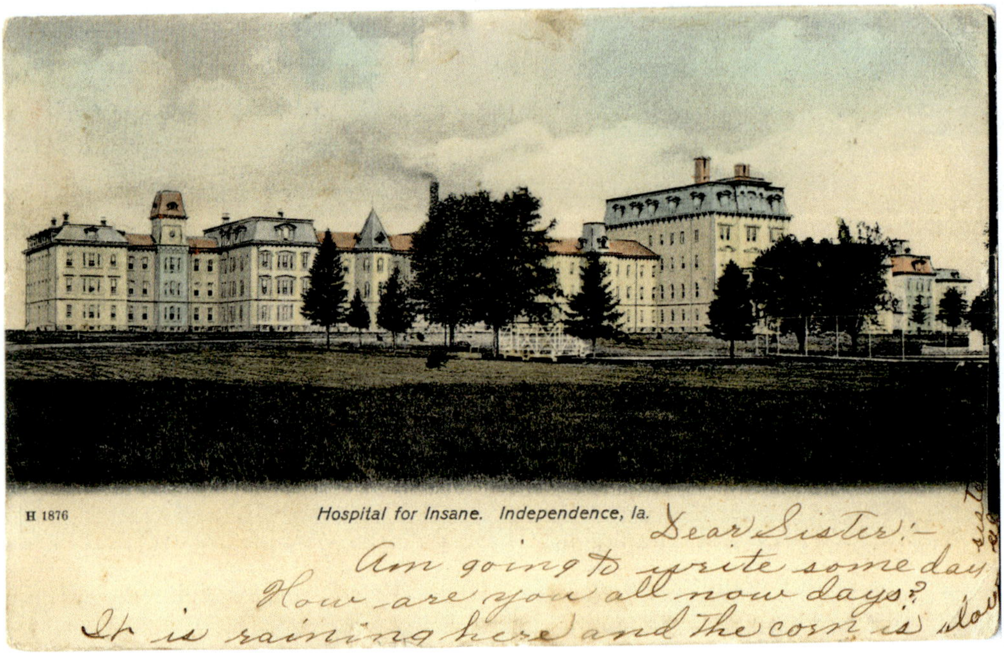
H 1876
Hospital for Insane. Independence, Ia.
Dear Sister:-
Am going to write some day
How are you all now days?
It is raining here and the corn is

Figure 132

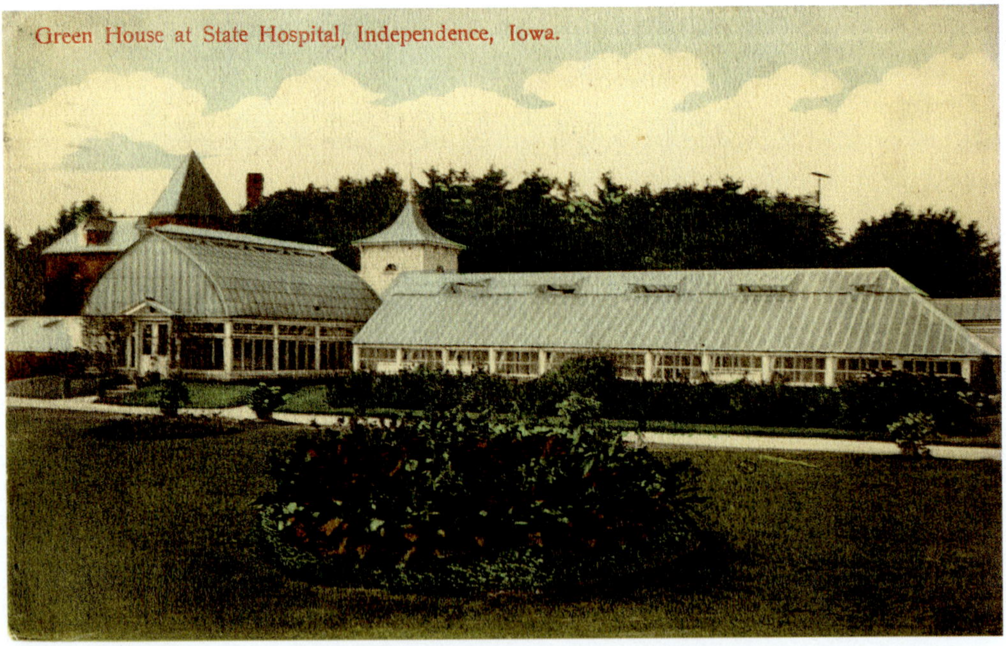
Green House at State Hospital, Independence, Iowa.

Figure 133

Illinois Southern Hospital for the Insane
Anna, Illinois, 1875

Opened as the Illinois Southern Hospital for the Insane (figure 134) in 1875, this facility included a four-story administration building with two adjoining wings and a three-story annex with four wings, two for men and two for women. A 100-bed infirmary housed patients with physical illnesses. The facility also included a cottage for tuberculosis patients.

In 1881, a fire completely destroyed the north wing of the main building (figure 135) and in 1895, another fire destroyed the center of the administration building and the south wing. Both were eventually replaced. By 1914, the facility (figure 136) cared for approximately 1,744 patients.

Two stories of the original administration building still stand along with remnants of the wings. The facility now operates as the Choate Mental Health and Development Center.

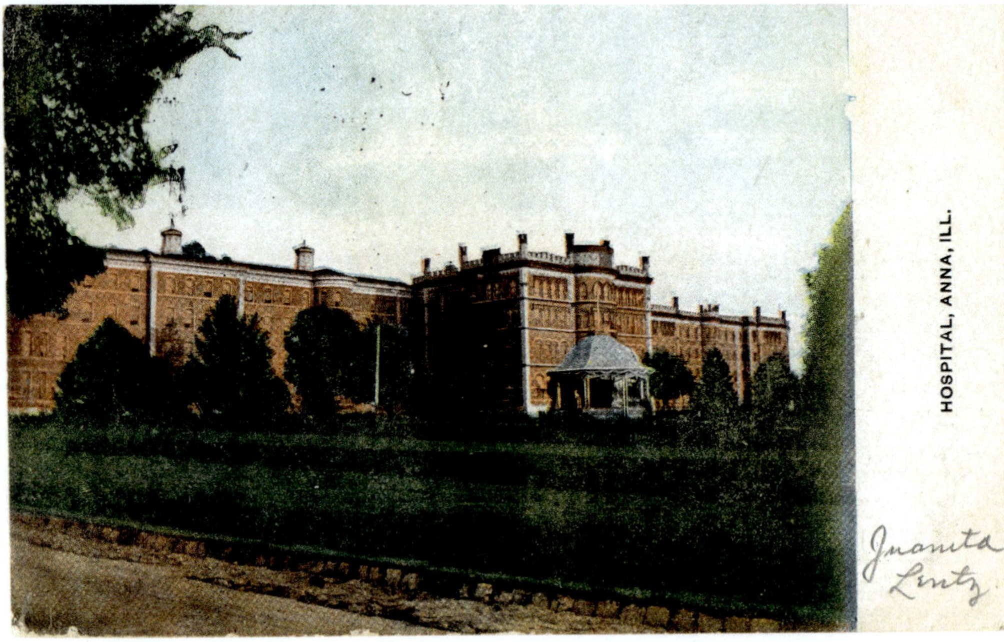
HOSPITAL, ANNA, ILL.
Juanita Lentz

Figure 134

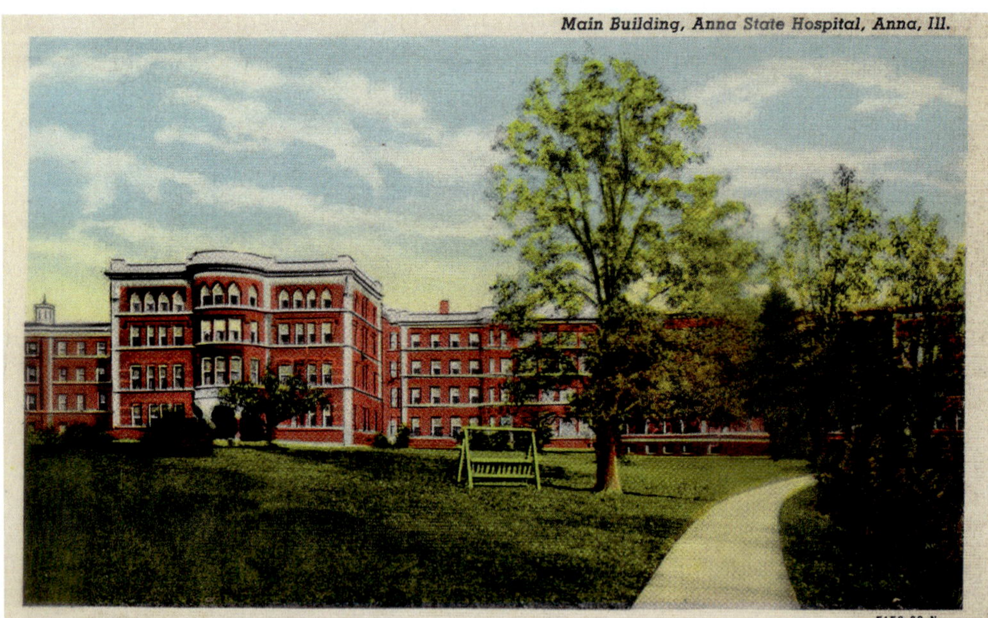
Main Building, Anna State Hospital, Anna, Ill.
5152-29-N

Figure 135

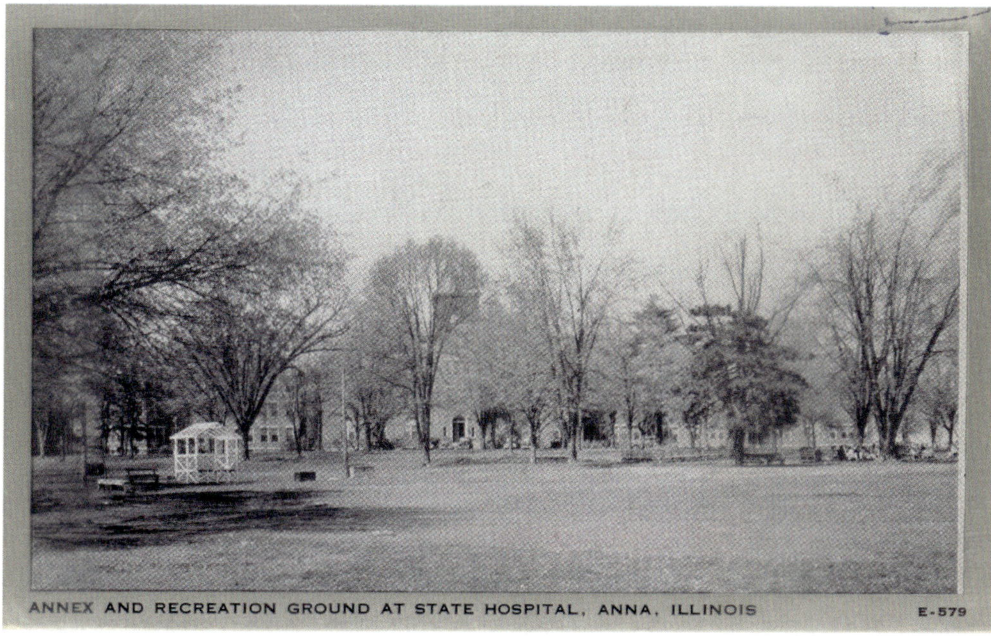
ANNEX AND RECREATION GROUND AT STATE HOSPITAL, ANNA, ILLINOIS
E-579

Figure 136

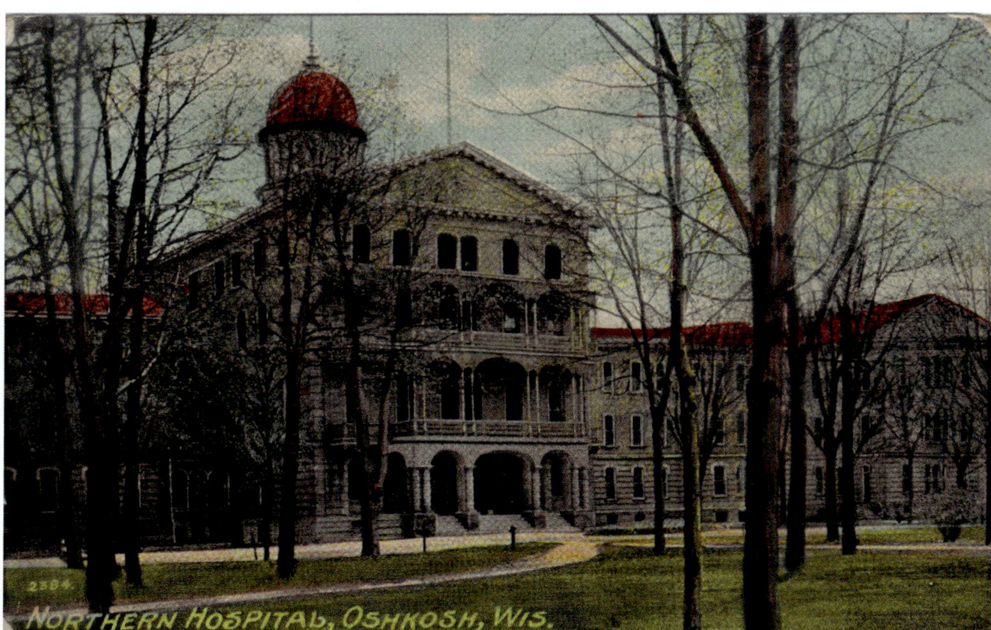
2384
NORTHERN HOSPITAL, OSHKOSH, WIS.

Figure 137

Northern Hospital for the Insane
Winnebago, Wisconsin, 1873

The Northern Hospital for the Insane (figure 137) admitted its first patient in 1873. This was the second state hospital for the mentally ill in Wisconsin and by 1881, both exceeded their capacity.

The Kirkbride building (figure 139) included a central administration building with four wings facing north and south. It was situated on the railroad, providing train service between Oshkosh and the western shore of Lake Winnebago.

The postcard in figure 138 shows a rare view of the interior of the facility's dining room.

The facility now operates under the name of the Winnebago Mental Health Institute. The original buildings have been demolished.

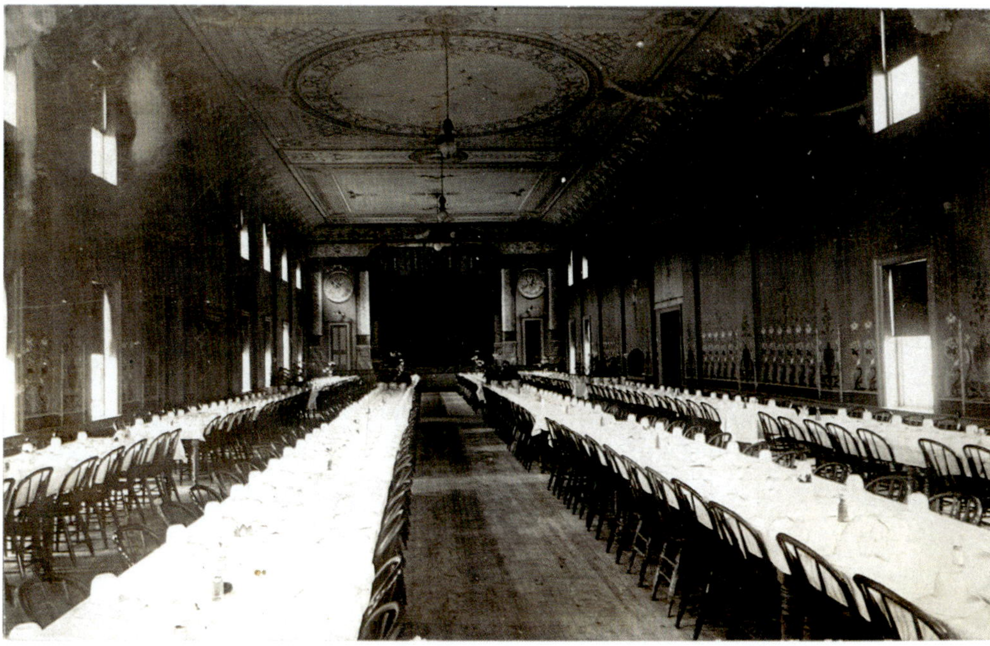

Figure 138

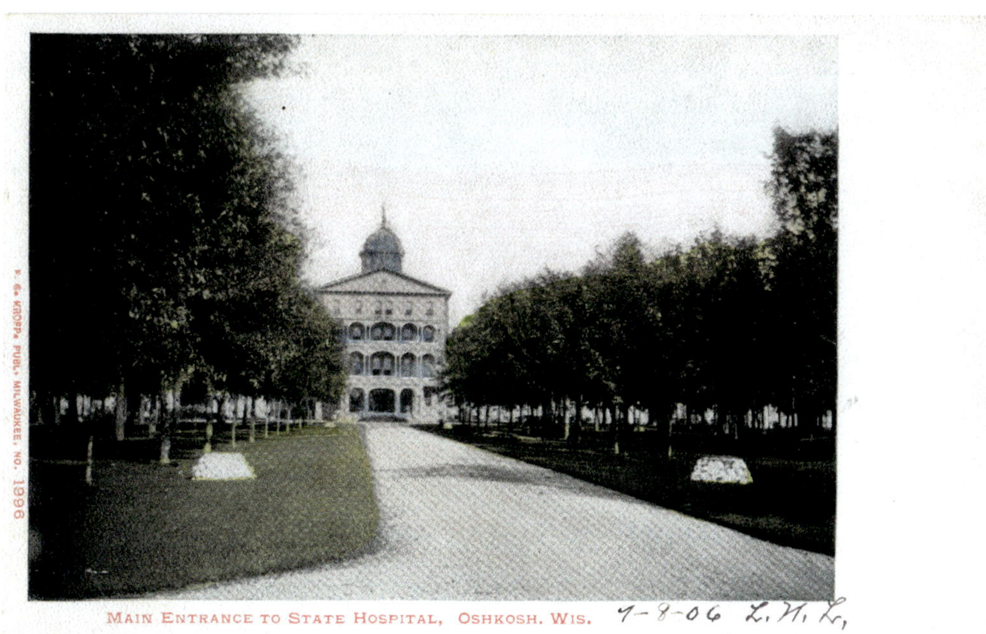
E. C. KROPP, PUBL., MILWAUKEE, NO. 1996
MAIN ENTRANCE TO STATE HOSPITAL, OSHKOSH, WIS.
9-8-06 L. M. L.

Figure 139

Central Kentucky Lunatic Asylum
Lakeland, Kentucky, 1873

The Central Kentucky Lunatic Asylum opened in 1873 in Lakeland, about 11 miles east of Louisville and accessible by rail lines that passed near the institution. The asylum had been a state house of reform for juvenile delinquents until 1873.

The postcard on the top of the next page (figure 140) shows a date of 1904, but the same image was also used for postcards produced years later.

This administration building (figure 141) was centrally located with three-story wings extending from either side with bedrooms or small dormitories on both sides. A new wing was added in 1890, consisting of five wards and a general dining room that could accommodate 225 patients. The facility included a large farm that eventually grew from 240 to 580 acres.

By 1900, an industrial and amusement building (figure 142) was completed with a sewing room, billiard rooms, a dance hall, and a chapel. Isolated cottages could house 50 to 200 patients. A separate "tuberculosis shack" (Thirty-Seventh Report and Fourth Report, n.d.) could house 24 patients.

The original buildings have been demolished and Central State Hospital continues to operate on the same site.

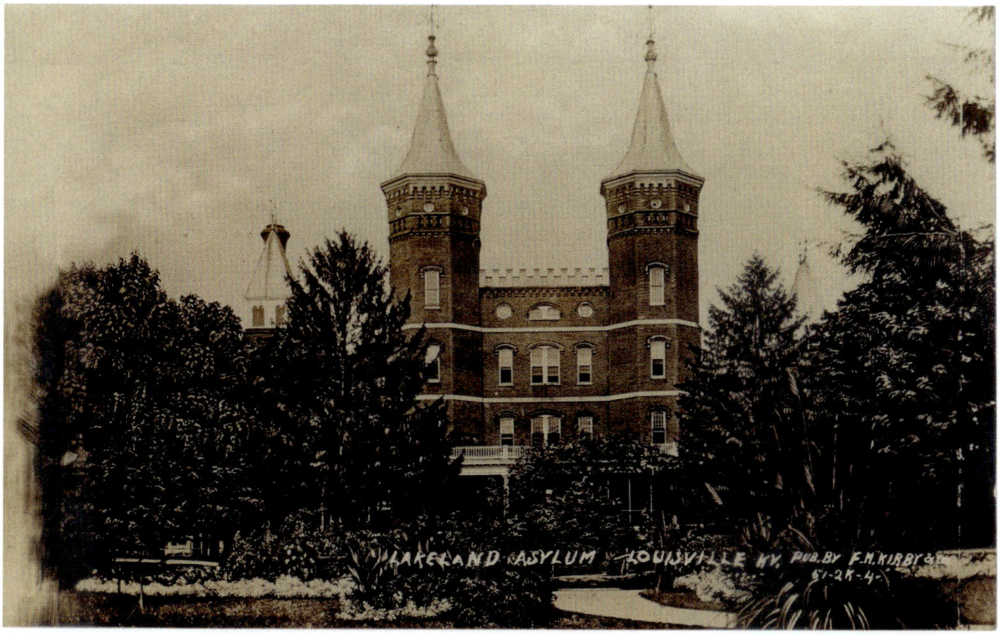

Figure 140

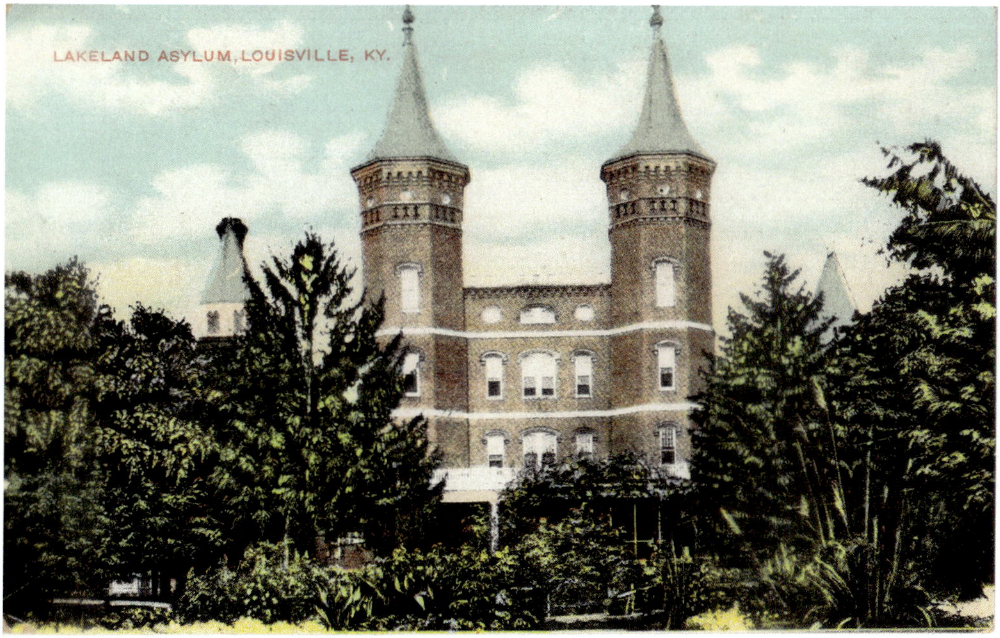

Figure 141

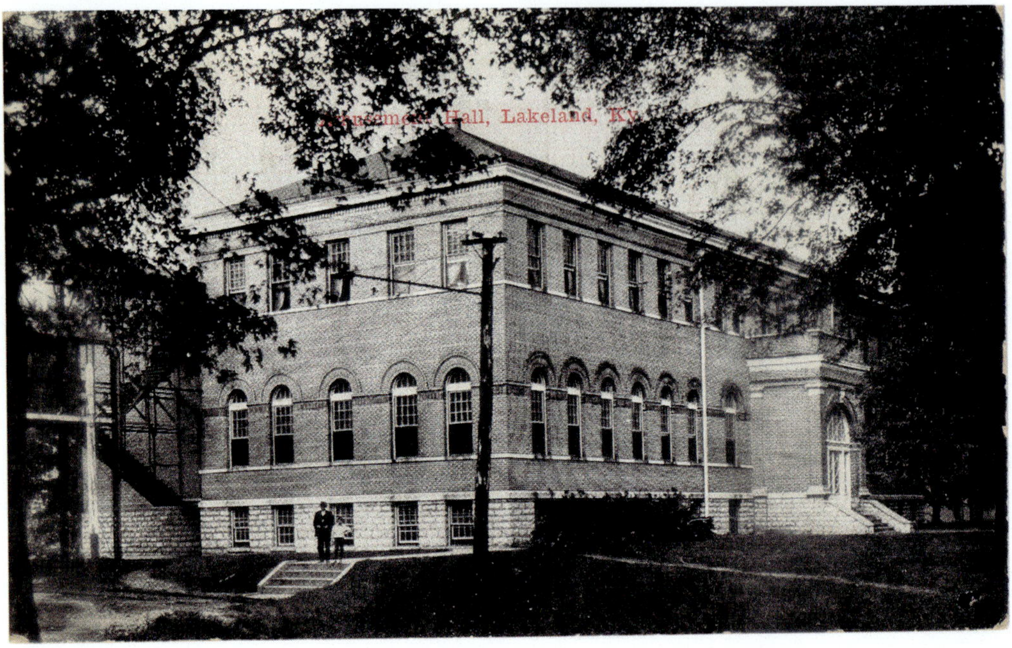

Figure 142

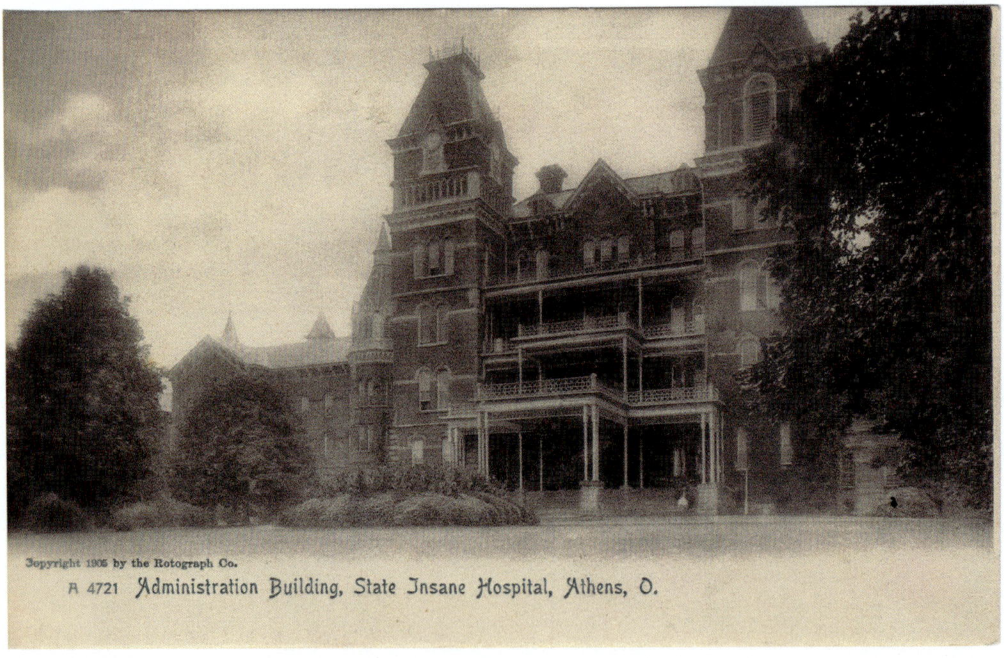

Figure 143

Athens Lunatic Asylum
Athens, Ohio, 1874

The Athens Lunatic Asylum opened in 1874. The fourth asylum in Ohio, Athens was a classic Kirkbride design with a four-story administration building (figures 143 and 144) and wings extending to the northeast and the southeast. The first superintendent of this facility was one of the earliest advocates of ending restraint of patients. However, reports indicate that by 1880, patients in this facility were again being restrained, with staff arguing that freedom from restraints resulted in too much destruction of property.

Initially situated on 141 acres of land, the facility eventually occupied more than 1,000 acres and included expansive gardens and grounds (figures 145 and 146).

Cottages for tuberculosis patients (figure 147) were added in 1911. The walls included a great deal of glass to permit maximum fresh air and sunshine. They were located north of the main buildings and connected by wire-screened corridors.

The original site of this facility was purchased by Ohio University. Several of the original buildings, including the Kirkbride building, have been well preserved and repurposed.

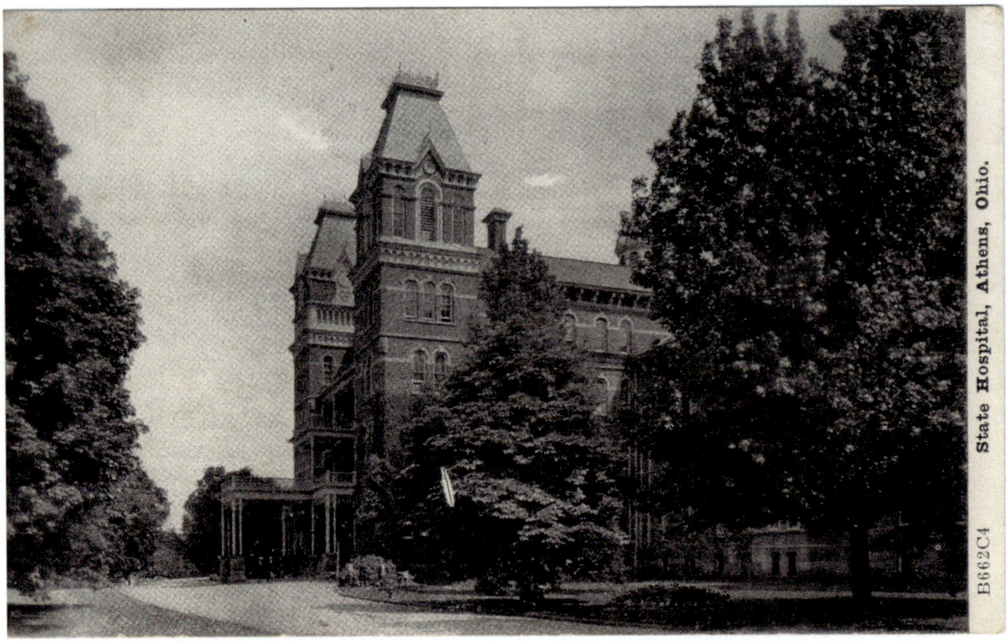

Figure 144

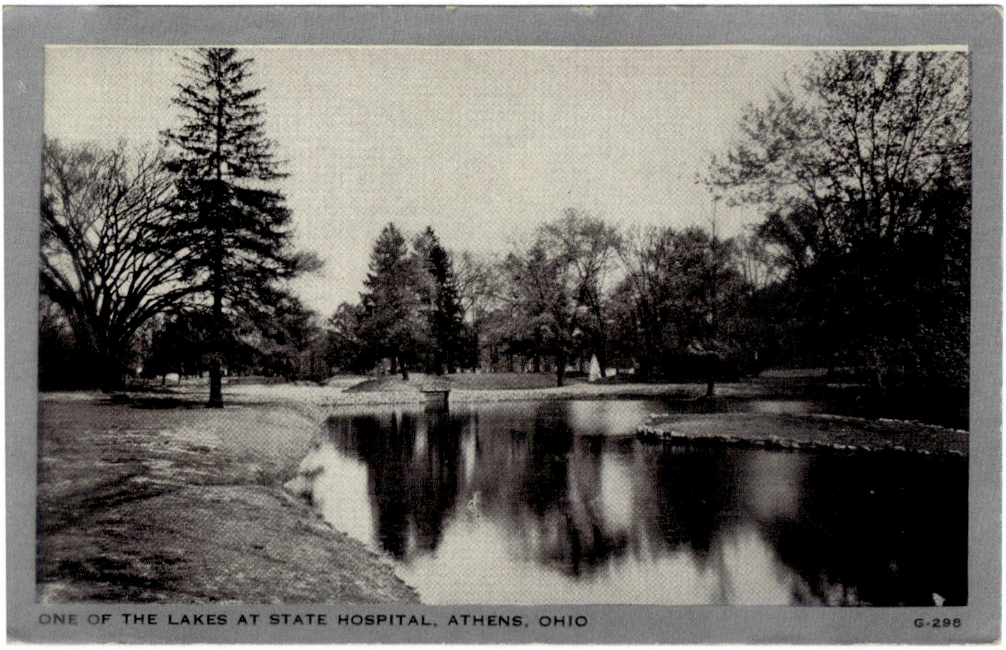

Figure 145

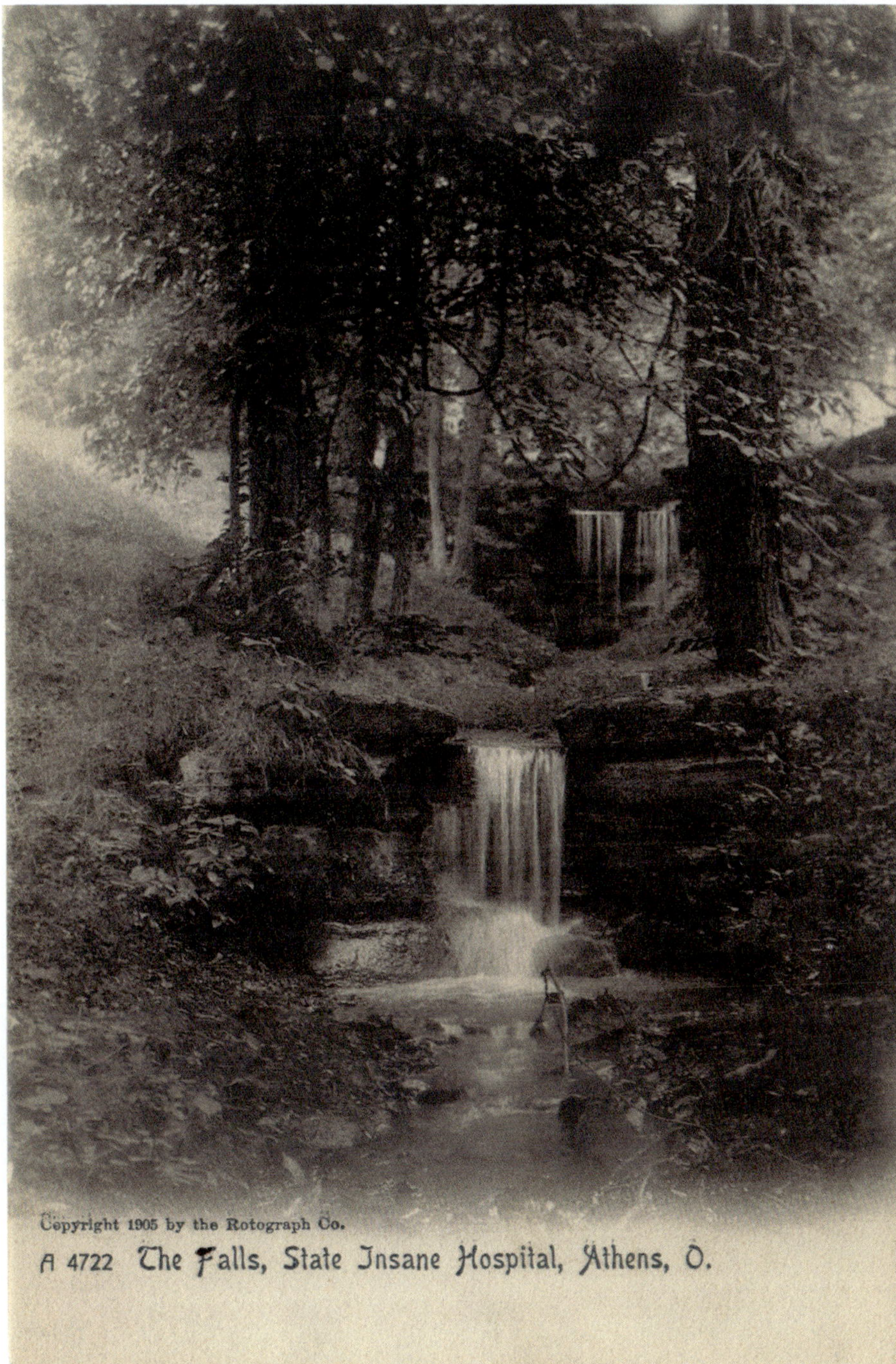
Copyright 1905 by the Rotograph Co.
A 4722 The Falls, State Insane Hospital, Athens, O.

Figure 146

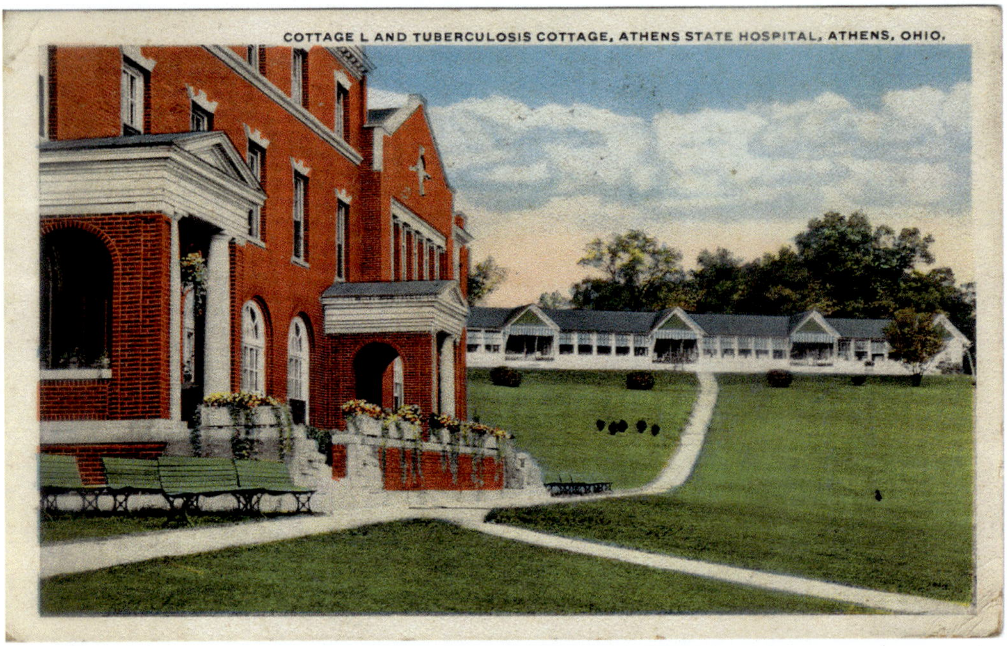
COTTAGE L AND TUBERCULOSIS COTTAGE, ATHENS STATE HOSPITAL, ATHENS, OHIO.

Figure 147

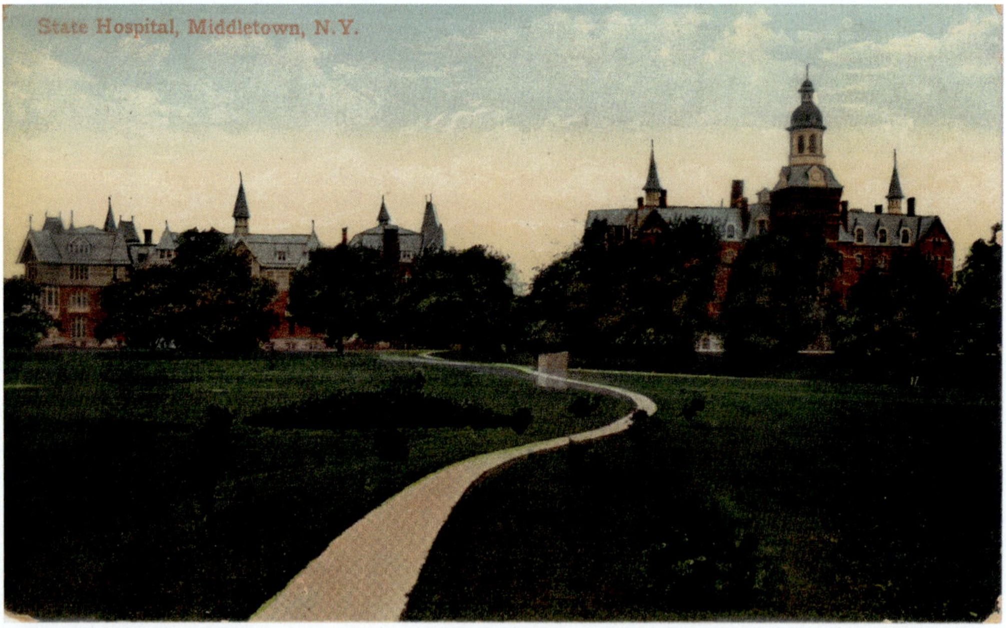
State Hospital, Middletown, N.Y.

Figure 148

State Homeopathic Asylum for the Insane
Middletown, New York, 1874

The State Homeopathic Asylum for the Insane (figures 148 and 149) in Middletown, New York opened in 1874 as the first institution in the United States using the homeopathic system of medicine. At a time when the use of patient restraints was highly criticized, homeopathic medicine seemed an attractive alternative. By 1889, the asylum housed 514 patients.

The facility (figure 150) consisted of a central four-story administrative building that included an attic and basement. Four pavilion buildings were eventually connected to it via corridors. In the early 1900s, several buildings and amenities were added including a new surgical and clinical pavilion, a building to care for acute patients, a reception room, a reading room, and a bowling alley.

The nurses' building was completed in 1910, next to the West Group building that was erected in 1908 for 500 chronically ill patients. The nurse's building was T-shaped and three stories high. Unmarried men occupied one end, unmarried women occupied the other, and married couples occupied the center wing.

By 1910 the average population was over 2,000. A staff house (figure 151) was added that year, designed to provide room for seven physicians. Each physician had a separate bedroom and a library.

The postcard in figure 152 includes an actual image rather than an illustration. The sender writes to her aunt in 1907, "Hospital work is a new idea for your old neice [*sic*]."

The facility was renamed Middletown Psychiatric Center and closed in 2006. Some of the original buildings remain, but they have not been maintained.

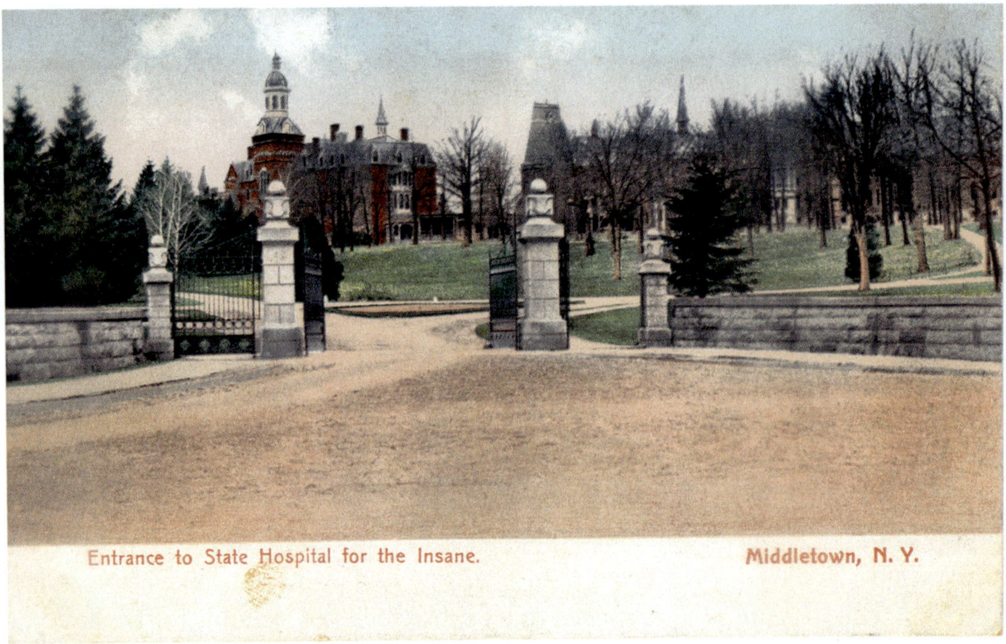
Entrance to State Hospital for the Insane.
Middletown, N. Y.

Figure 149

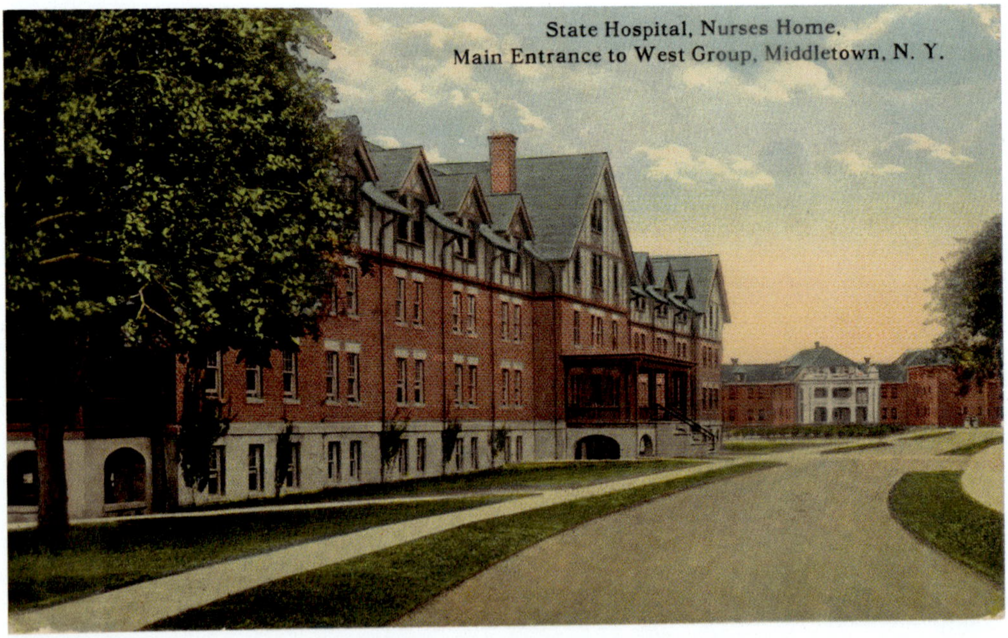
State Hospital, Nurses Home,
Main Entrance to West Group, Middletown, N. Y.

Figure 150

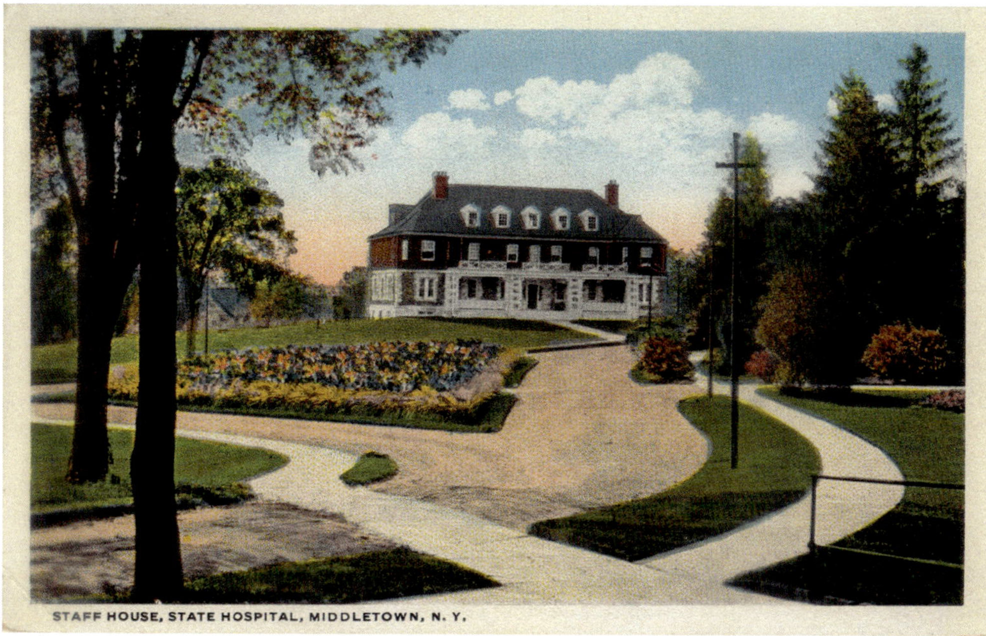

Figure 151

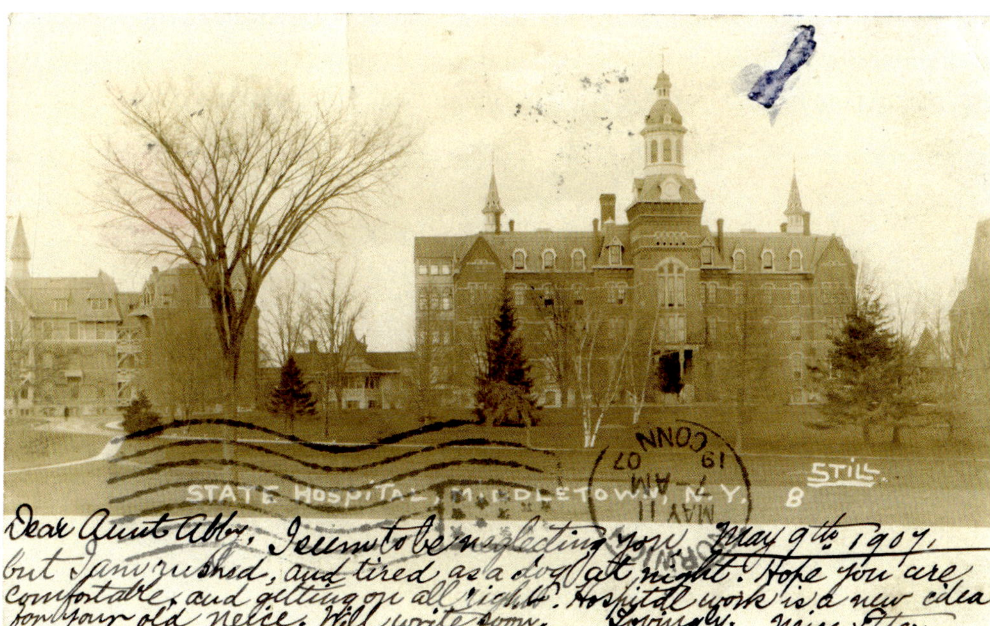

Figure 152

State Hospital for the Insane No. 2
St. Joseph, Missouri, 1874

State Hospital for the Insane No. 2 (figure 153) opened in 1874 with 25 patients. The facility contained 32 dormitories to accommodate 275 patients and was quickly filled to capacity.

On the night of January 25, 1879, a fire significantly damaged this Kirkbride structure (figure 154). Patients were housed in temporary lodgings that included the local courthouse and a medical hospital. Local community members contributed money and clothing for patients and the facility was reopened in 1880. By 1914, there were 1,629 patients.

The asylum changed names several times over the years, eventually becoming the Northwest Missouri Psychiatric Rehabilitation Center, located across the street from its original site. That facility has closed and a correctional facility now occupies the site, making use of a surviving portion of the original Kirkbride structure.

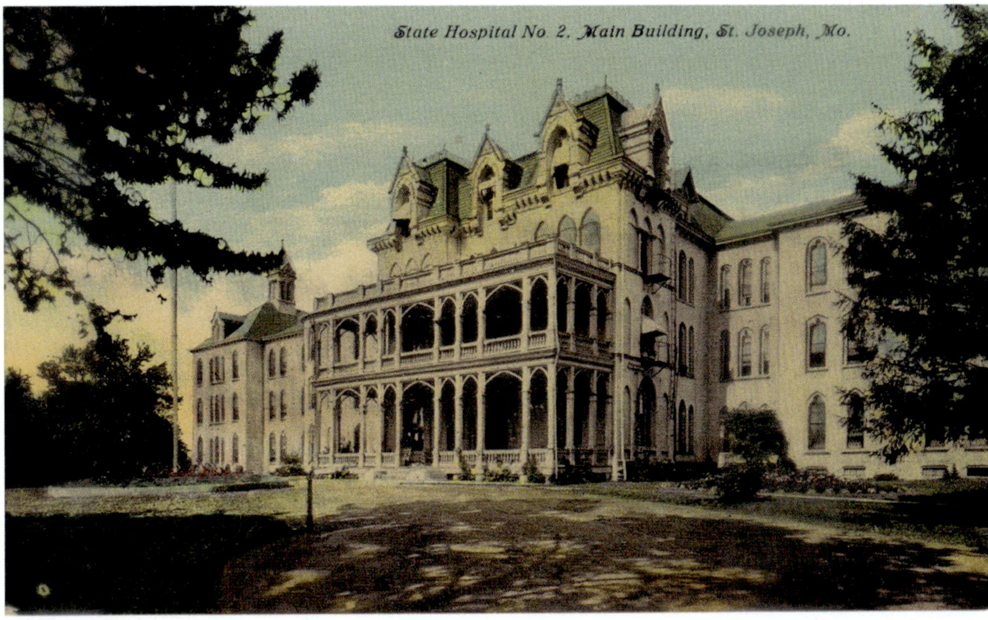
State Hospital No. 2. Main Building, St. Joseph, Mo.

Figure 153

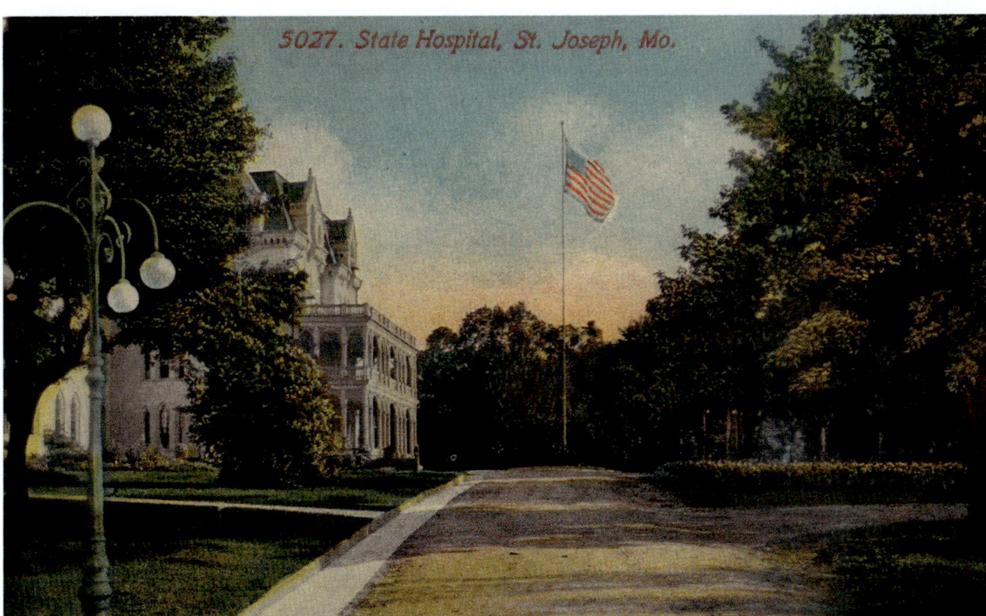
5027. State Hospital, St. Joseph, Mo.

Figure 154

State Hospital for the Insane
Imola, California, 1875

The State Hospital for the Insane at Napa, California was opened in 1875. Due to the rapid increase in population, the first state asylum at Stockton had become quickly overcrowded and a second California hospital was needed. The Napa hospital was built following the Kirkbride plan (figure 155), with a central building flanked by north and south wings for male and female patients.

Cottages were added to the site in later years. A tailor shop and sewing room were the main sources of industrial work for the patients, while a carpenter shop, mill, tin shop, dairy, and vegetable patch helped make the hospital self-sufficient. By 1915, the hospital cared for 2,136 patients. The postcard in figure 156, postmarked 1907, provides a description and advertisement of the hospital.

This facility continues to operate as Napa State Hospital, but the original buildings have been demolished.

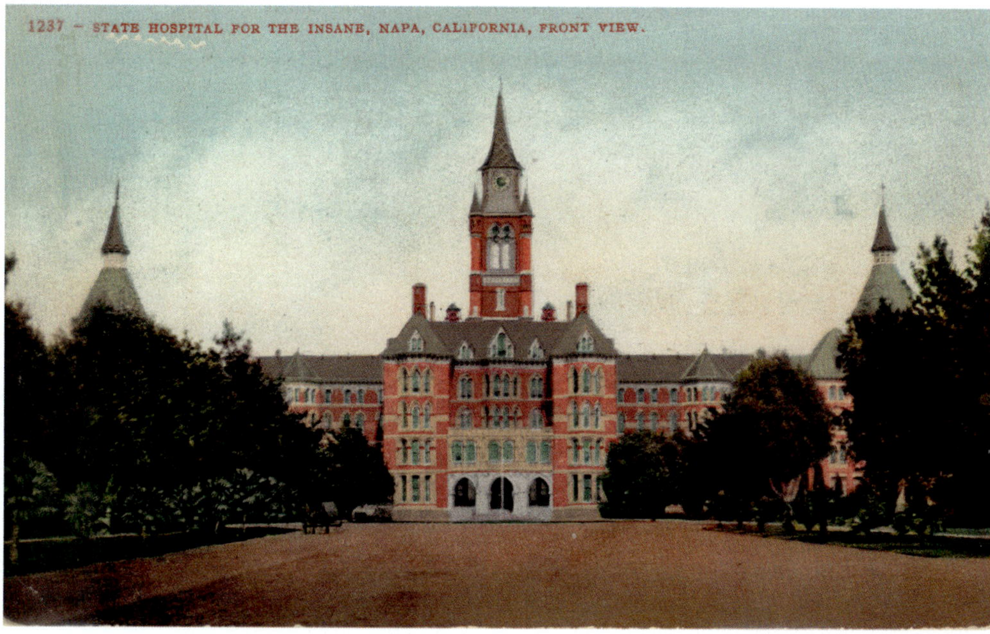
1237 – STATE HOSPITAL FOR THE INSANE, NAPA, CALIFORNIA, FRONT VIEW.

Figure 155

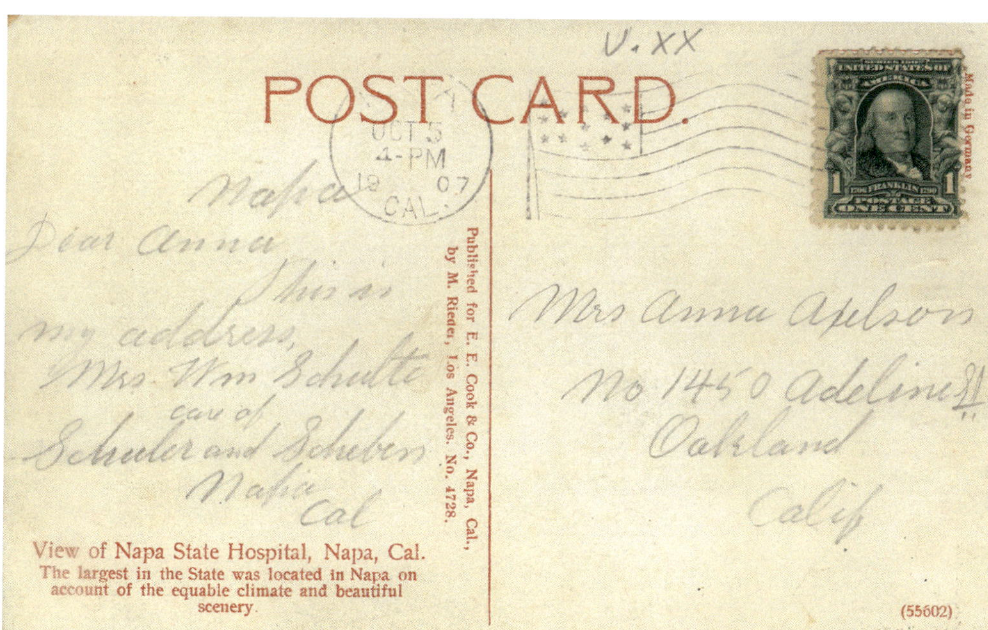

Figure 156

New Jersey State Hospital for the Insane
Greystone Park, New Jersey, 1876

The New Jersey State Hospital for the Insane opened in 1876 to relieve crowding at the first state facility in Trenton. Nearly 300 patients were transferred from Trenton to Morris Plains and by 1911, the hospital was very crowded, housing more than 2,500 patients.

Built on the Kirkbride plan, the hospital's main building was completed in 1899 and was constructed out of local greystone. The central building included wards on the upper floors for employees, while the two adjoining wings provided 40 wards for patients. The figure 157 provides an interior view of one of the hospital wards.

Renamed the Greystone Park Psychiatric Hospital, this facility was relocated in 2008. The original Kirkbride building has survived and the state is exploring the feasibility of redevelopment options.

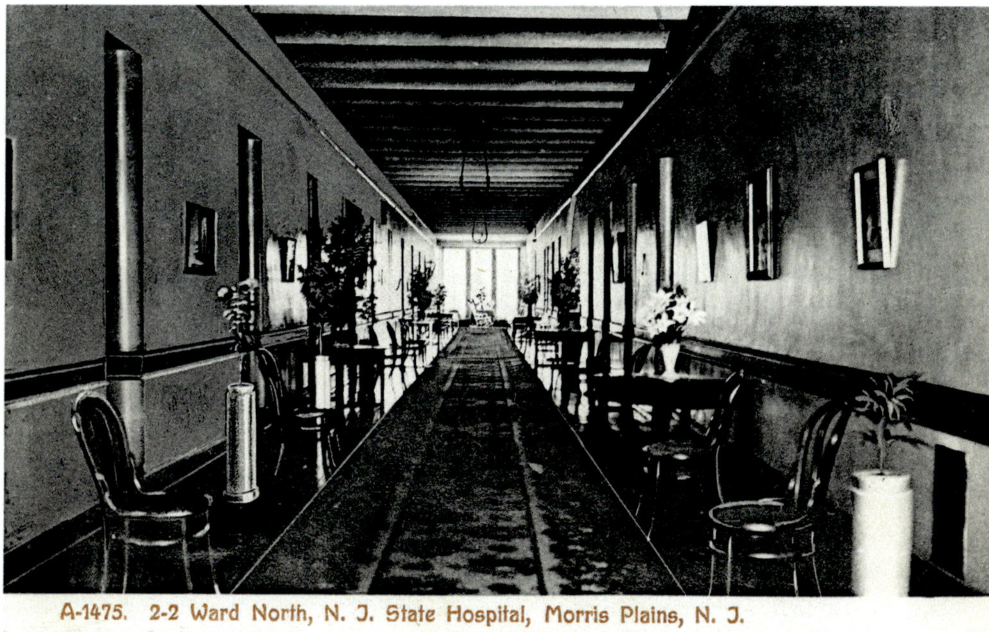
A-1475. 2-2 Ward North, N. J. State Hospital, Morris Plains, N. J.

Figure 157

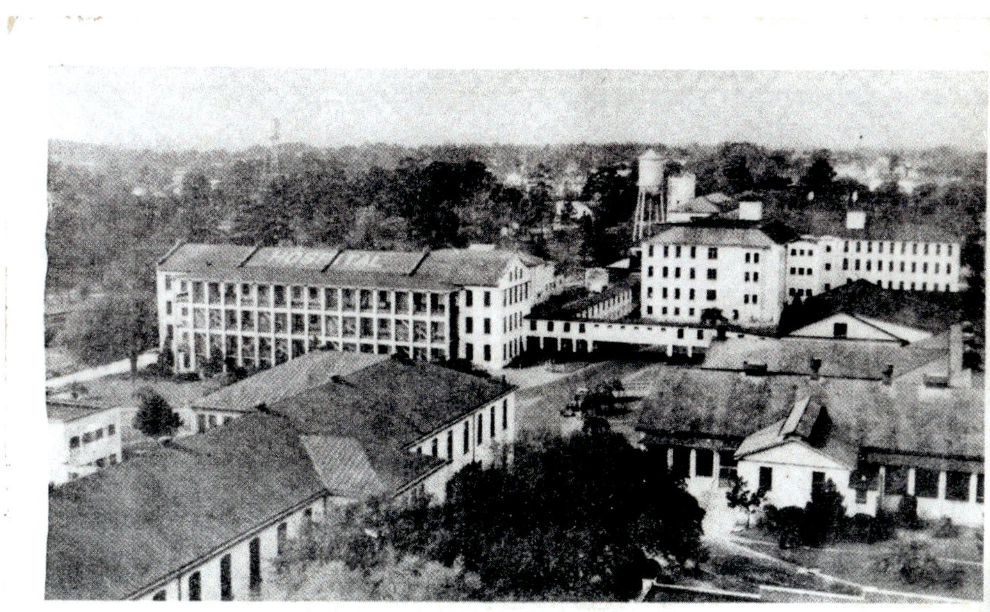

Figure 158

Florida State Hospital for the Insane
Chattahoochee, Florida, 1877

Florida State Hospital for the Insane opened in 1877. The original building was erected in 1834 as a government arsenal. After the Civil War, it was sold to the state authorities to be used as a state prison. When the prison was abolished in 1877, the building was converted to a state hospital. The institution was located about a mile from the Apalachicola River, within a few hundred yards of the Georgia line.

Patients suffering chronic mental illnesses were separated from patients with acute illnesses. Sewing, farming, working in the carpenter shop, gardening, and doing work in the dairy farm were common tasks for patients. Recreation included theater performances and weekly dances. The hospital aimed to provide one nurse for every ten patients. By 1914, the institution had 1,210 patients.

The postcard in figure 158 shows the wards for white male patients.

A nursing school was established in 1919. By 1940, there were 95 nurses at the hospital. The postcard in figure 159 shows the nurses' home, which has been reported to have been destroyed by fire in 1937.

The 1954 postcard (figure 160) provides a more recent view.

Florida State Hospital still operates on the original site and the officer's quarters, established in an arsenal, are still in used as the hospital's main administration building.

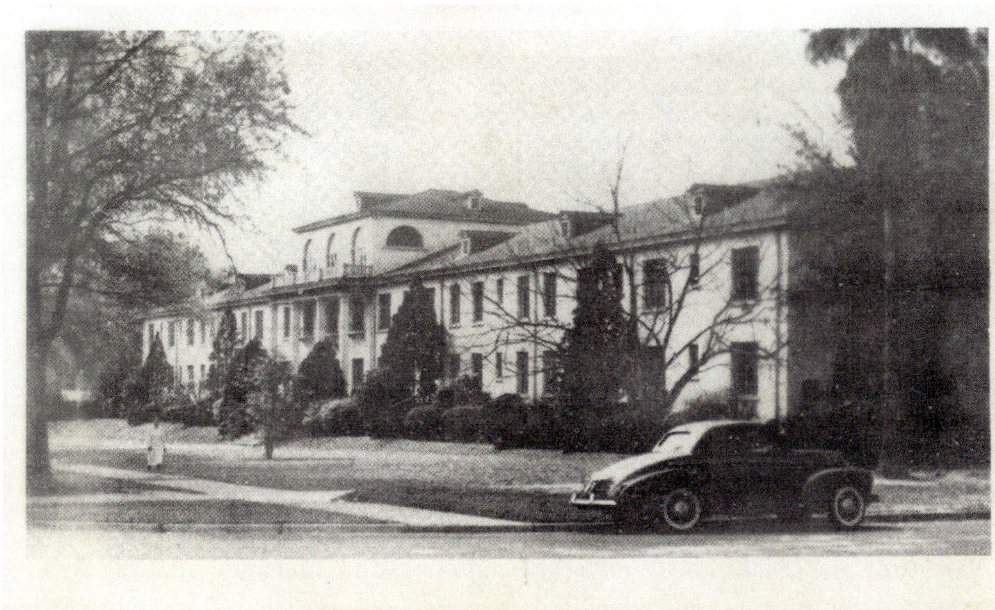

Figure 159

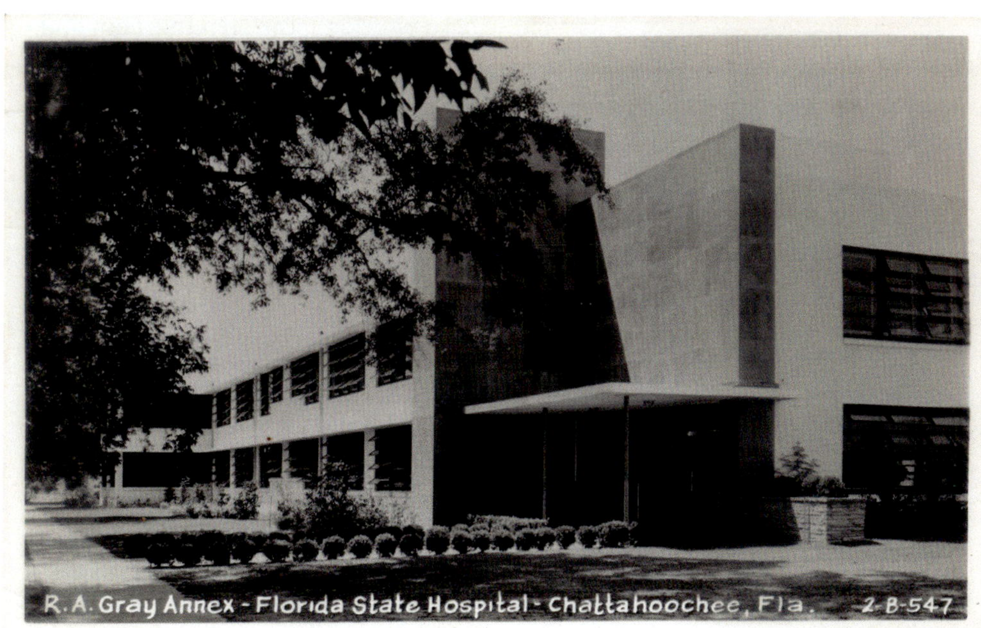
R. A. Gray Annex - Florida State Hospital - Chattahoochee, Fla. 2-B-547

Figure 160

Grafton State Hospital
North Grafton, Massachusetts, 1877

Grafton State Hospital was established in 1901, initially as a farm colony for the chronically ill patients housed at the Worcester State Asylum. The Grafton site occupied 700 acres of land, providing more room for patient housing, and also providing vast outdoor space for a farm operated by the patients.

In 1912, the Grafton hospital became administratively separate from the Worcester asylum. By 1945, it occupied more than 1,200 acres and cared for more than 1,700 patients.

The administration building, erected in 1913, and the auditorium, built in 1931, are shown in figure 161, a postcard from the 1930s or 1940s.

This facility closed in 1973 as part of the deinstitutionalization movement and the site was repurposed as the Tufts University Cummings School of Veterinary Medicine. Several of the buildings still stand and most have been renovated and are in use.

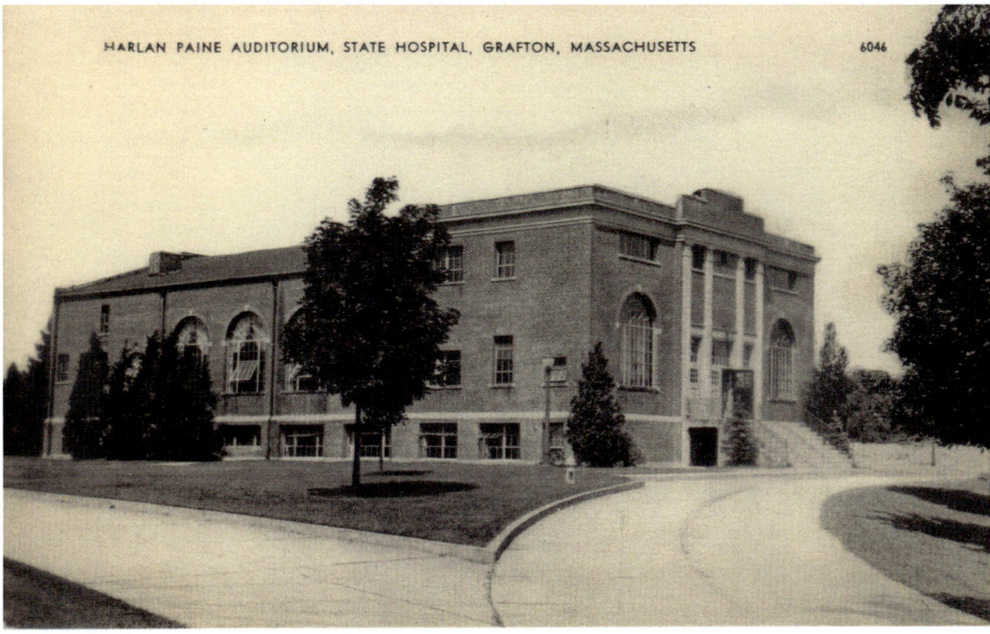
HARLAN PAINE AUDITORIUM, STATE HOSPITAL, GRAFTON, MASSACHUSETTS
6046

Figure 161

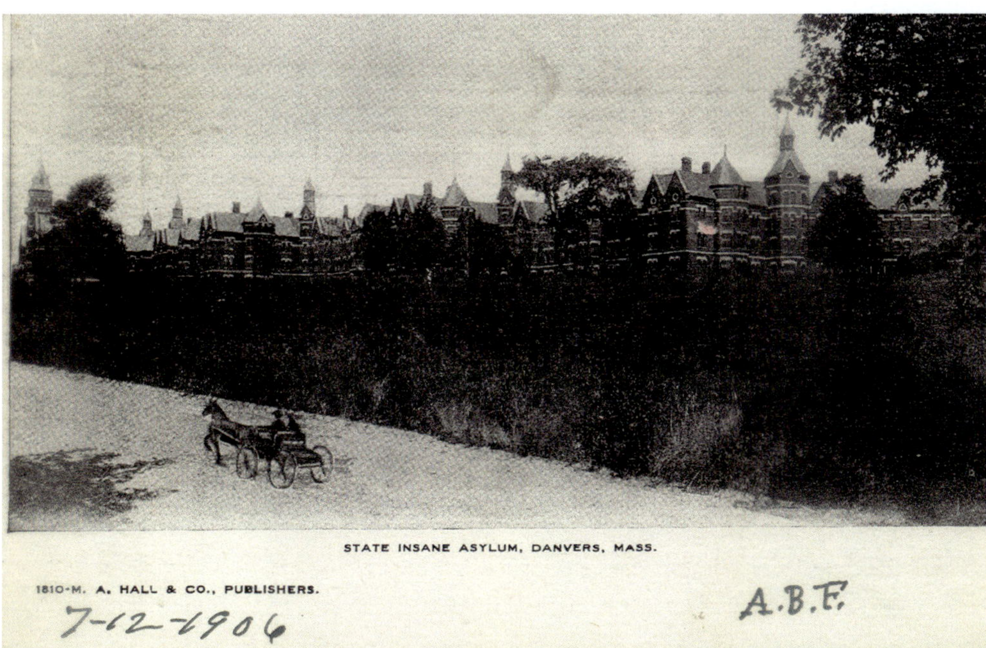
STATE INSANE ASYLUM, DANVERS, MASS.
1810-M. A. HALL & CO., PUBLISHERS.
7-12-1906
A.B.F.

Figure 162

State Lunatic Hospital
Hathorne, Massachusetts, 1878

The State Lunatic Hospital in Danvers was opened in 1878 to provide room for the state's growing population of mentally ill citizens. The Kirkbride structure was 700,000 square feet in more than 40 buildings on the property. The beauty of the building (figures 162 and 163) attracted approximately 12,000 visitors per year by 1880.

The reverse of the postcard from figure 163 (shown in figure 164) shows an advertisement for the hospital.

A colony, Middleton Colony, was added in 1903 to house chronically ill female patients (figure 165). Farm work was done by men and women were employed in housekeeping and laundry work for the colony.

The hospital closed in 1992. Small portions of the original Kirkbride buildings have been preserved and renovated and are currently in use as apartment buildings.

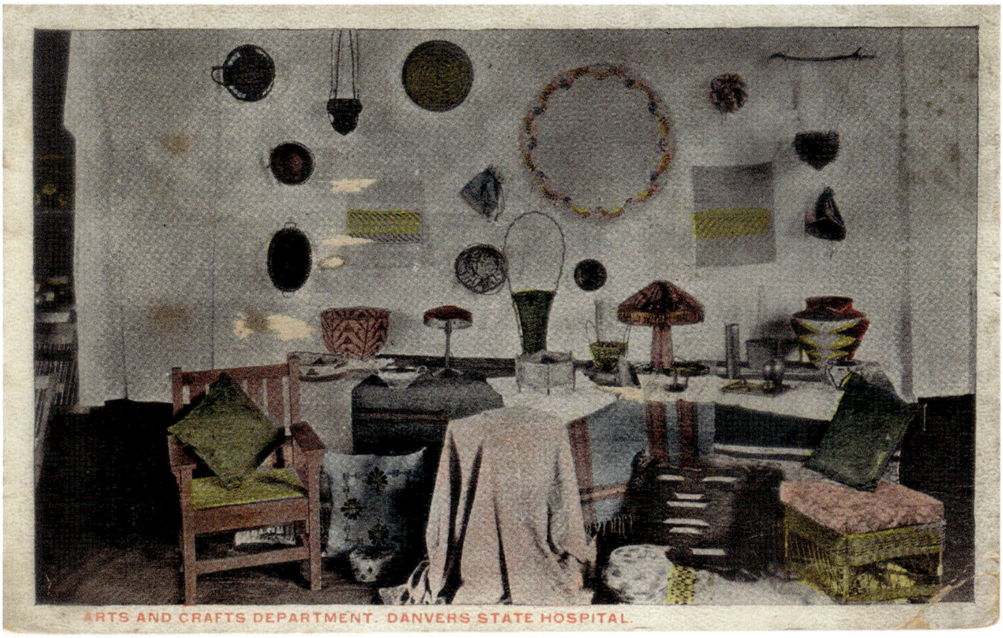

Figure 163

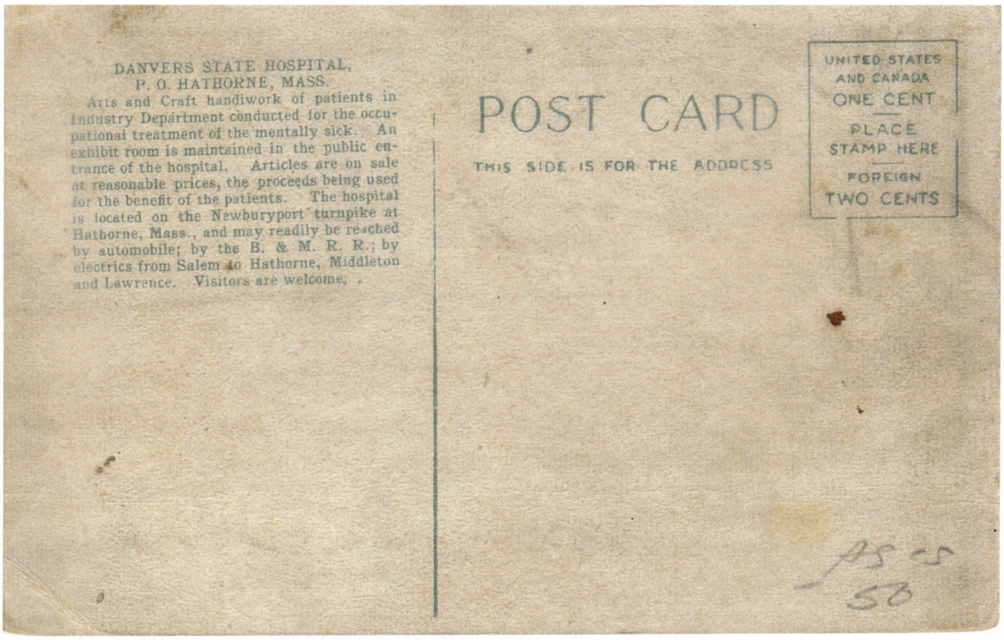

Figure 164

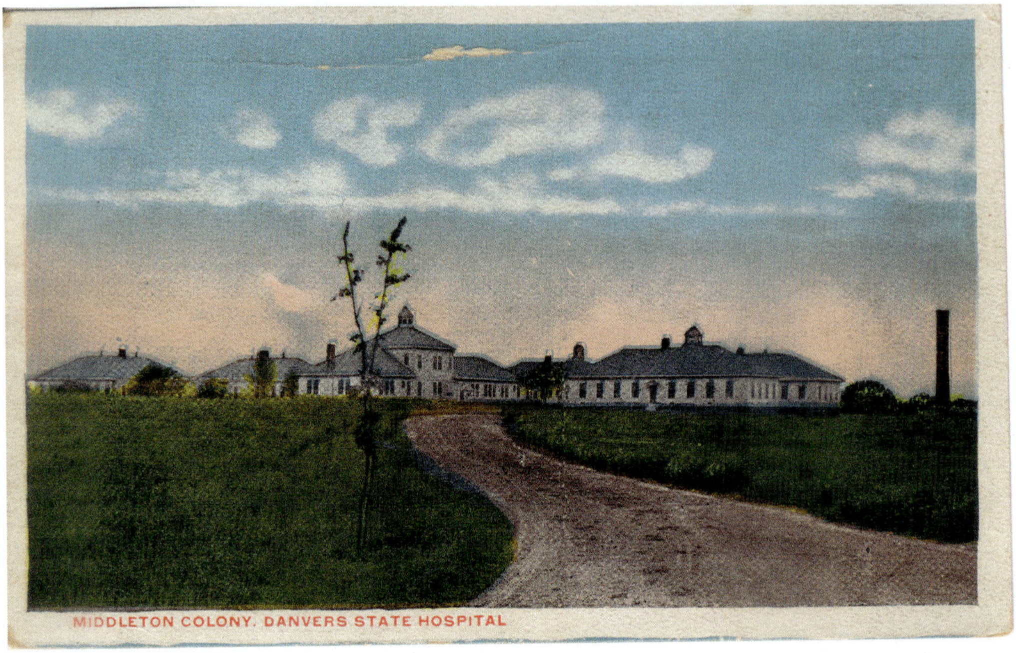

Figure 165

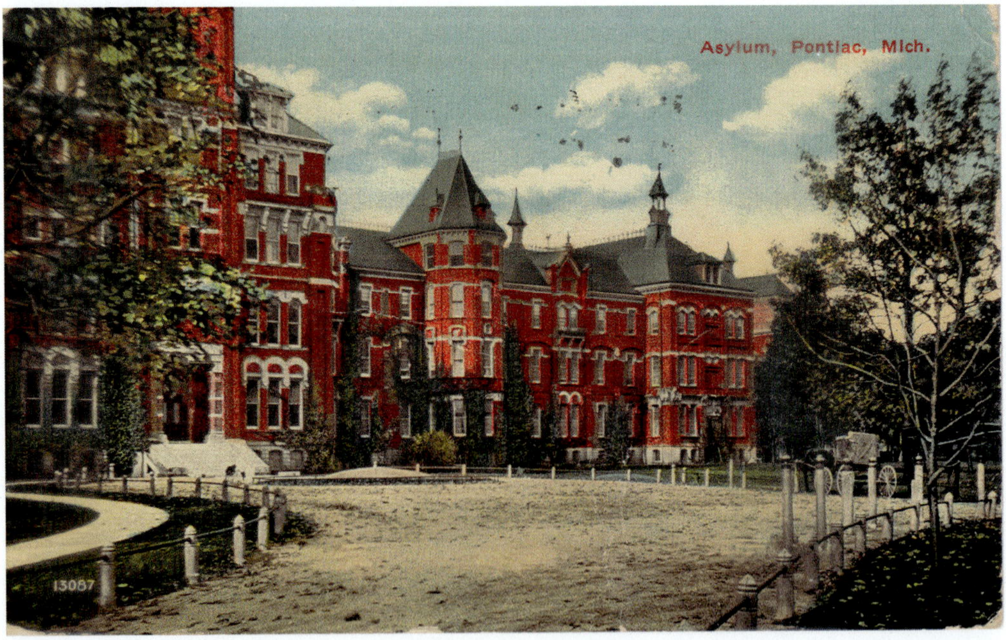

Figure 166

Eastern Michigan Asylum
Pontiac, Michigan, 1878

The Eastern Michigan Asylum in Pontiac, Michigan was opened in 1878. The second state hospital in Michigan, the Kirkbride building (figure 166) included space for cooking, heating, power, workshops, and laundry.

By 1882, two new wings had been added and, less than ten years later, the interior of the administration building was badly damaged by fire, along with adjoining halls. The damage was repaired the same year.

In 1891, a second fire, which began in the attic of the administration building, destroyed the interior of that building and damaged adjoining wings. By the next autumn the damage had been repaired with the addition of some fire-proofing measures. In 1907, several additions were made including the erection of a new chapel and assembly hall and by 1915, a new men's building was completed and occupied.

The postcard in figure 167, postmarked 1925, shows the administration building and wings. The lawn sign states, "The grounds and walks are private. VISITORS must not trespass." This policy differed from that of other institutions, where visitors were often encouraged.

The next postcard (figure 168), from the 1920s, provides a view of a hallway in the asylum.

In 1973, the facility was operating as the Clinton Valley Center, which eventually closed in 1997. All of the original buildings were demolished by 2000.

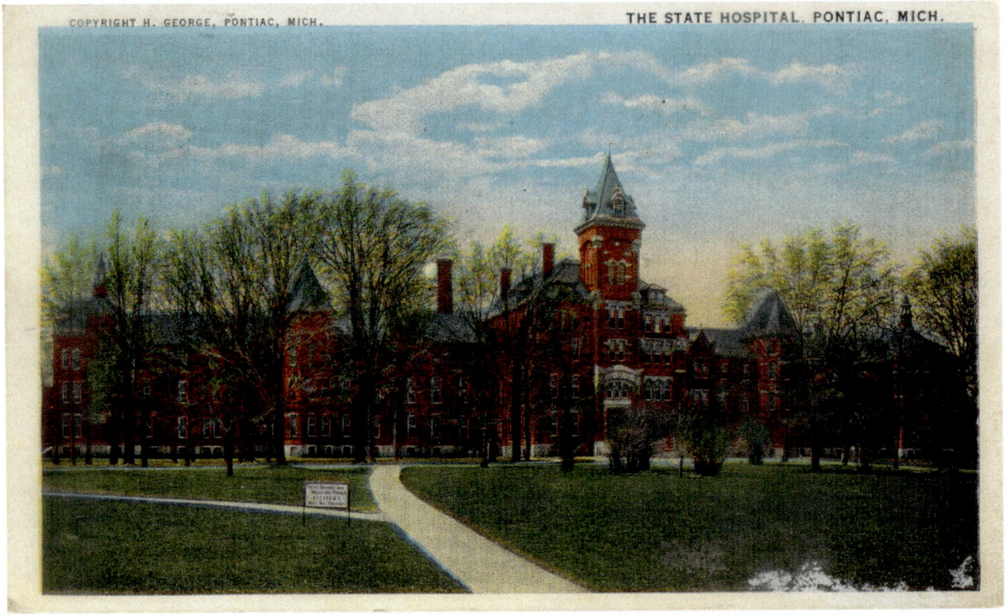

Figure 167

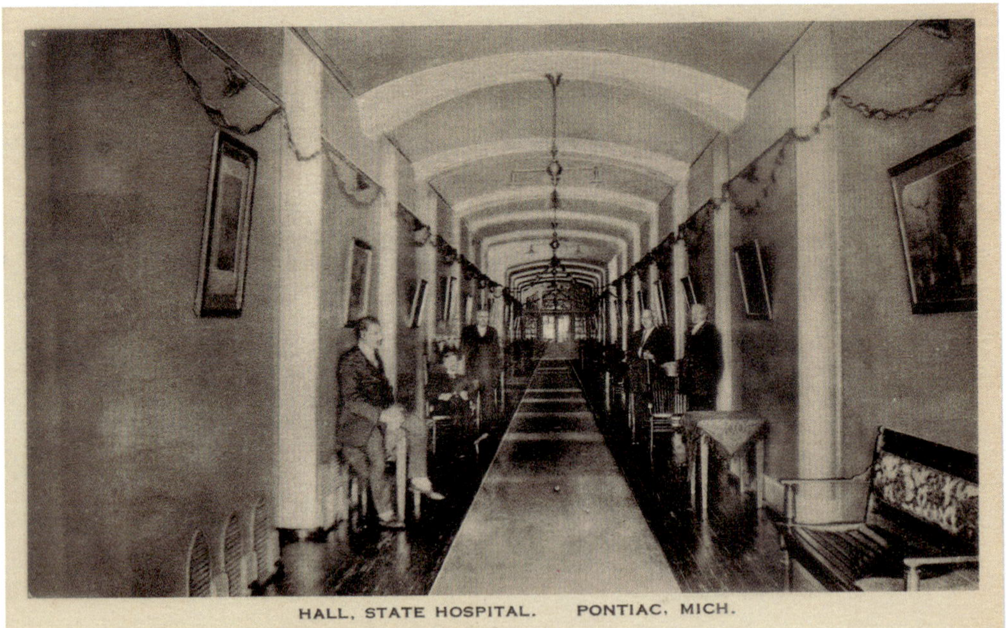

Figure 168

Topeka Insane Asylum
Topeka, Kansas, 1879

The Topeka Insane Asylum, located two miles west of the Kansas State Capitol building on a 240-acre tract of land, accepted its first patient in June 1879. The facility included six modified Kirkbride buildings, each three stories high and capable of housing 140 patients. A large custodial building was also opened for male patients. The postcard in figure 169, postmarked 1910, shows the central administrative building.

A reception hospital for the treatment of acute and curable cases was eventually added to the facility. It was equipped with surgical, electrical, and hydrotherapeutic equipment, along with a clinical laboratory.

By 1901, the official name of the institution changed from the Topeka Insane Asylum to the Topeka State Hospital (figure 170). Four years later, the original board of charities was discontinued and a board of control took charge of the institution. By 1914, the facility had 540 beds.

The 1908 postcard in figure 171 provides a photograph (rather than an illustration) of the facility.

The Topeka State Hospital closed in 1997 and the central building was demolished in 2010.

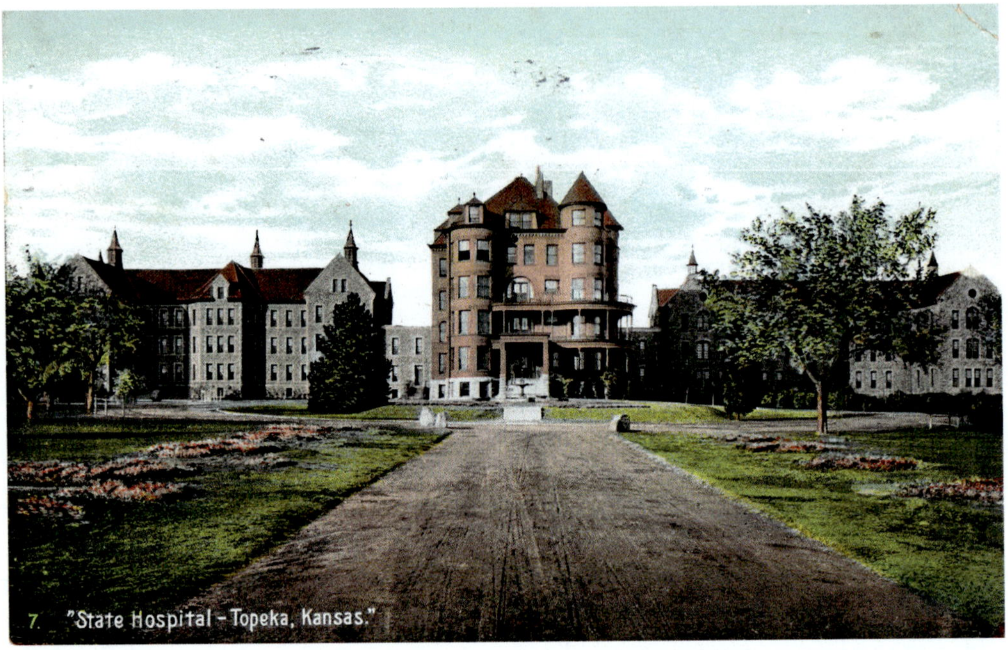

Figure 169

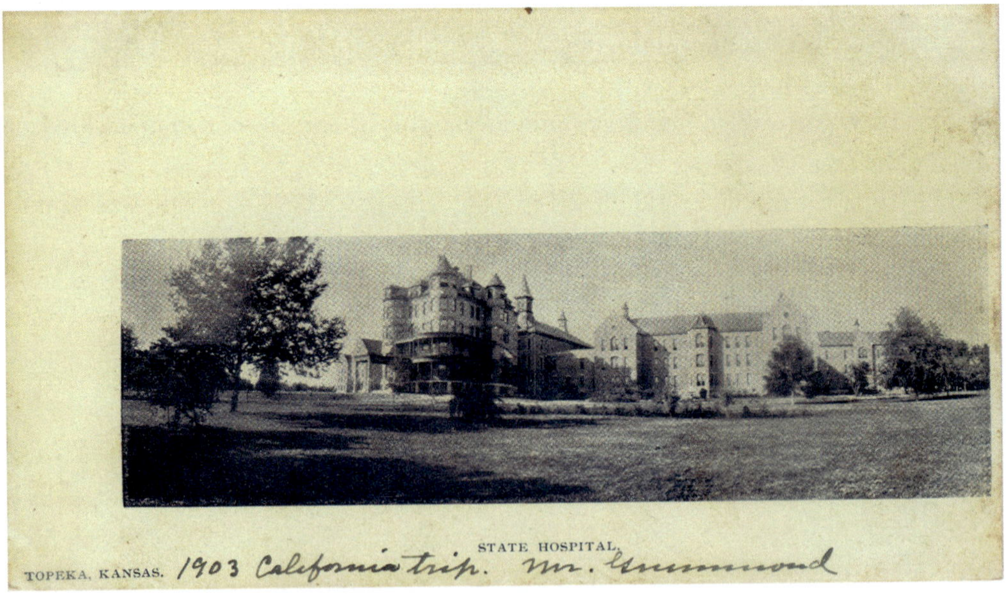

Figure 170

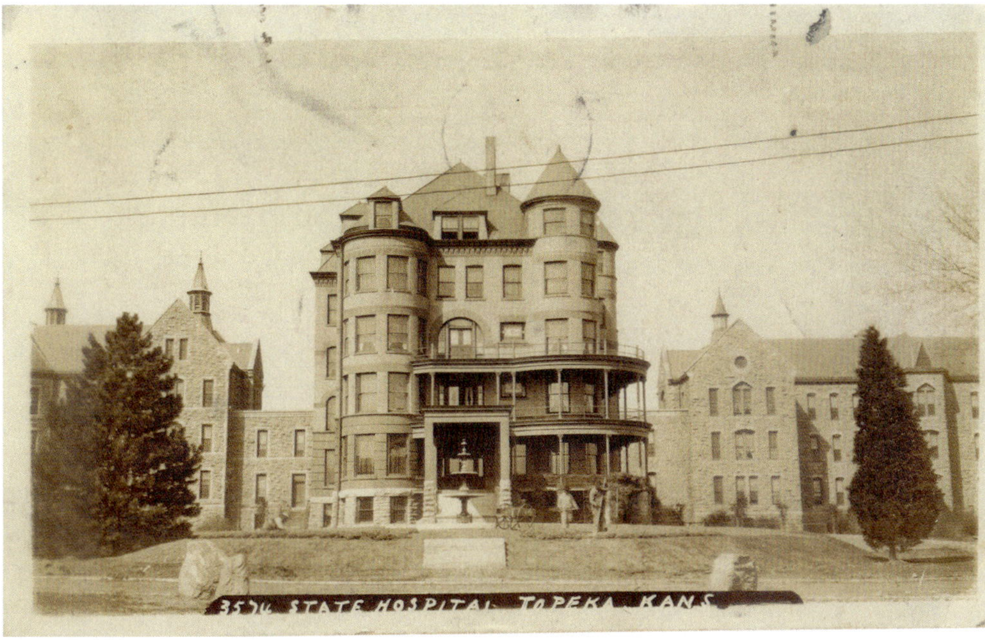
3574 STATE HOSPITAL TOPEKA KANS.

Figure 171

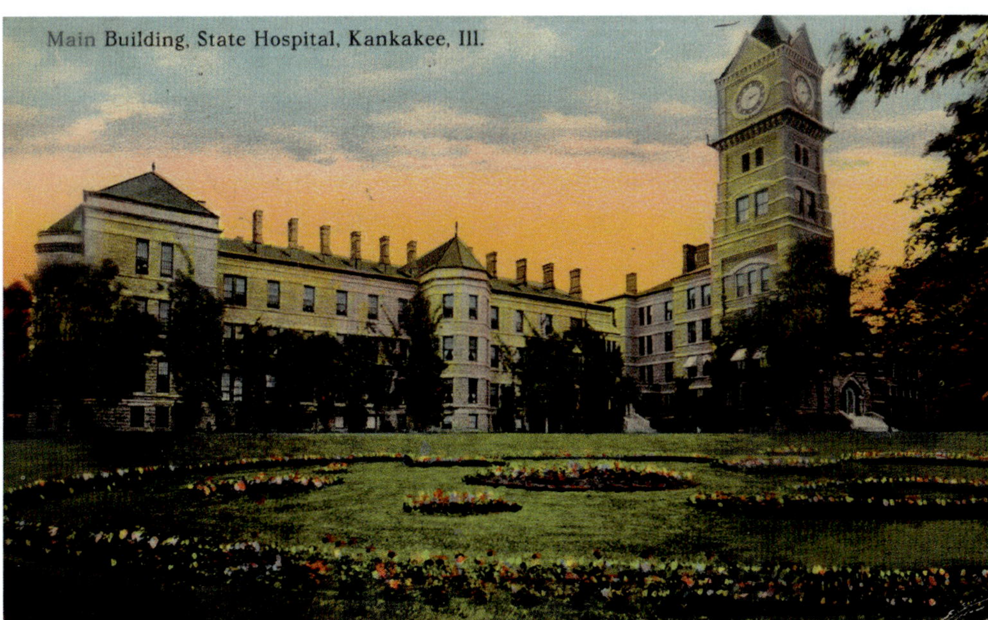
Main Building, State Hospital, Kankakee, Ill.

Figure 172

Illinois Eastern Hospital for the Insane
Kankakee, Illinois, 1879

The Illinois Eastern Hospital for the Insane (figure 172) opened in 1879 in Kankakee, Illinois. Kankakee was among the first facilities in the US to use detached wards—also known as the "cottage system"—to house patients. Most institutions at this time followed the Kirkbride plan of architecture, providing long wards attached to a central administrative building. At Kankakee, a central three-story building (figure 173) containing a large marble clock face was surrounded by smaller buildings for patients. Each of these buildings stood detached with no fences, no enclosures, and no connecting corridors.

In January, 1885, a fire destroyed one of the hospital's infirmaries (figure 174) and resulted in six deaths. The legislature then approved funds for a fire department, fire escapes, and fireproofing. By the following year, the number of patients had reached 1,500 and buildings for 1,000 additional patients were completed.

Patients engaged in various kinds of employment, including manufacturing brooms, baskets, mattresses, and harnesses. A patient with engraving skills made cards and stationary for the institution. An 840-acre farm also served as a source for patient work.

The facility now operates as the Shapiro Developmental Center. The original clock tower has been preserved.

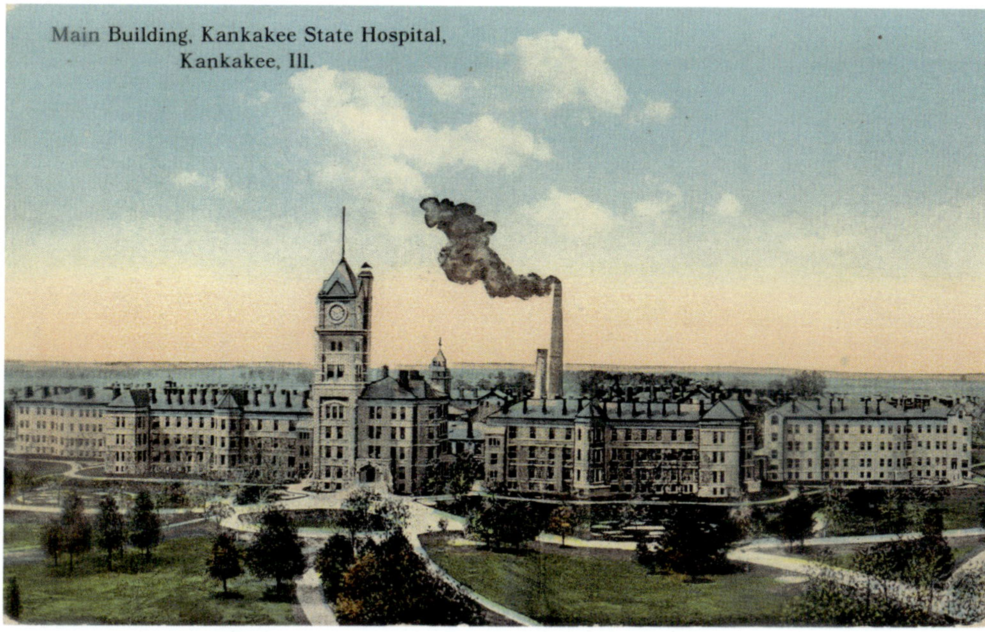
Main Building, Kankakee State Hospital,
Kankakee, Ill.

Figure 173

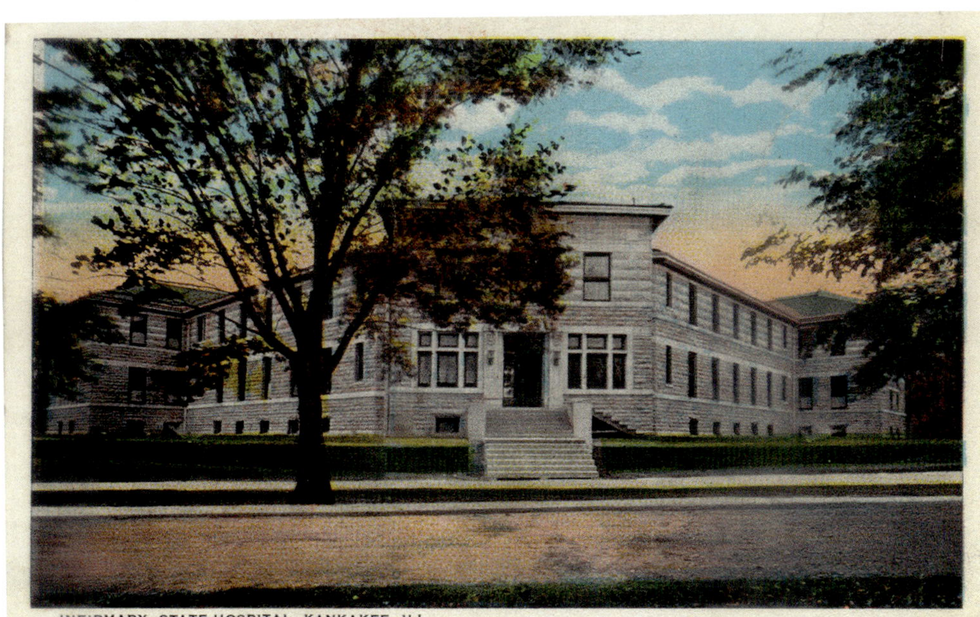
INFIRMARY, STATE HOSPITAL, KANKAKEE, ILL.

Figure 174

Second Minnesota Hospital for the Insane
Rochester, Minnesota, 1879

The Second Minnesota Hospital for the Insane, later renamed the Rochester State Hospital, opened in 1879 on 160 acres a mile from Rochester. The building was incomplete when the first patients were accepted, consisting of a center building and a small wing for 100 male patients that were transferred from other facilities. The building was hastily completed and 100 female patients were then received. Another large extension on the men's side accommodated 200 more patients and similar wings were later added for women, raising the capacity of the facility to 600 (figures 175 and 176).

The next two postcards of this facility (figures 177 and 178), sent before 1907, show the grounds and a larger view of the facility.

By 1914, the facility occupied 1,720 acres, and housed 1,121 patients. The original Kirkbride building was demolished in 1964 and the hospital closed in 1982.

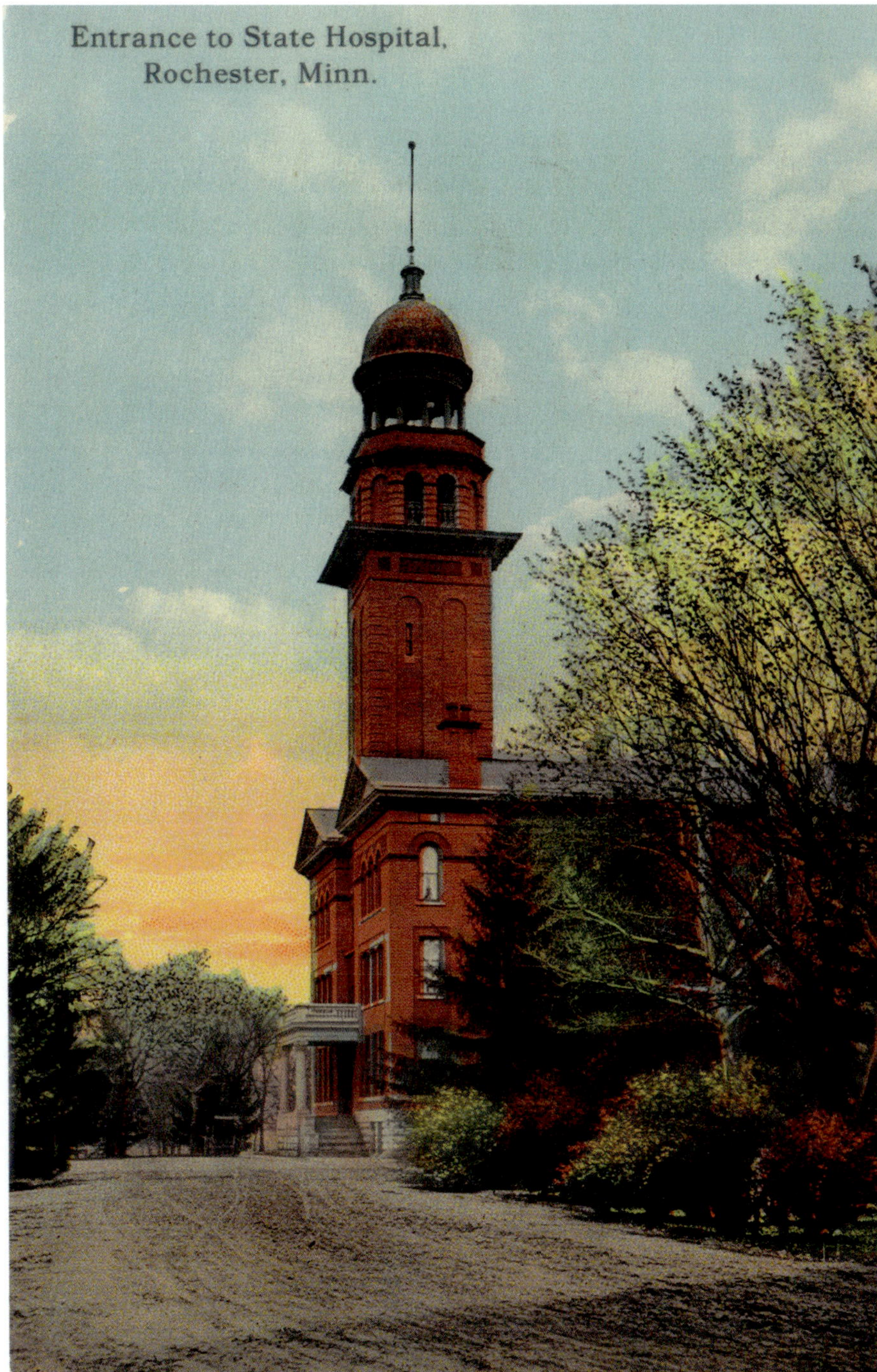

Figure 175

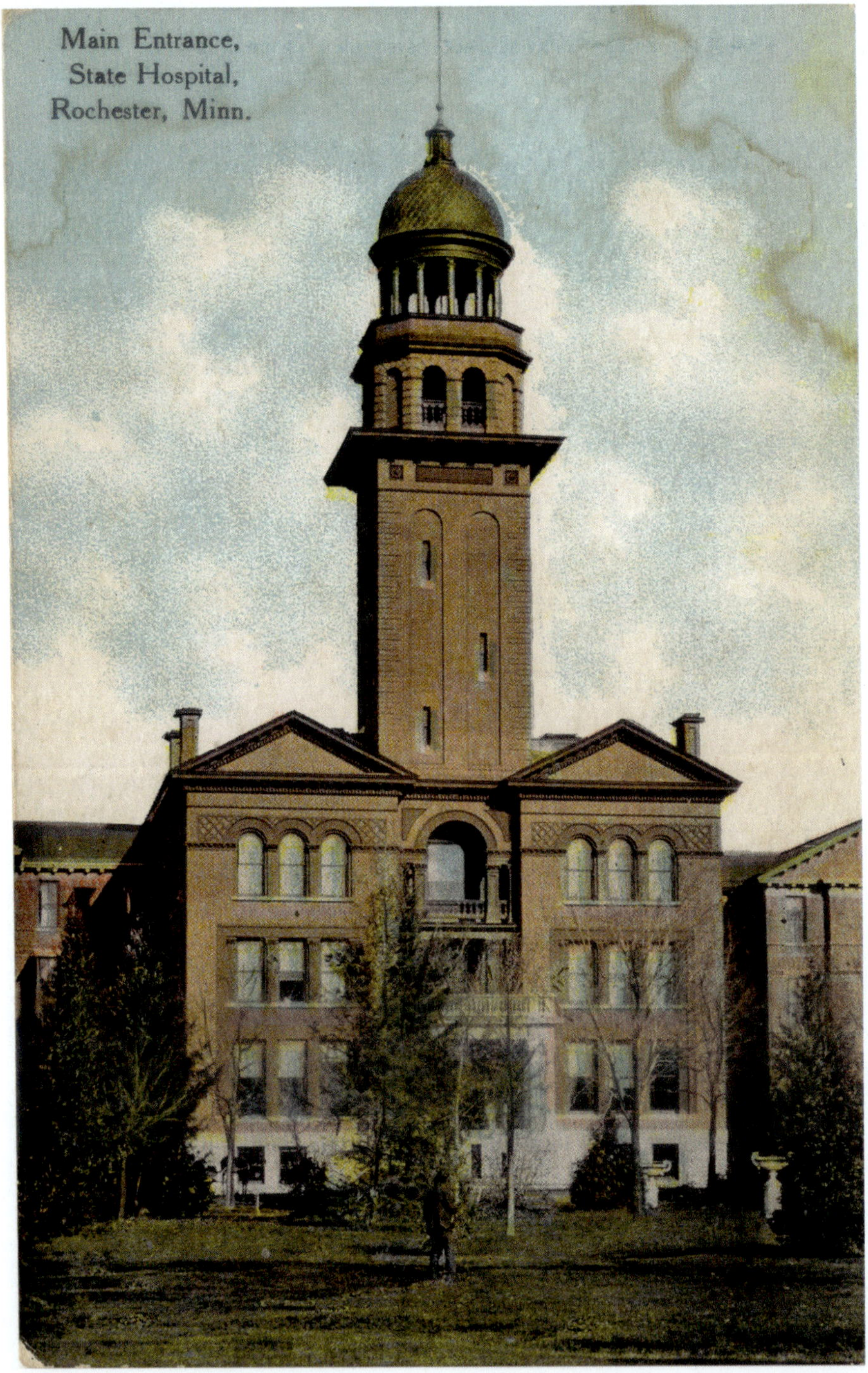

Figure 176

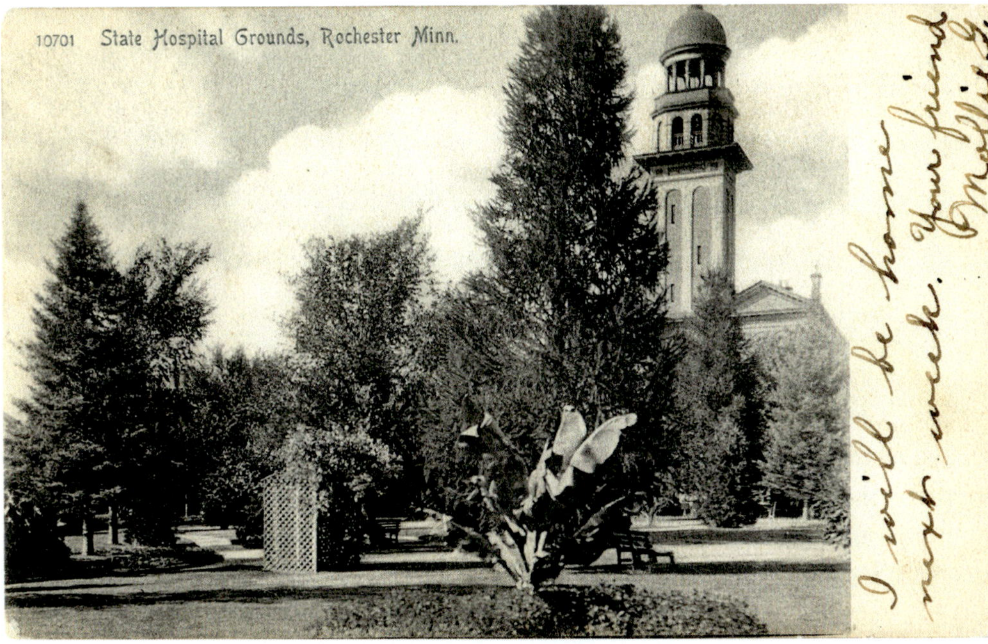

Figure 177

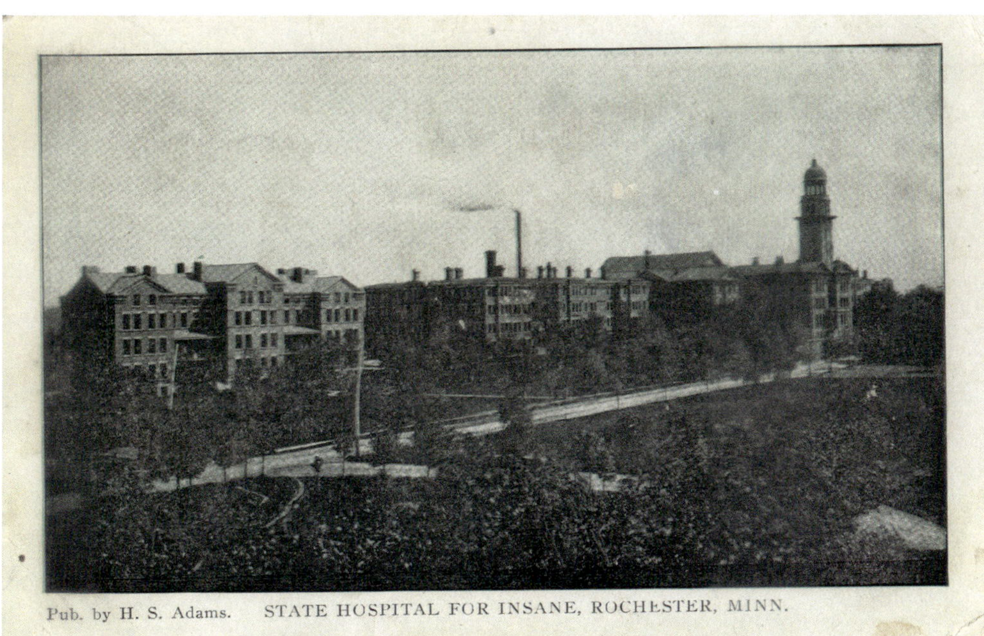

Figure 178

Dakota Hospital for the Insane
Yankton, South Dakota, 1879

The Dakota Hospital for the Insane, later renamed the Yankton State Hospital, opened in 1879. The original building (figure 179) was a large frame one-story building with two wings extending off the back side of the building. In 1882, the original building was completely destroyed by fire. The main building for the facility was still being built at that time, and patients and staff moved into that building while it was under construction. By 1880, the Kirkbride facility consisted of 640 acres, housing a central administration building with 12 wards.

It is interesting to note that of the surviving 20 postcards of this state hospital, none are in color and all are early authentic photographs rather than illustrations. Ten of these photos depict the park (figures 180–183 are a few of them).

A receiving hospital for female patients was built in 1907. It included parlors, sleeping quarters, and treatment rooms.

In the annual reports of the asylum, the superintendent drew attention to the grand furnishings of the women's hospital (figures 184–187), including the oak furnishings and the marble staircase.

The facility now operates as the Human Services Center on the original site. Several of the original buildings remain.

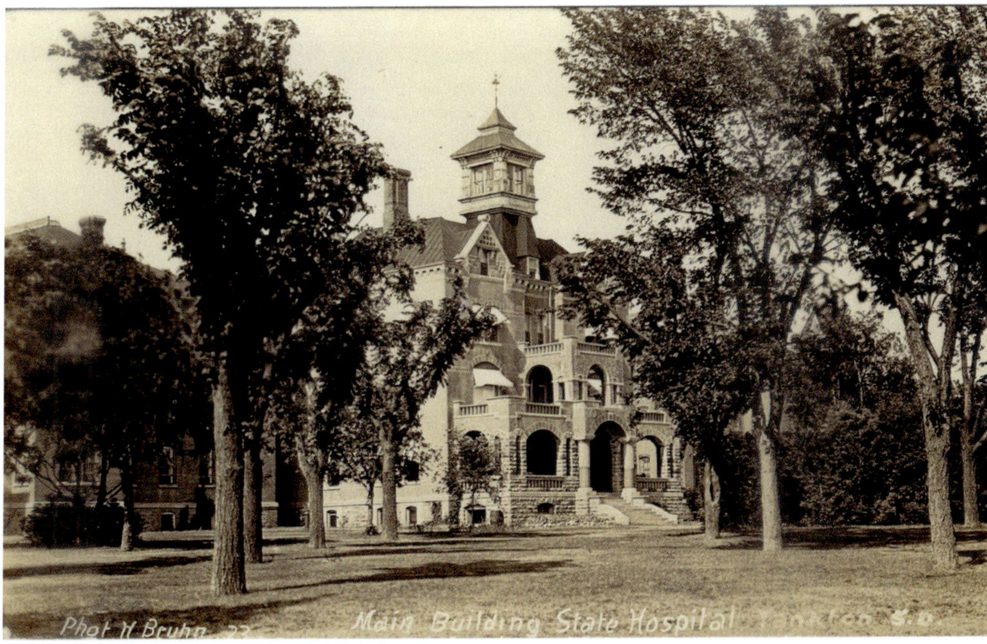

Figure 179

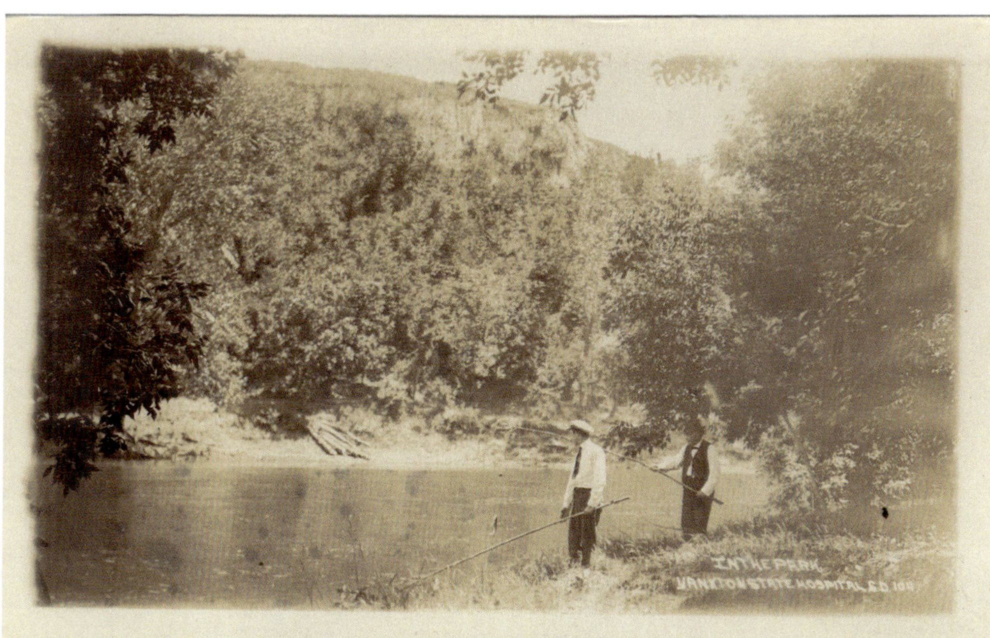

Figure 180

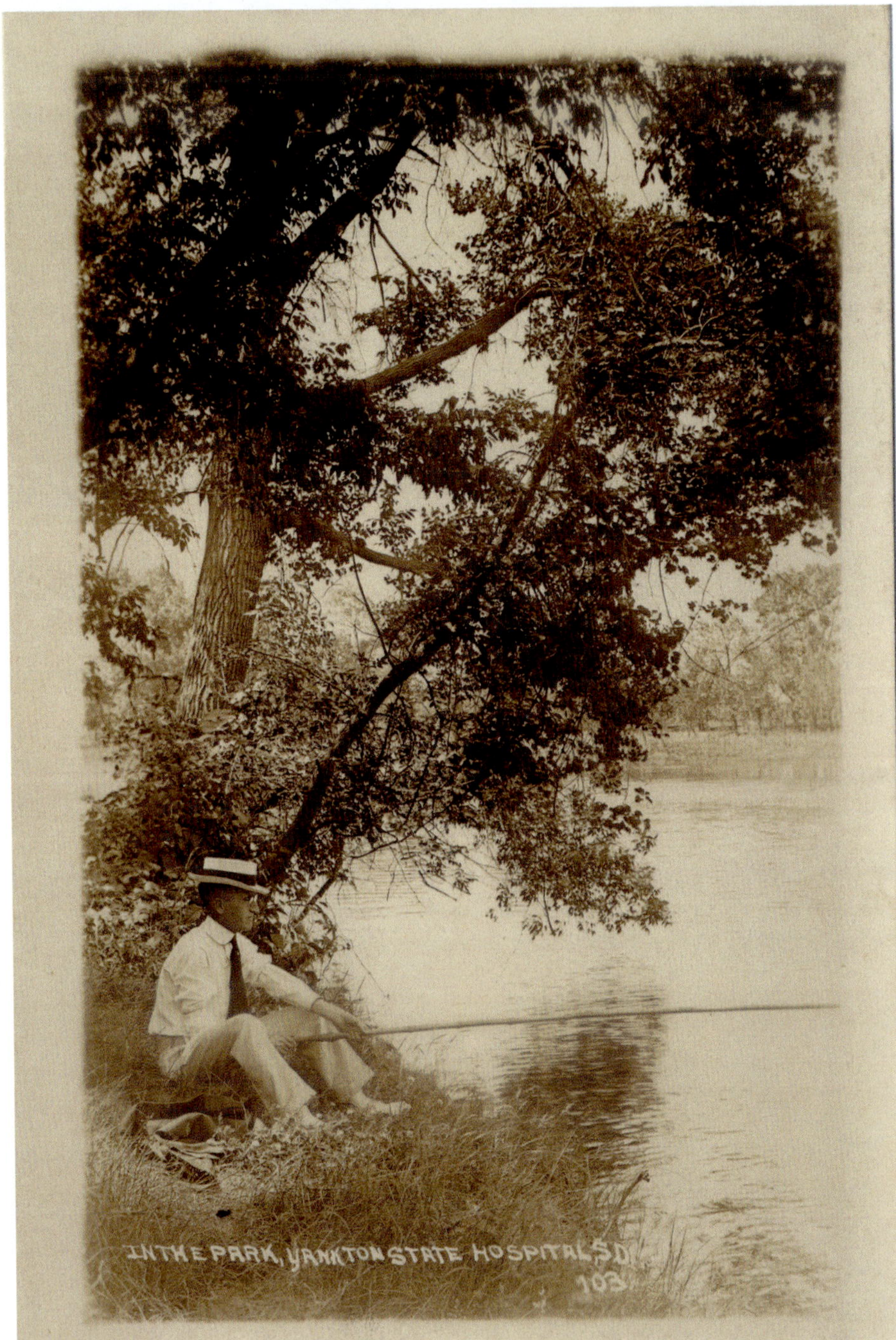

Figure 181

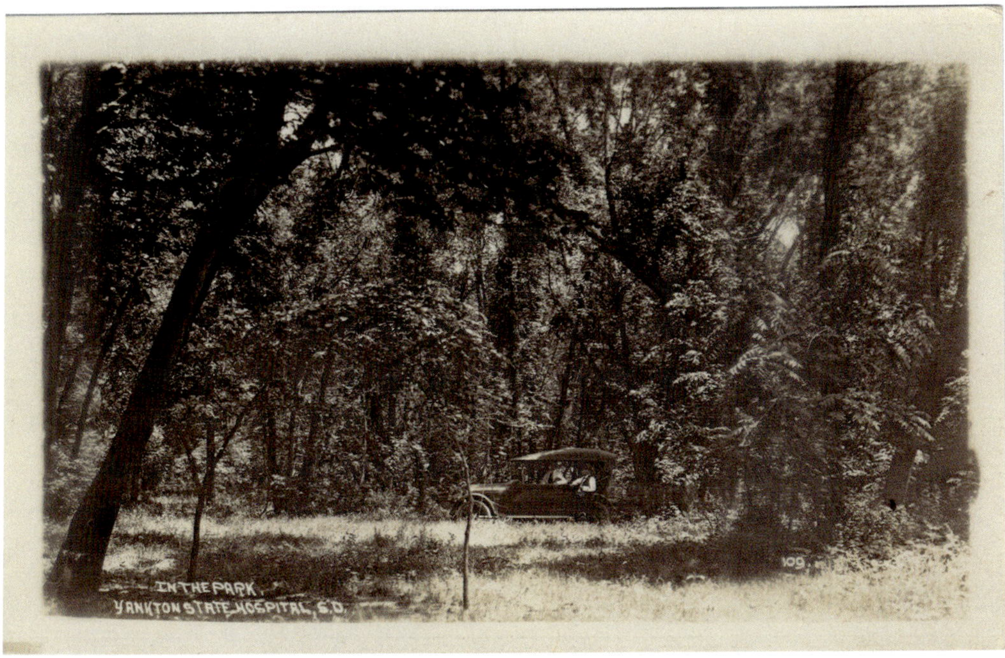

Figure 182

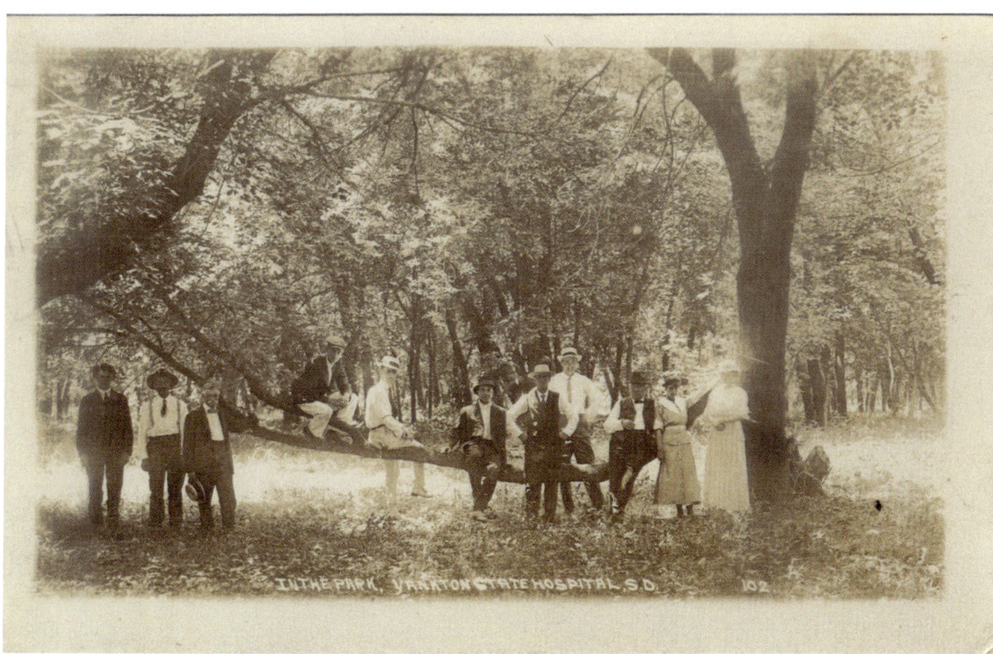

Figure 183

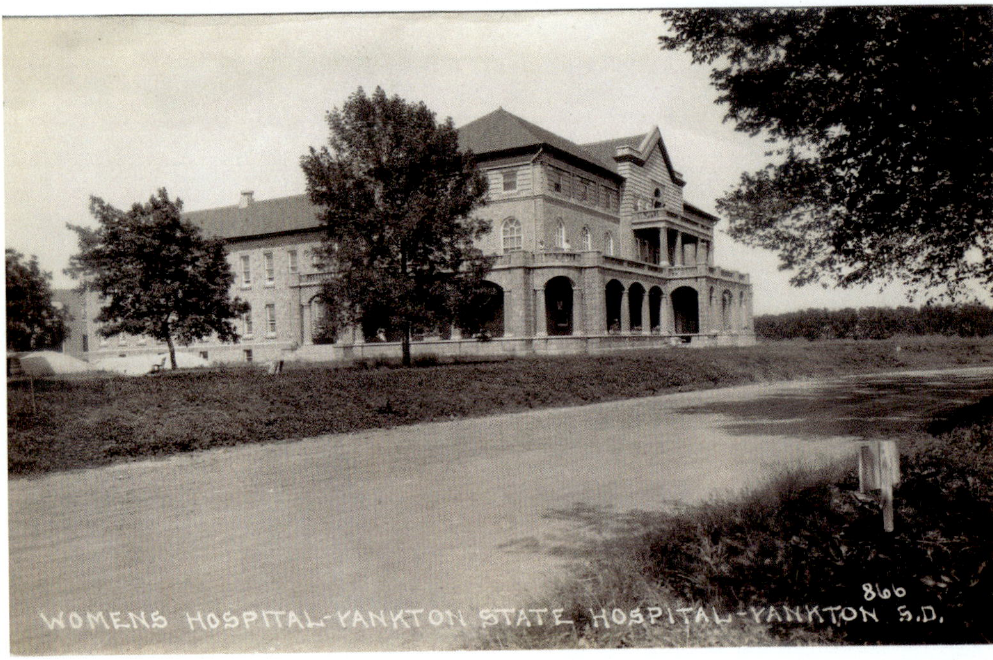
866
WOMENS HOSPITAL-YANKTON STATE HOSPITAL-YANKTON S.D.

Figure 184

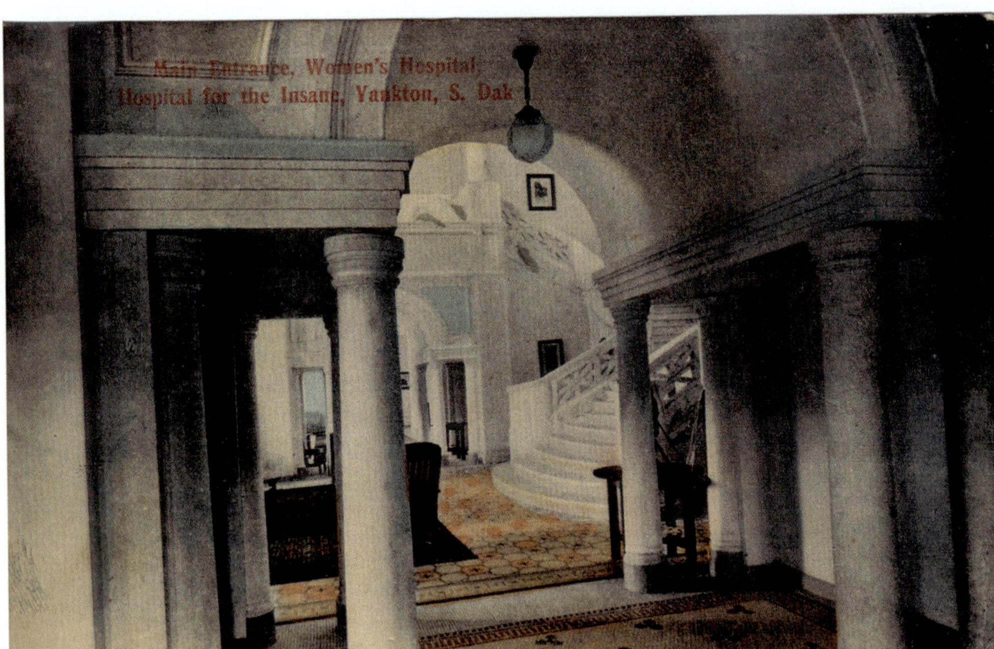
Main Entrance, Women's Hospital
Hospital for the Insane, Yankton, S. Dak

Figure 185

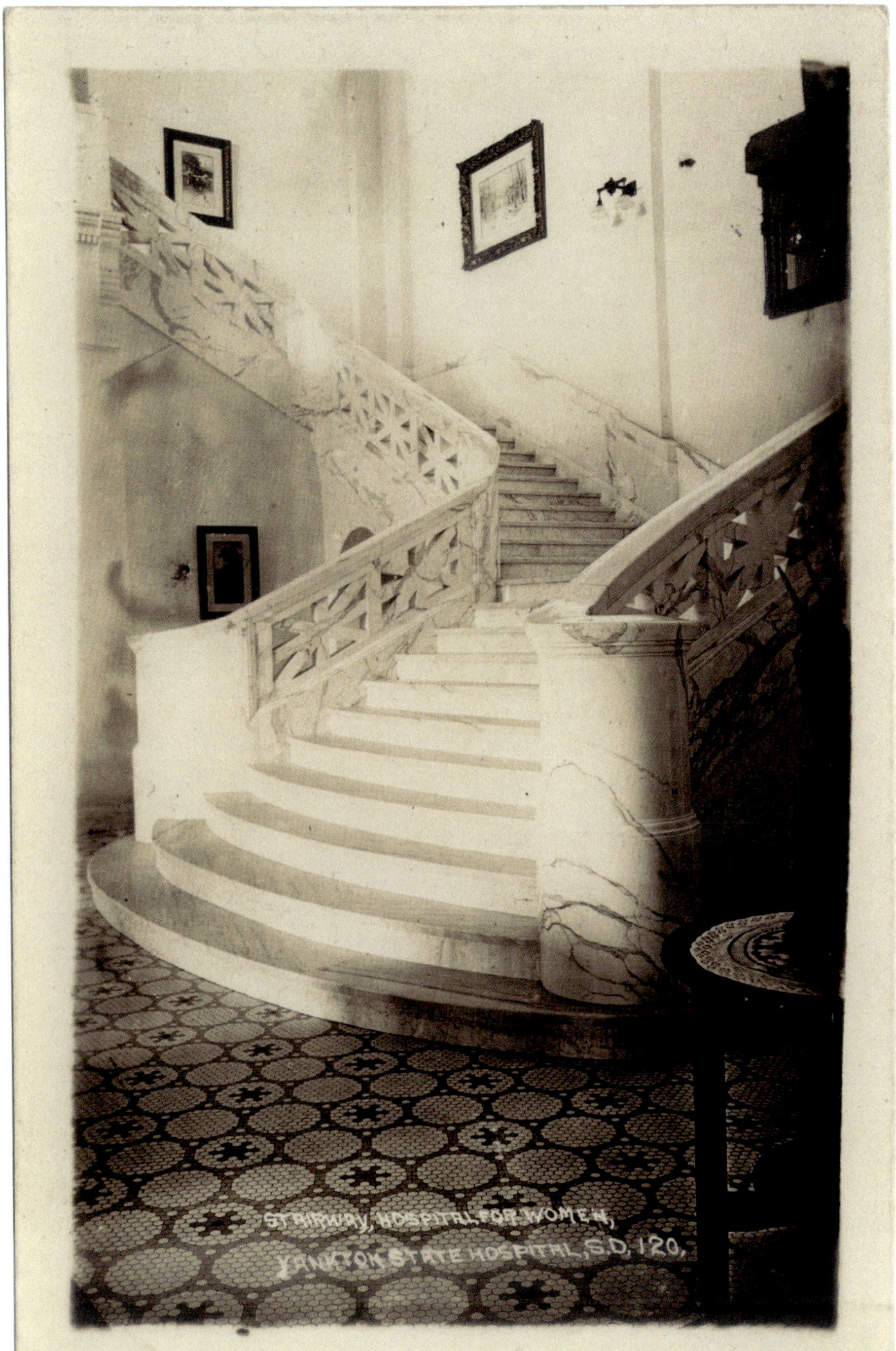

Figure 186

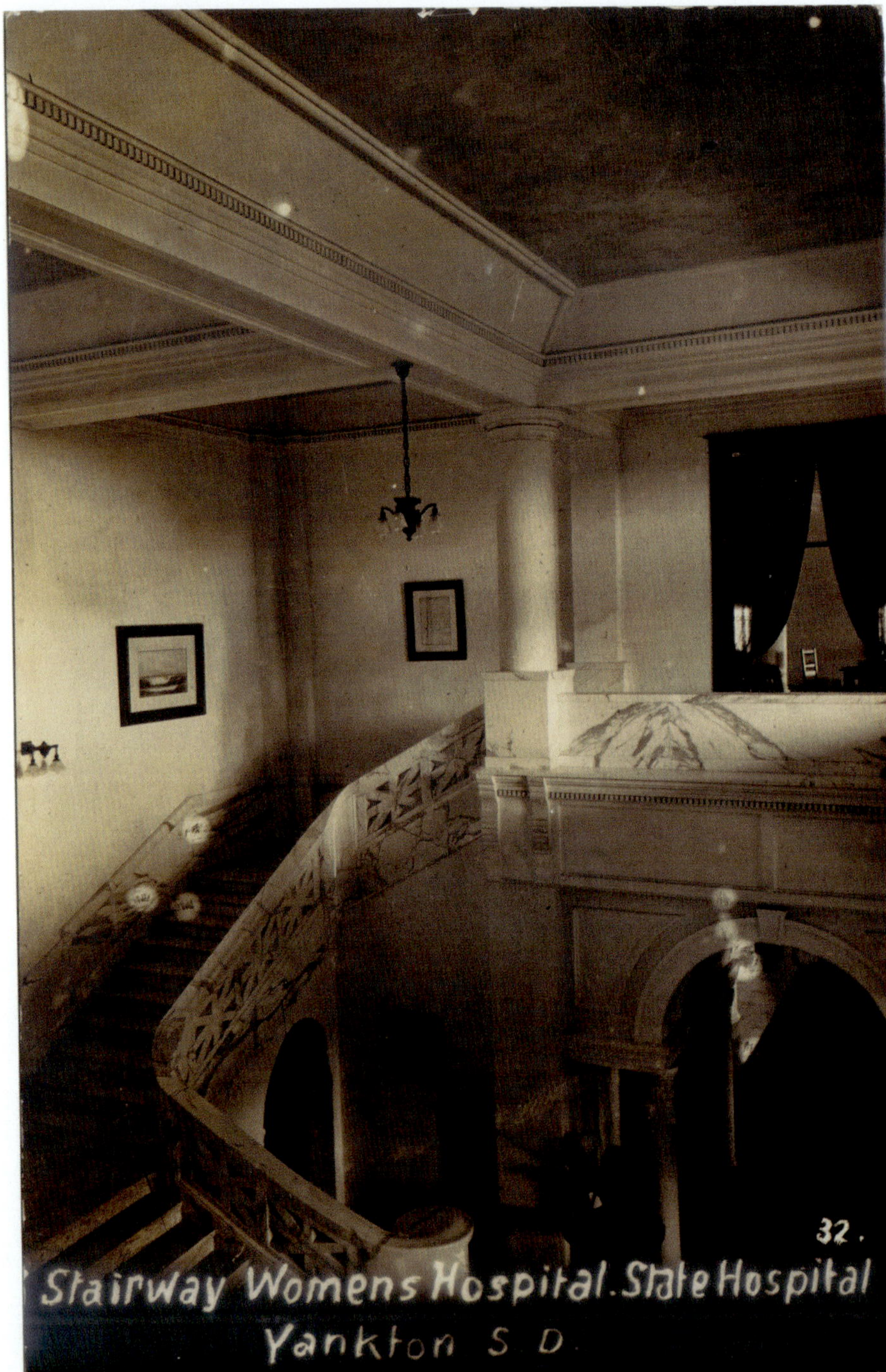

Figure 187

Buffalo State Asylum for the Insane
Buffalo, New York, 1880

The Buffalo State Asylum for the Insane in Buffalo, New York was opened in 1880, though construction on the grand Kirkbride facility (figure 188) was not completed until the 1890s. The Kirkbride plan allowed the addition of wings as needed, and the asylum grew extensively. According to reports from the early 1900s, medical officers had to walk one and a half miles to reach the end of the furthest ward from the administration building.

In 1883, instruction for women attendants at this facility began and by 1886, a class of seven had graduated.

The Buffalo Psychiatric Center operates in new facilities on the original grounds of the hospital. The original Kirkbride structure has been preserved and options for reuse of the building are being considered.

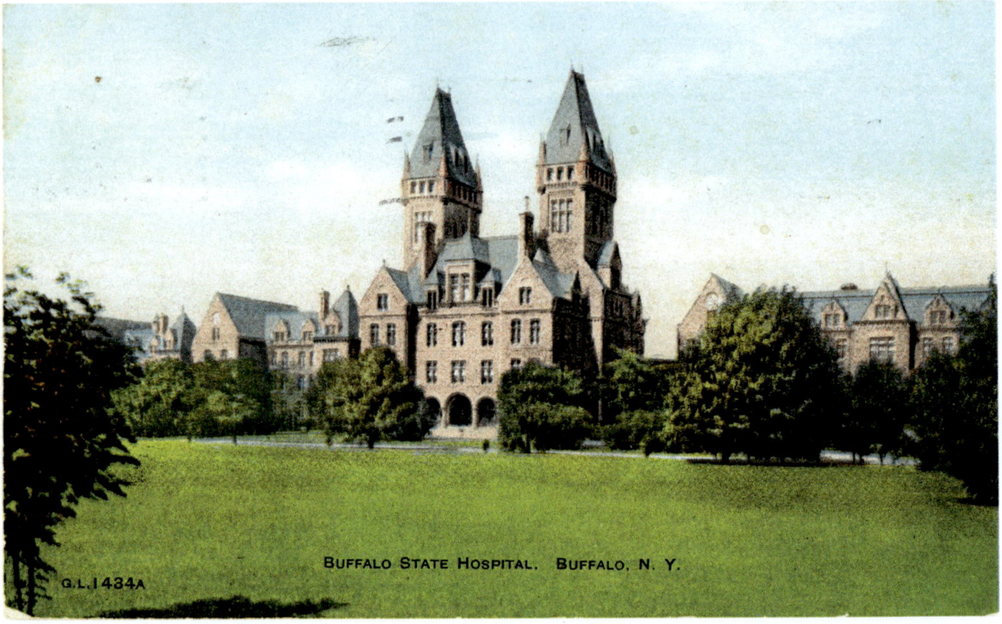

Figure 188

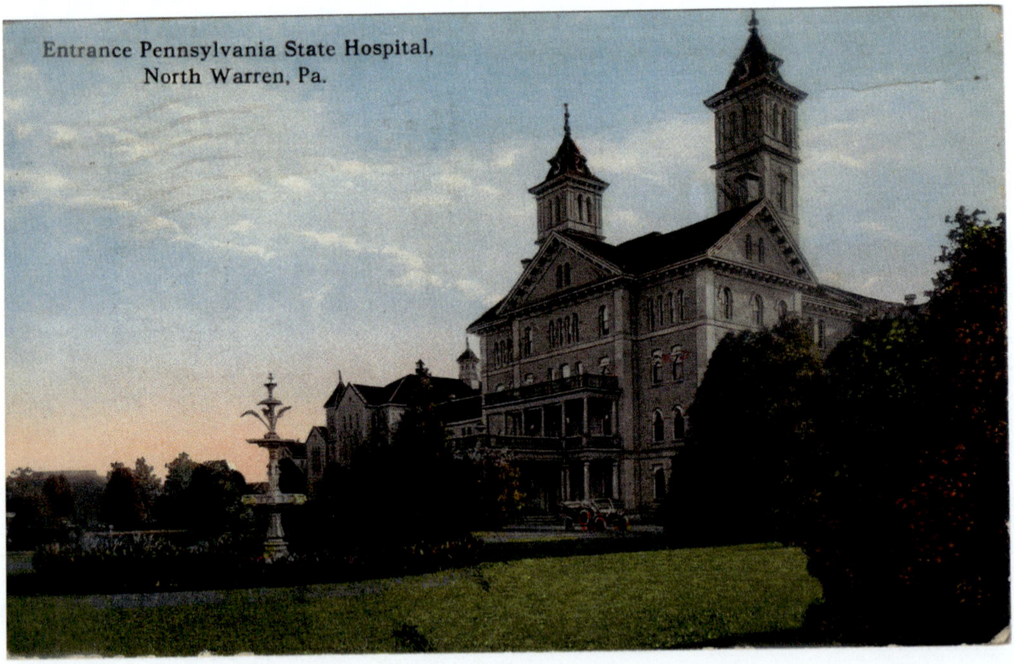

Figure 189

State Hospital for the Insane
Warren, Pennsylvania, 1880

The State Hospital for the Insane was opened in October of 1880 as the third state mental institution in Pennsylvania. A site at Warren was chosen to provide care for patients in the northwestern part of the state. Overcrowding was still a significant problem in Pennsylvania hospitals a decade later, resulting in the decision to treat acute cases of mental illness in state hospitals, while sending those with chronic mental illness to farm colonies.

The original buildings included a main center building with three horizontal sections on each side connected to the center by parallel wings. They were built about 1,600 feet from the Conewago Creek bank. Other buildings were slowly added and by 1912, there were 28 buildings. By 1914, the hospital had a capacity of 1,282 and the average population was 1,350.

The views of the entrance to the hospital in figures 189–190 are from 1910. The outing grounds are pictured in figure 191.

This facility continues to operate in the original buildings as Warren State Hospital.

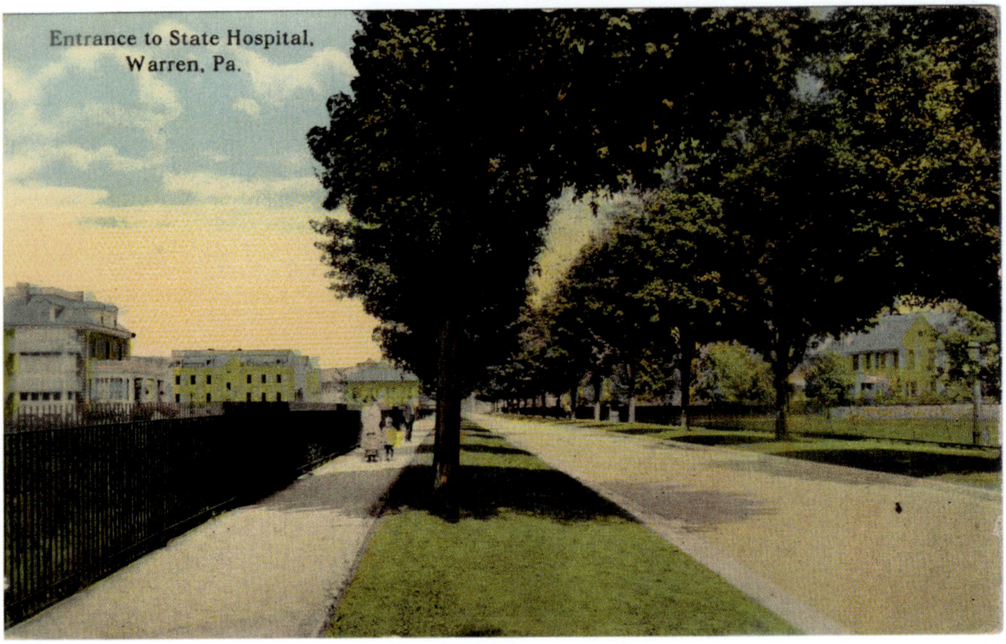
Entrance to State Hospital,
Warren, Pa.

Figure 190

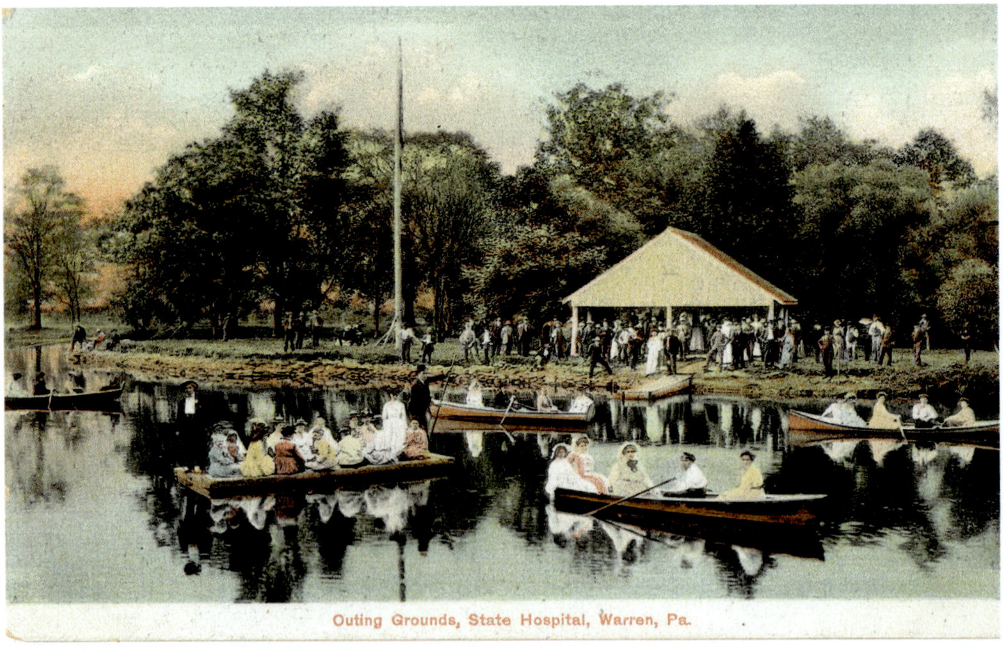
Outing Grounds, State Hospital, Warren, Pa.

Figure 191

State Hospital for the Insane of the Southeastern District of Pennsylvania
Norristown, Pennsylvania, 1880

The State Hospital for the Insane of the Southeastern District of Pennsylvania opened in July 1880. The original capacity was established at 704 patients, but by October 1882, there were 859 patients. The facility included eight wards, physically detached from the administration building but connected to it through basement corridors. It also included a chapel, a kitchen, a boiler house, and laundry.

The 1910 image in figure 192 shows the administration building. The building was designed to be less ornate than some, with the hopes of avoiding unnecessary costs.

The entrance gate and guard house are depicted on the postcard in figure 193, postmarked 1911.

Figure 194 shows the modern assembly hall that was built in 1909. The lower floor had a dance hall. The upper floor contained an auditorium for chapel services and assembly of patients, with theater seats for 1,200 patients.

In the early 1900s, a fire at the hospital badly damaged one of the wards (figures 195 and 196).

The female nurses' home (figure 197), which was built in 1904, had a capacity of 110 nurses. A home for male nurses was built shortly after.

This facility continues to operate as Norristown State Hospital. The administration building still stands, but is in a state of disrepair and has been abandoned.

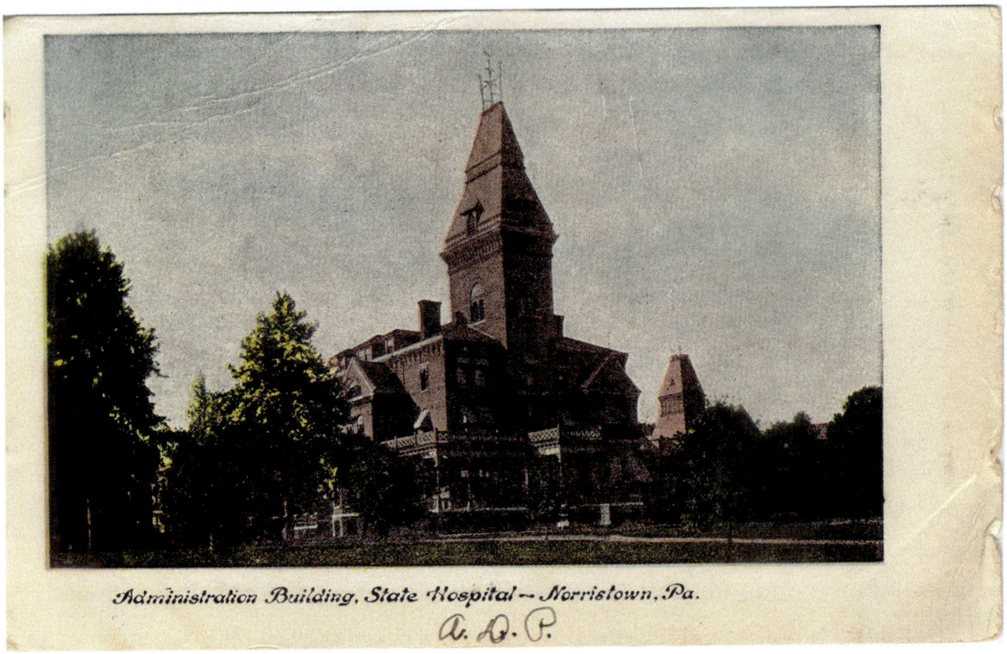
Administration Building, State Hospital — Norristown, Pa.
A. D. P.

Figure 192

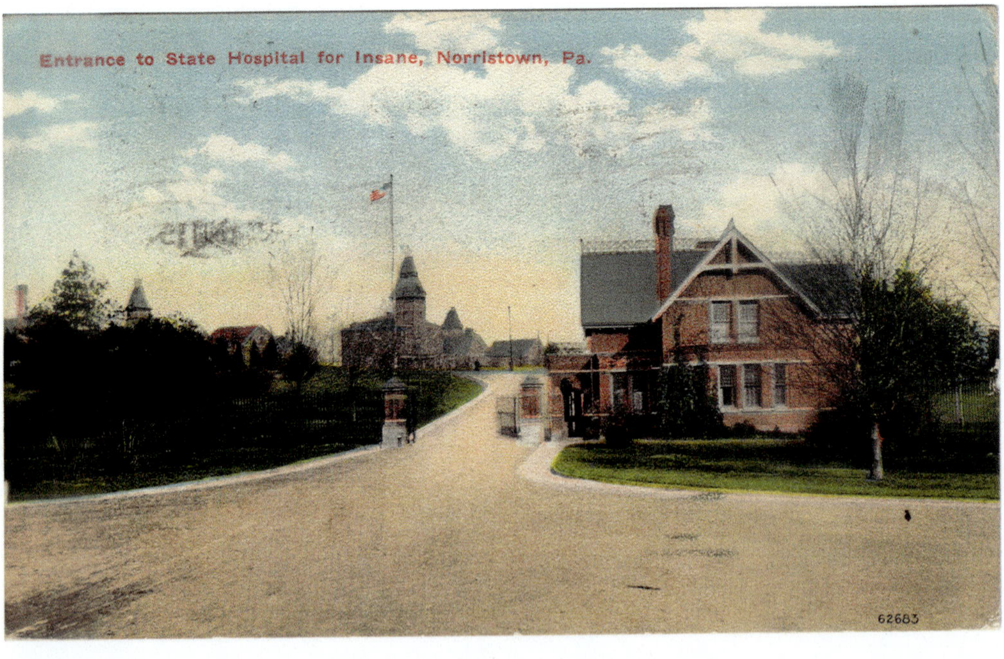
Entrance to State Hospital for Insane, Norristown, Pa.
62683

Figure 193

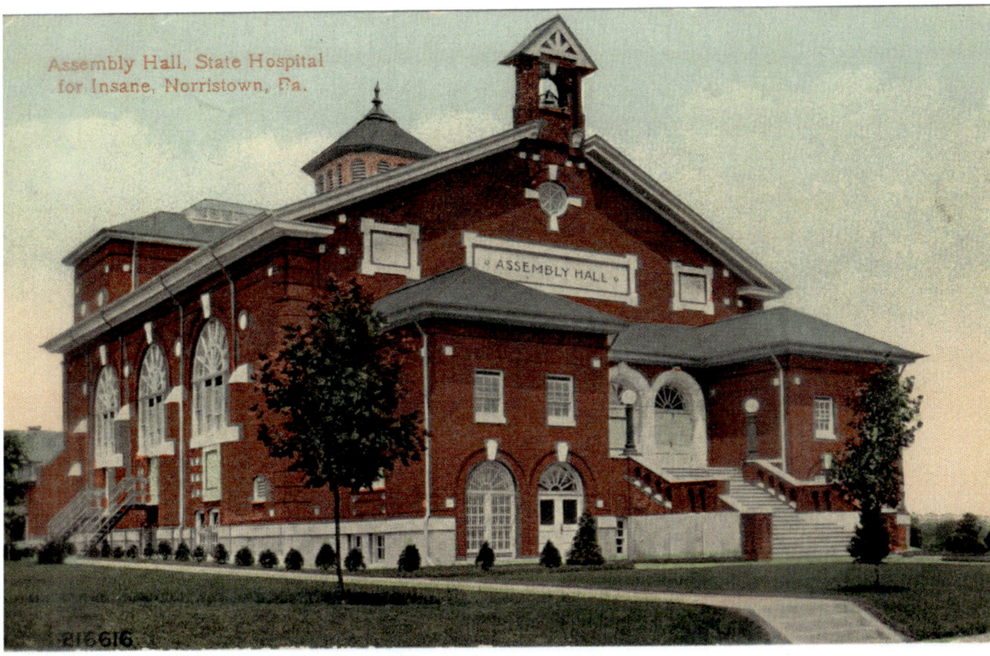
Assembly Hall, State Hospital
for Insane, Norristown, Pa.
ASSEMBLY HALL
216616

Figure 194

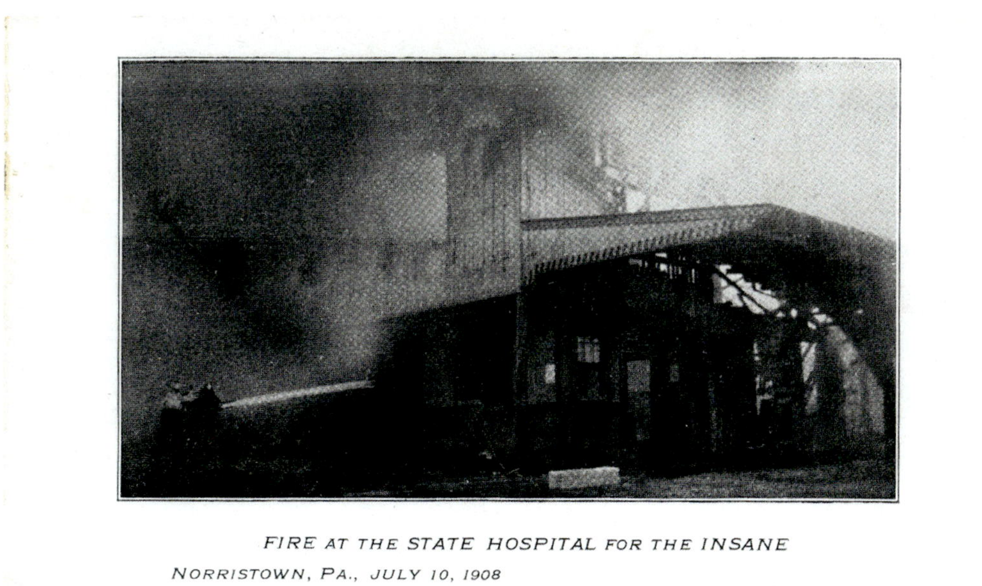

Figure 195

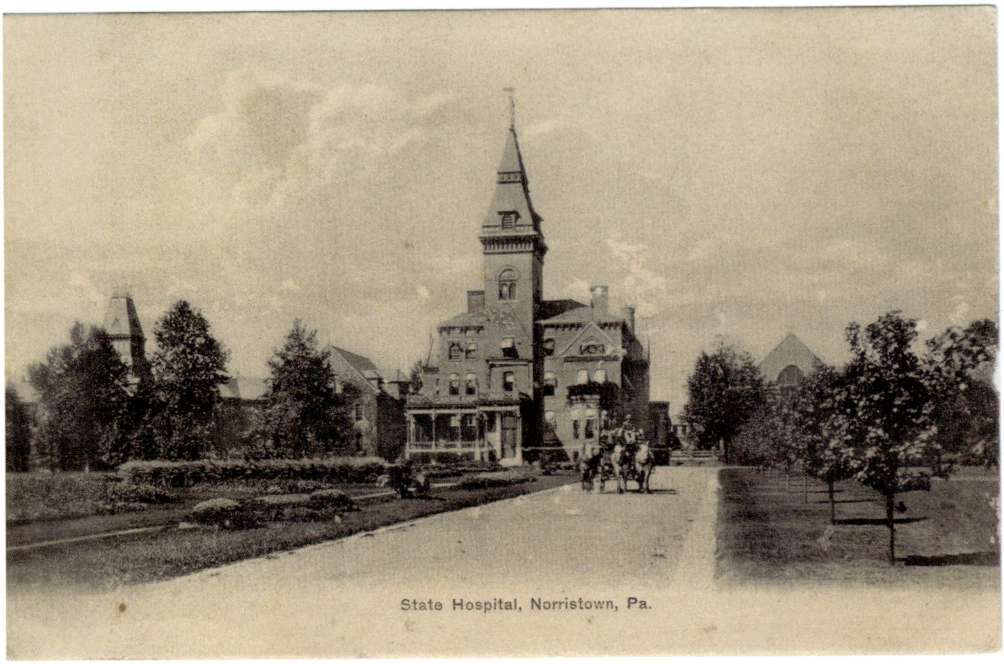

Figure 196

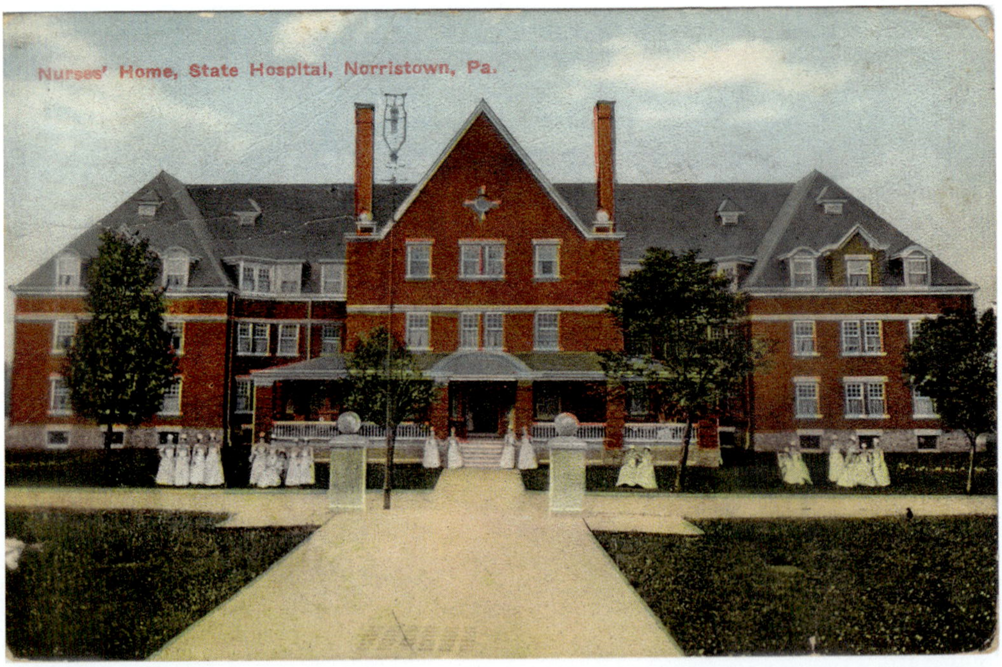

Figure 197

Asylum for Colored Insane
Goldsboro, North Carolina, 1880

The Asylum for Colored Insane opened in Goldsboro on August 1, 1880, to care for mentally ill African Americans in the state of North Carolina. A 170-acre farm served as the site for the asylum. The first buildings consisted of a four-story brick building and an adjoining three-story building to accommodate patients. When the facility opened, it accommodated 70 patients. Additions were made over the next several years and by 1913, there were 763 patients.

There were no postcards of this facility in the author's collection. The facility now operates as a psychiatric hospital called Cherry Hospital. An on-site museum exploring the hospital's history has been established.

New York State Inebriate Asylum
Binghamton, New York, 1881

This large Gothic Revival structure (figure 198) was opened in 1864 as the New York State Inebriate Asylum, the first public building erected specifically as a place to treat alcoholism. After controversy over leadership and spending, the Inebriate Asylum closed in 1879. The state provided funding to remodel the building for reuse as the Binghamton Asylum for the Chronic Insane. The first patients were 298 individuals transferred from asylums at Utica, Poughkeepsie, and Middletown. The facility was renamed Binghamton State Hospital in 1890.

The hospital grew quickly. Additional buildings and services included a training school for nurses, additions to the grounds and farm, larger wards and hospitals for patients, a summer camp for convalescent patients, and an assembly hall. Patients were entertained by a brass band organized by the employees and weekly dances were held. A choir consisting of employees and patients provided music for Sunday services and on the wards.

By 1913, there were 2,000 patients and nearly 500 employees.

The postcard in figure 199, postmarked 1910, shows the expansive grounds of the asylum, including rolling lawns, trees, and walkways.

A semi-circular drive (figure 200) served as the main entrance.

The original Kirkbride structure closed in 1993 but remains standing on the campus of the Greater Binghamton Health Center. It is currently being renovated to serve as part of the campus of the State University of New York Upstate Medical University. Local residents commonly refer to the large Gothic Revival structure as "the castle."

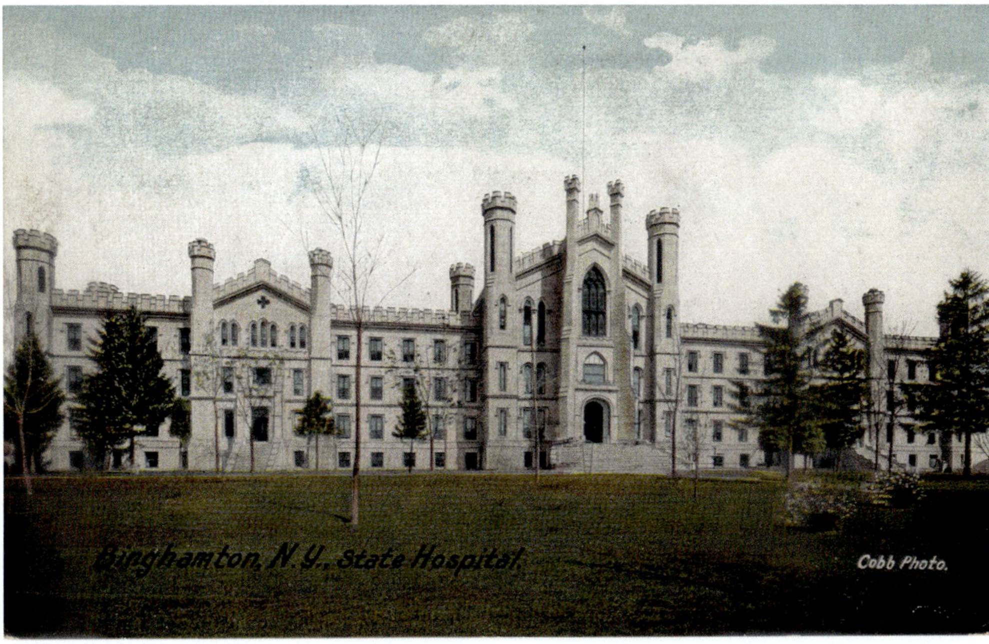
Binghamton, N.Y., State Hospital
Cobb Photo.

Figure 198

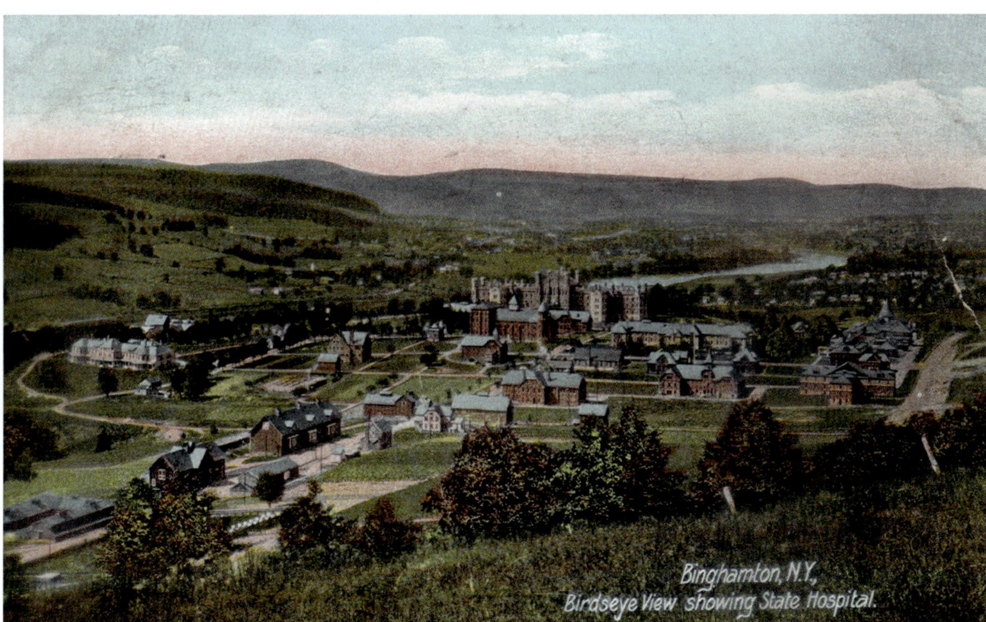
Binghamton, N.Y.,
Birdseye View showing State Hospital.

Figure 199

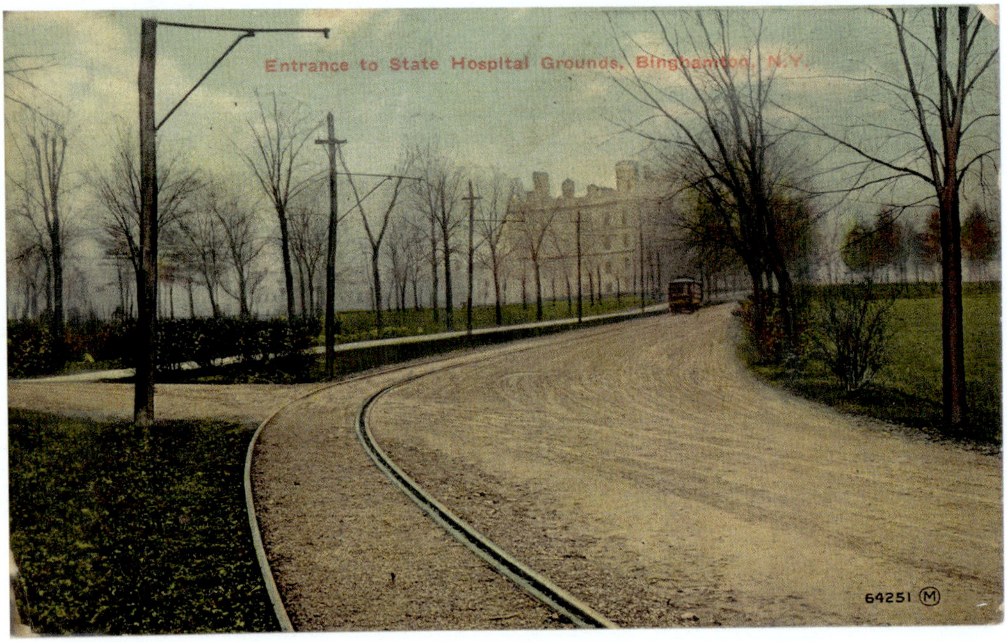

Figure 200

Nevada Insane Asylum
Sparks, Nevada, 1882

The Nevada Insane Asylum opened in 1882, receiving its first patients from a private asylum at Stockton, California. Later renamed Nevada State Hospital, the original building was three stories, built to accommodate 160 patients. The main building was enlarged in 1895 for male patients and another building was added for female patients. By 1912, the population was 242.

The asylum operated a large working farm where patients worked under supervision. There were no images of this facility in the author's collection, though a postcard may be found at the University of Nevada's Special Collections.

In 2011, the hospital's cemetery, with patient graves dating to 1882, was rededicated and preserved. The facility is now known as Northern Nevada Adult Mental Health Services.

Western North Carolina Insane Asylum
North Carolina, 1883

The Western North Carolina Insane Asylum opened in 1883, providing some relief for other overcrowded asylums in North Carolina. Within the first two years, 252 patients were received. By 1897, the institution had the capacity to care for 785 patients.

Patients helped to build the grounds and roads of the facility and by 1893, the hospital occupied more than 331 acres. The facility included a bowling alley, a billiard room, a greenhouse, a golf course, and a farm colony.

The facility was renamed State Hospital at Morganton (figure 201) in 1890 and again renamed Broughton Hospital in 1959. Broughton Hospital continues to occupy the same site and the original Kirkbride buildings have survived.

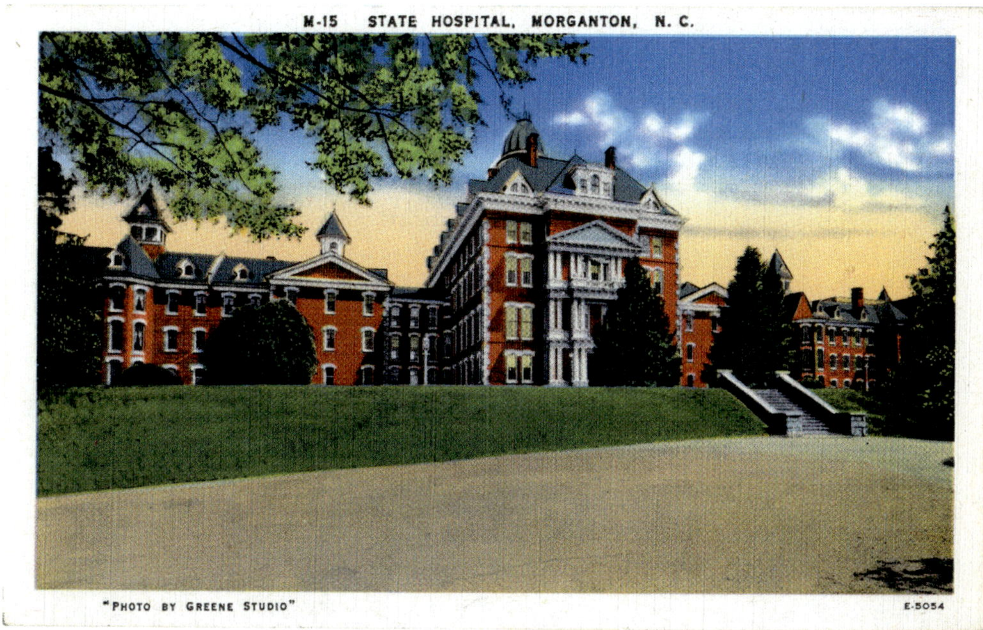
M-15 STATE HOSPITAL, MORGANTON, N. C.
"PHOTO BY GREENE STUDIO"
E-5054

Figure 201

Colorado State Insane Asylum
Pueblo, Colorado, 1883

Originally named the Colorado State Insane Asylum, the facility initially cared for less than 15 patients, but by 1961, more than 6,000 patients resided there. The site occupied 300 acres of land and later included a 5,000-acre dairy farm.

A temporary cottage was erected for female patients until a more substantial building could be erected. The permanent building for women (figure 203) was not finished until 1888 and an administration building was completed in 1892. By 1894, a two-story cottage for 70 men was completed and by 1909, three more cottages were opened for 300 patients.

The postcard in figure 202 shows the main administration building.

In 1917, the facility's name was changed to Colorado State Hospital and in 1991, it became known as the Colorado Mental Health Institute at Pueblo. It continues to operate under this name while the current status of the original buildings is unknown. A museum displaying items from the history of the facility operates in the superintendent's residence, built in 1934.

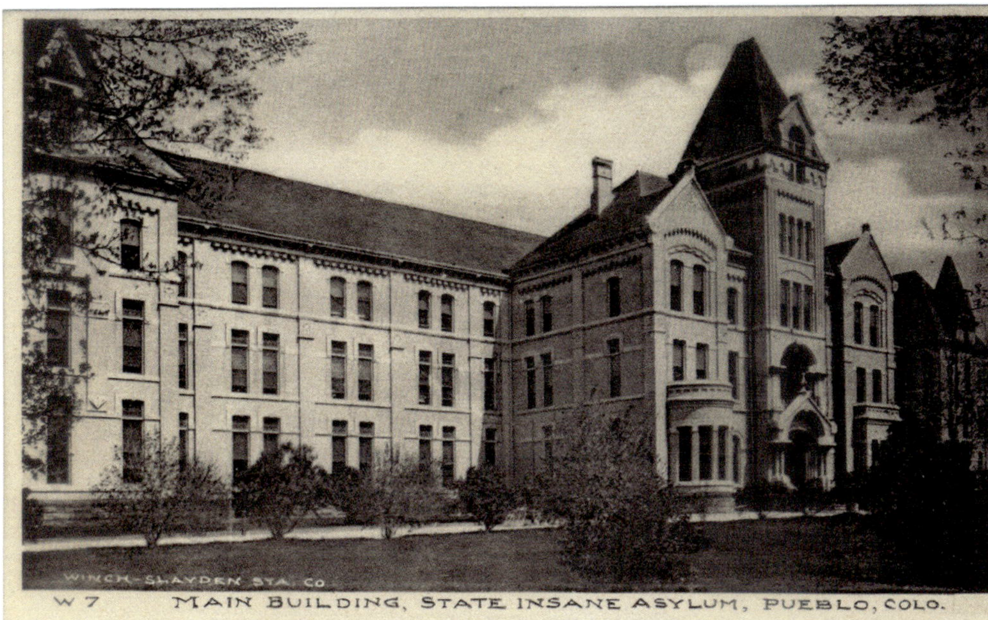
WINCH-SLAYDEN STA. CO.
W 7 MAIN BUILDING, STATE INSANE ASYLUM, PUEBLO, COLO.

Figure 202

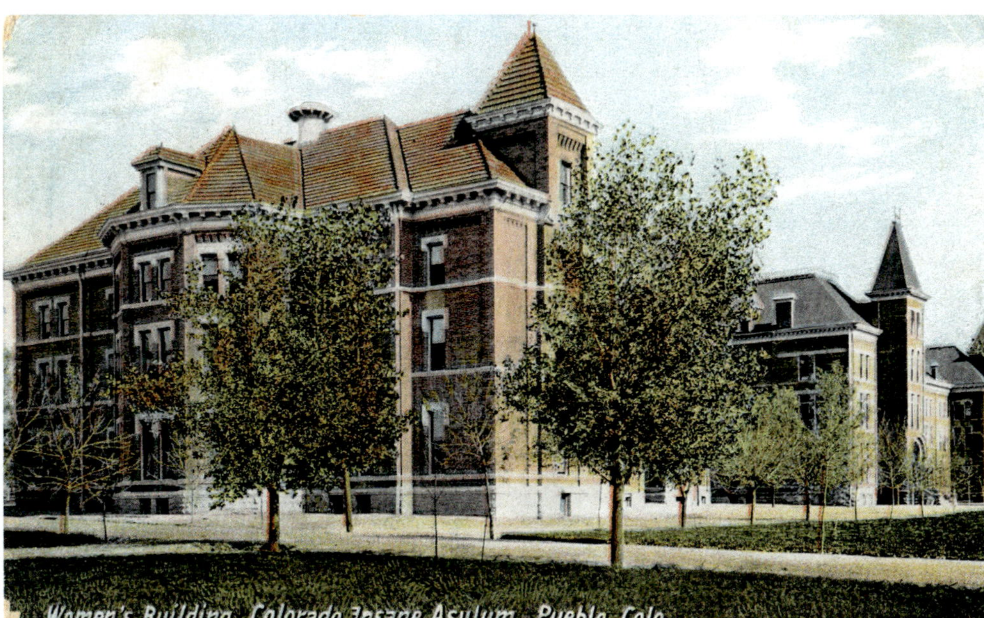
Women's Building, Colorado Insane Asylum - Pueblo, Colo.

Figure 203

Oregon State Insane Asylum
Salem, Oregon, 1883

The Oregon State Insane Asylum (figure 204) opened in 1883. While the original building had a capacity for 412 patients, 370 patients were immediately transferred by train from an asylum in Portland. The building included a four-story central administration building with attached wings containing a total of 18 wards. Additions to the facility included an auditorium, amusement hall, and a pathology laboratory. By 1914, the capacity had increased to 1,525 patients.

The facility originally occupied 107 acres with 61 additional acres added within two years. Patients worked on the farm and in the gardens (figure 205).

The following building, frequently called the "dome building" was constructed between 1910 and 1912. Patients were admitted here and medical procedures were also performed. The building featured in the top postcard on page 187 (figure 206) was called the receiving ward.

Oregon State Hospital continues to operate as a psychiatric hospital on the original site. The dome building is currently used by the state's Department of Corrections. The Kirkbride building is now home to a museum focused on the history of the hospital.

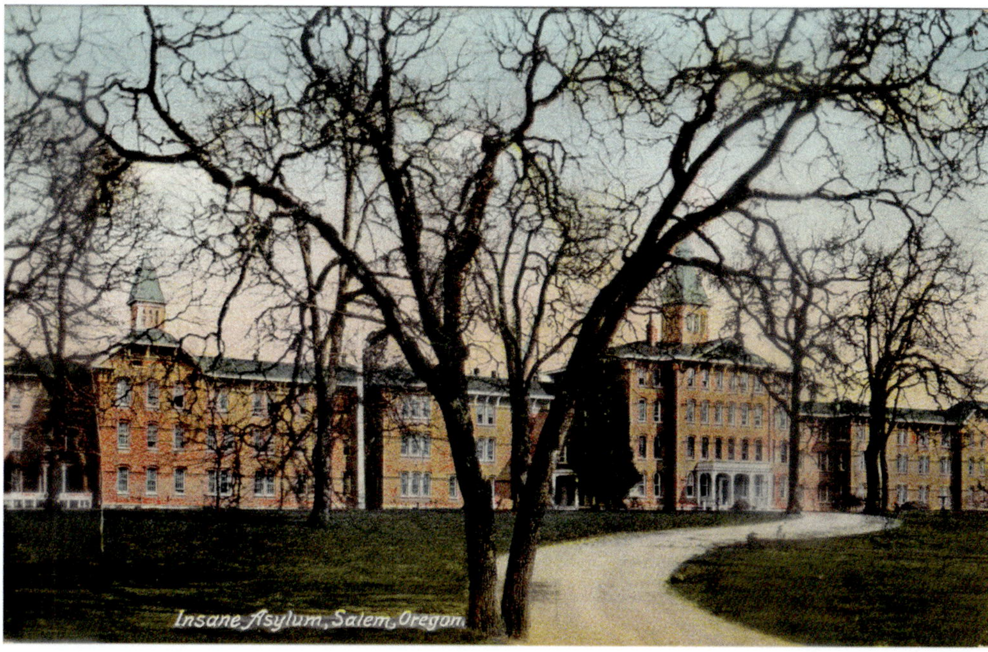

Figure 204

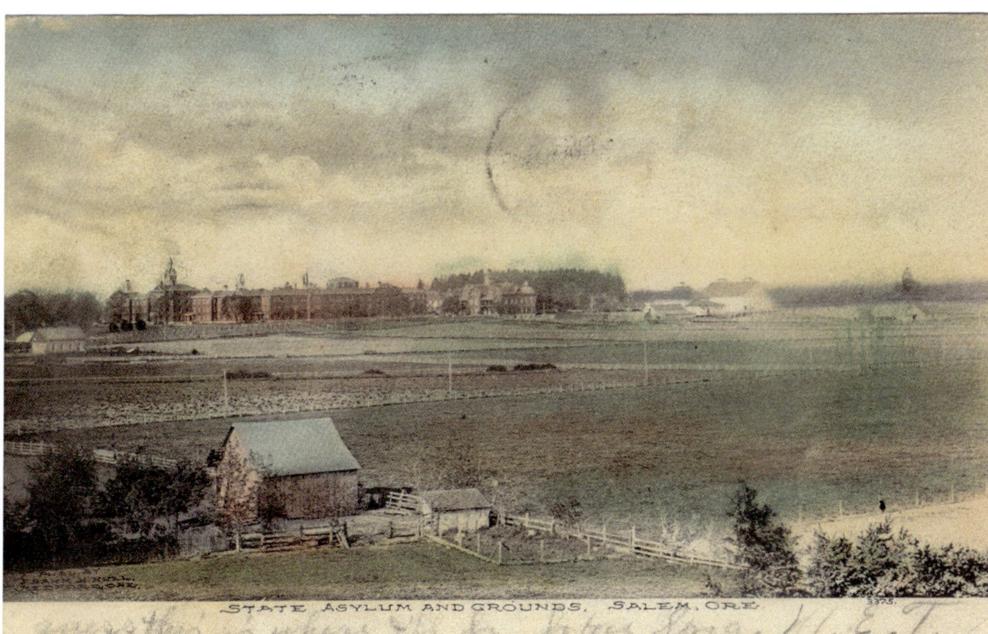

Figure 205

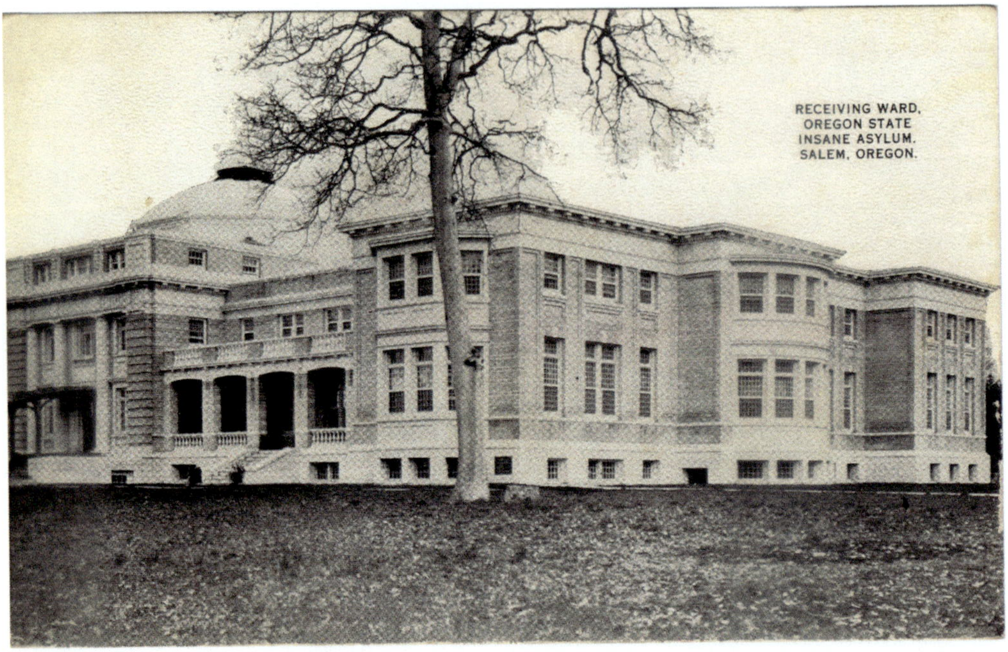
RECEIVING WARD,
OREGON STATE
INSANE ASYLUM.
SALEM, OREGON.

Figure 206

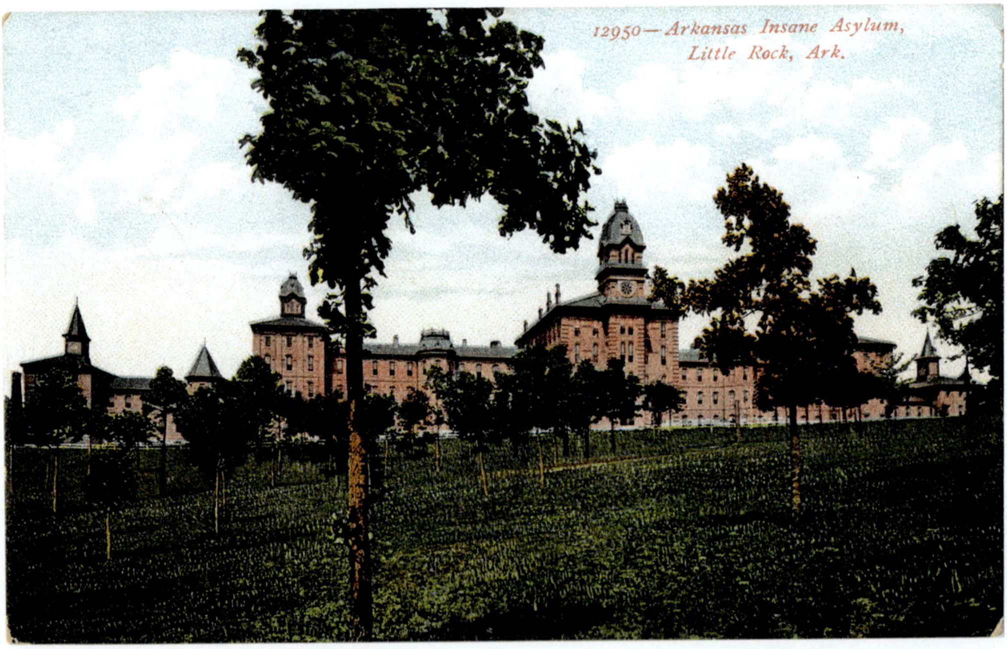
12950—Arkansas Insane Asylum,
Little Rock, Ark.

Figure 207

Arkansas Lunatic Asylum
Little Rock, Arkansas, 1883

The Arkansas Lunatic Asylum was the first state lunatic asylum for Arkansas residents. The original four-story building included a tower and three-story wings extending to the north and south, which included 212 rooms. A rear building contained the kitchen and laundry. Two years after opening, a new building was added to accommodate 200 patients, increasing the capacity of the building to 450 patients. Male patients were employed outdoors, while female patients were employed at sewing and other indoor activities.

The facility had a devastating year in 1894. There were 132 deaths with epidemics of erysipelas (a bacterial infection) and dysentery. In addition, a cyclone destroyed six wards and caused considerable damage to the center buildings and several smaller buildings. That same year, the springs that supplied water to the institution stopped functioning. Two years later, the laundry building was destroyed by fire. By 1900, it was determined that the property was in a state of disrepair and the buildings were systematically repaired. By 1914, the facility had 1,584 patients.

The postcard in figure 207 shows this facility in the early 1900s.

Arkansas State Hospital continues to operate as a psychiatric inpatient facility. The original buildings have been demolished and replaced.

Territorial Insane Asylum
Provo, Utah, 1885

The Territorial Insane Asylum (figure 208) was established in 1885, nestled at the foot of the mountains in Provo, Utah. Prior to the establishment of this facility, the mentally ill in Utah were housed in poorhouses, asylums in different counties, or private institutions funded by the patient's home county. The institution opened nine years before Utah became a state.

The main building (figure 209) was four stories with an attic and included a center building and two towers. The attached patients' buildings were four stories high, each with a tower and cupola. In 1901, two cottages were built, allowing space for 30 patients each; this was a significant change from the more common wards that housed large numbers of patients.

The asylum was separated from the town by the city dump, which was later turned into a city park (figures 210 and 211).

After several name changes, the facility became Utah State Hospital in 1927 and continues to operate as a mental health care facility in the same location. The original buildings have been demolished and replaced.

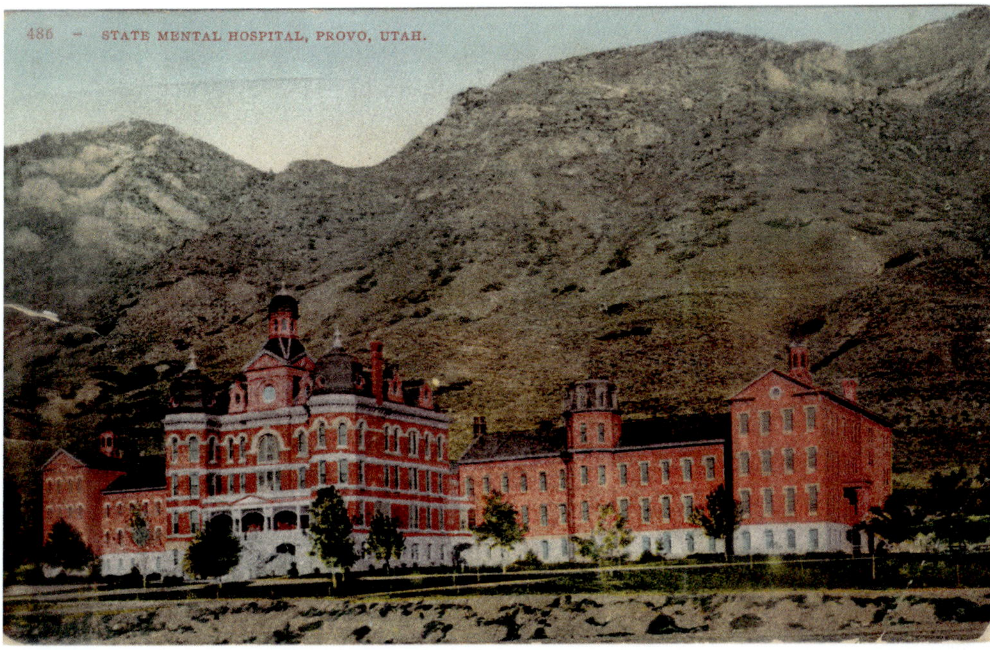

Figure 208

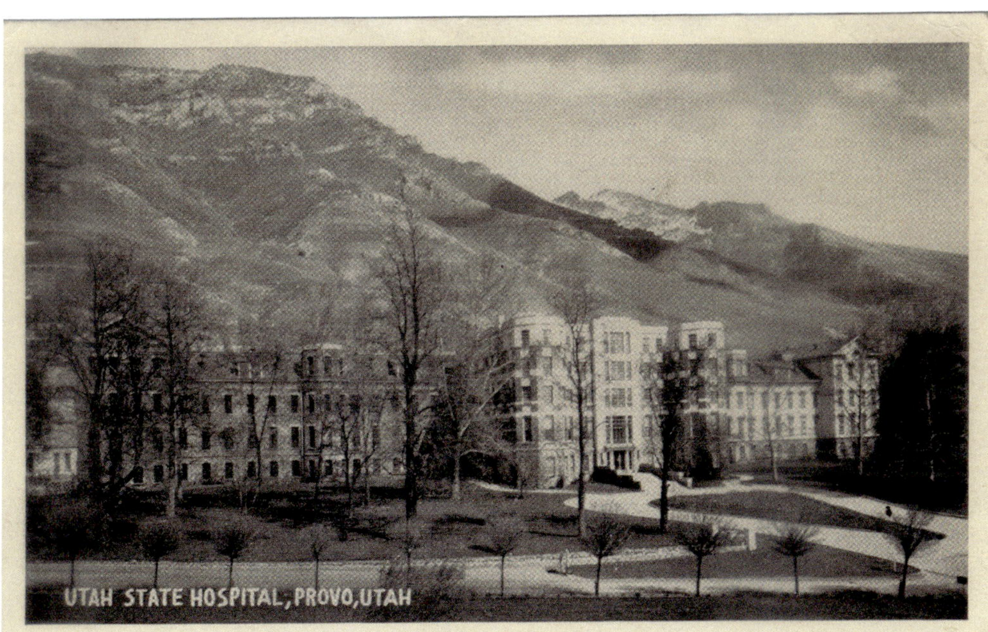

Figure 209

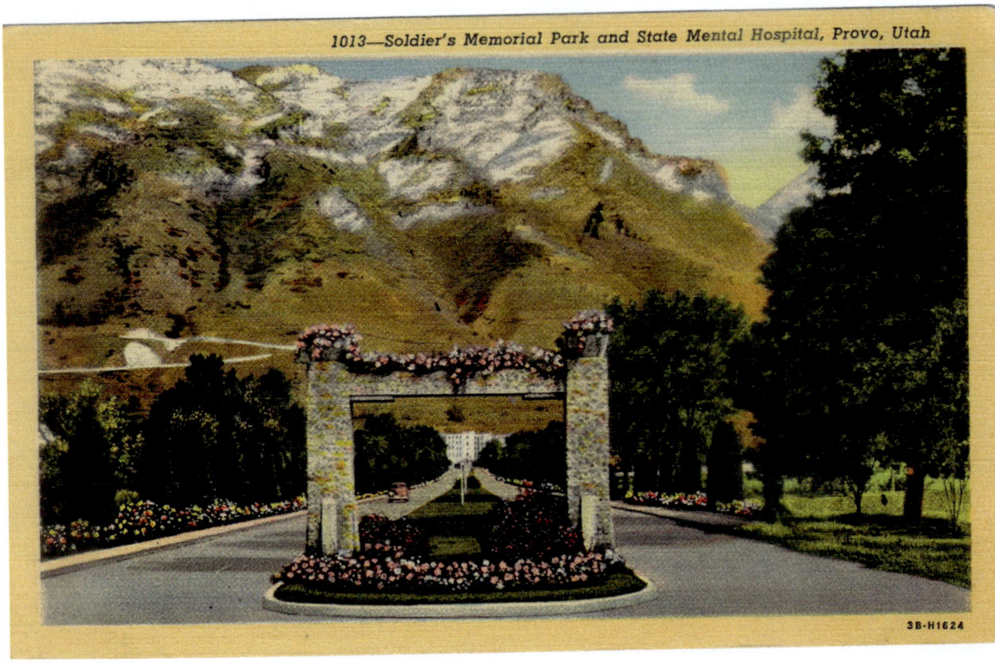
1013—Soldier's Memorial Park and State Mental Hospital, Provo, Utah
3B-H1624

Figure 210

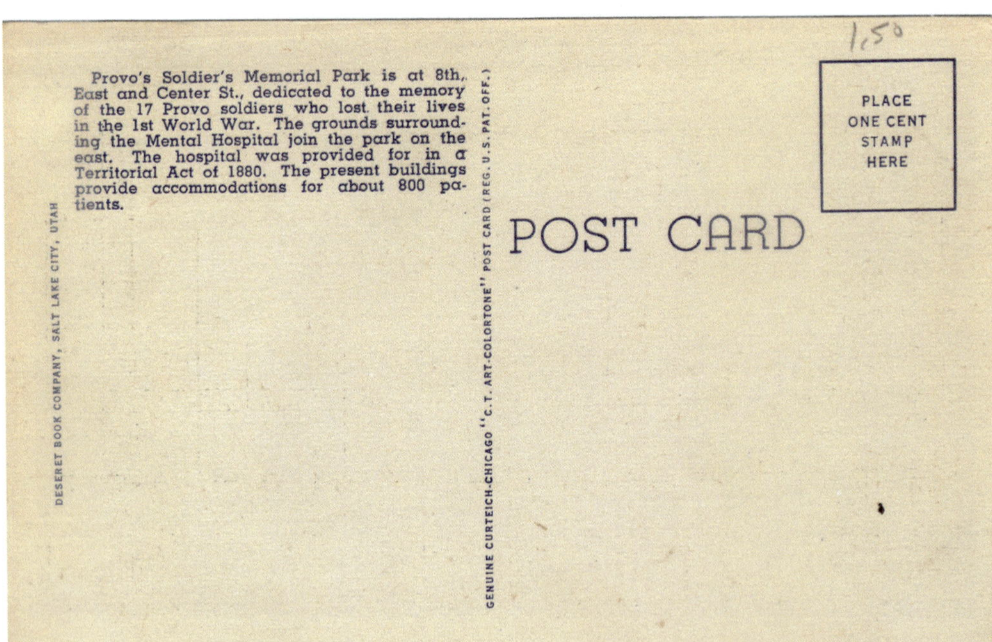

Figure 211

Northern Michigan Asylum
Traverse City, Michigan, 1885

The Northern Michigan Asylum, later renamed the Traverse City State Hospital, was opened about 1.5 miles from the city of Traverse. It was the third psychiatric facility opened in the state of Michigan.

The original Kirkbride building was designed to accommodate 500 patients. It contained 18 wards, nine for each sex, with its own dining room, restrooms, and an exit. The central administration building housed physicians and their families and other employees. By 1890, 12 cottages had been added to house tuberculosis patients and by 1906, a training school for nurses was established. A farm, established in 1885, grew to 729 acres.

The postcard in figure 212, postmarked 1908, provides a view of the facility.

The hospital closed in 1989, but many of the original buildings have been preserved and renovated. They are currently part of a larger complex that includes retail shops and eateries and serves as the setting for local markets and cultural events.

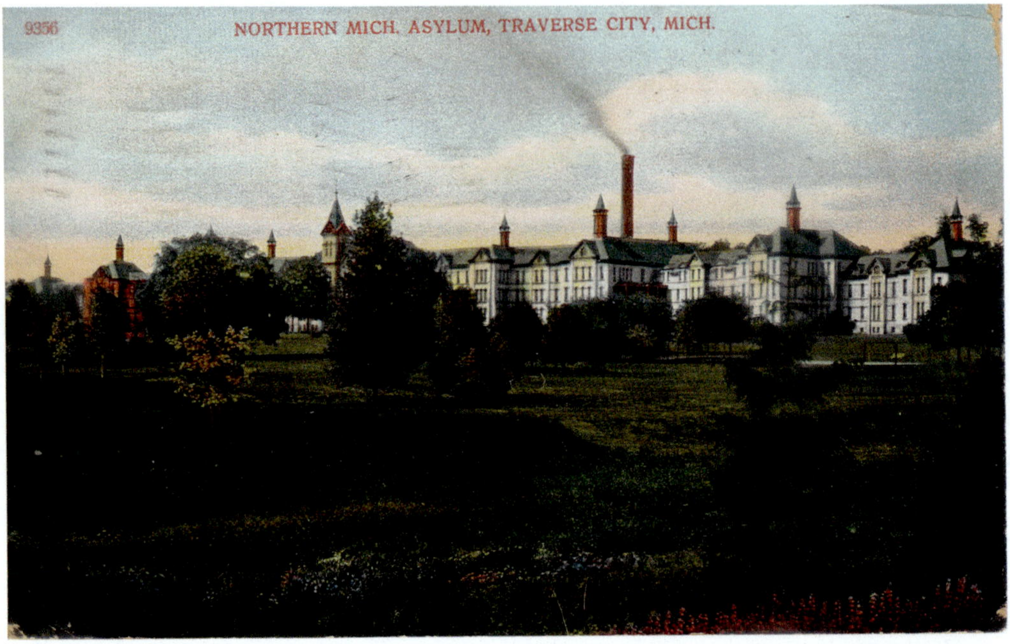
9356
NORTHERN MICH. ASYLUM, TRAVERSE CITY, MICH.

Figure 212

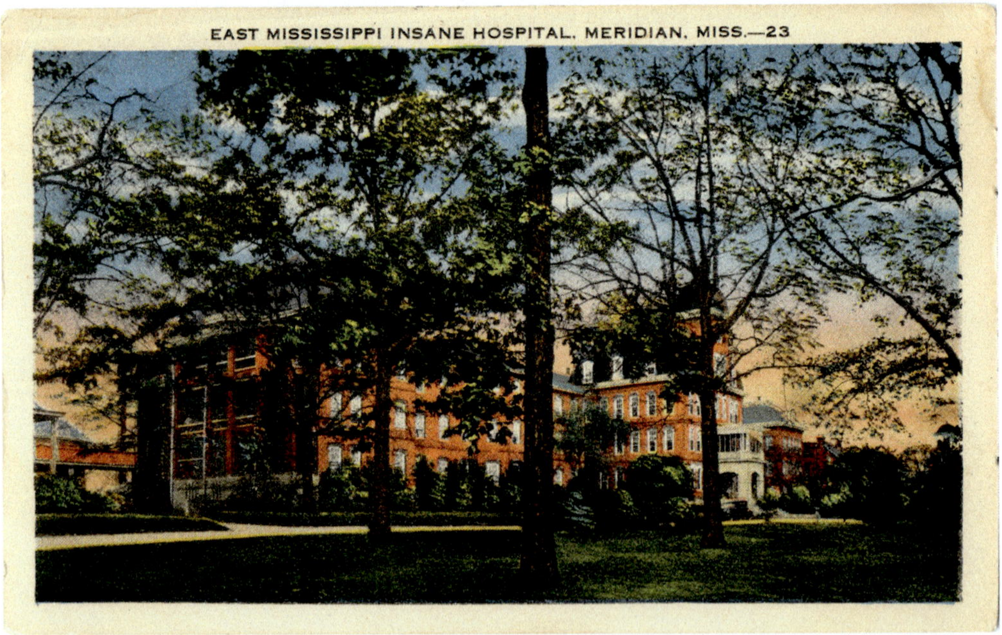
EAST MISSISSIPPI INSANE HOSPITAL, MERIDIAN, MISS.—23

Figure 213

East Mississippi Insane Asylum
Meridian, Mississippi, 1885

The East Mississippi State Insane Asylum (figure 213) opened in 1885 on 560 acres of land in Meridian, Mississippi. This was the second asylum established by the state of Mississippi, following advocacy efforts by Dorothea Dix.

This facility was built on the Kirkbride plan with a three-story administration building and two wings. It was designed to house 250 patients, but by 1913, it housed 640 patients. A medical building and patient cottages were added later.

The postcard in figure 214, postmarked 1922, shows a different view of the administration building and side buildings.

The figure 215 shows the "convalescent cottages," added around 1913 for recovering patients or those with less severe cases of mental illness.

Renamed in the 1930s, the East Mississippi State Hospital continues to operate as a mental health facility.

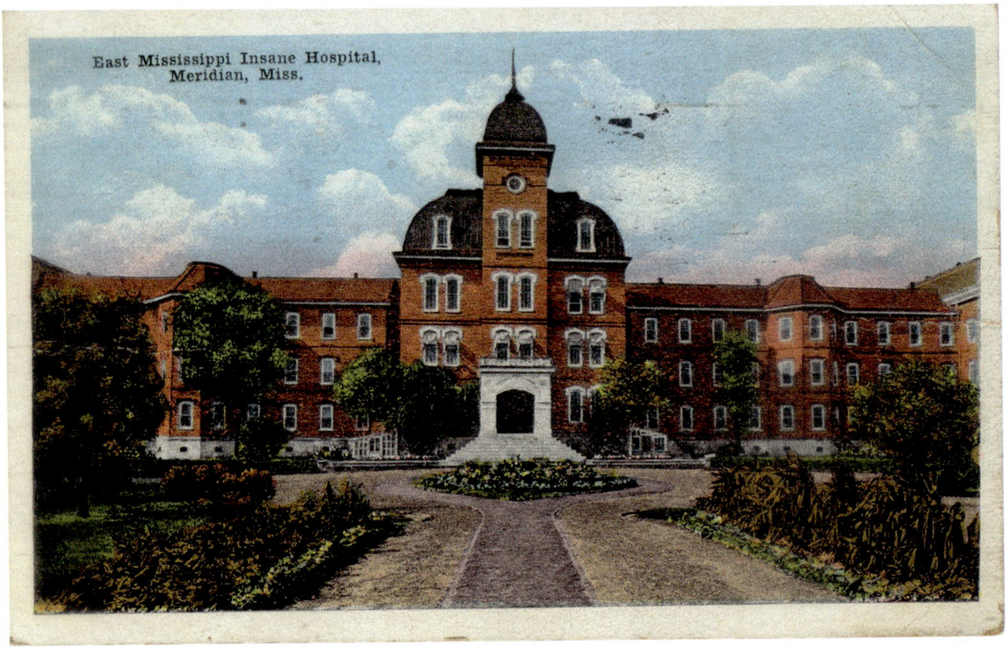
East Mississippi Insane Hospital,
Meridian, Miss.

Figure 214

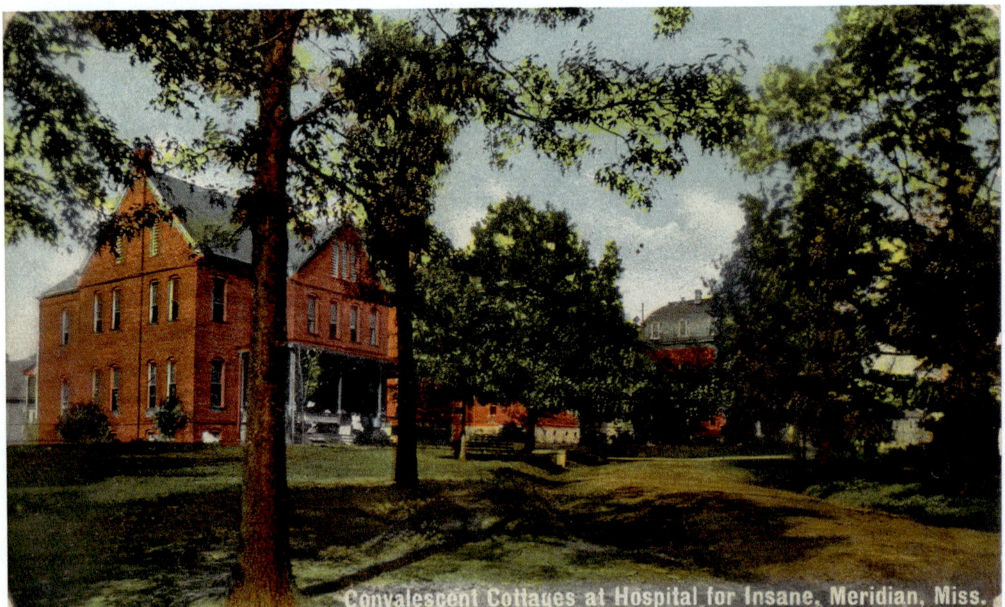
Convalescent Cottages at Hospital for Insane, Meridian, Miss.

Figure 215

Michigan Asylum for Insane Criminals
Ionia, Michigan, 1885

The Michigan Asylum for Insane Criminals, opened in 1885, began as an asylum for housing the criminally insane. The first buildings were physically connected with the state House of Corrections by walls. The asylum originally cared for 81 male patients who were later separated from prisoners and housed in separate facilities.

By 1890, the population had increased to 124 patients and overcrowding had become a problem. Eight acres that overlooked the original buildings were added, along with a cottage for 50 male patients. In the years that followed, several additional buildings were erected at the new location for patient housing and services.

The postcards in figures 216 and 217, postmarked 1912 and 1907 respectively, show the different parts of the facility.

A handwritten comment stated, "This is the north side, they keep me in the south."

The postcard in figure 218 shows another view of the buildings.

The postcard in figure 219, postmarked 1908, shows the superintendent's home.

The Ionia State Hospital closed in the 1970s and the original buildings have been demolished.

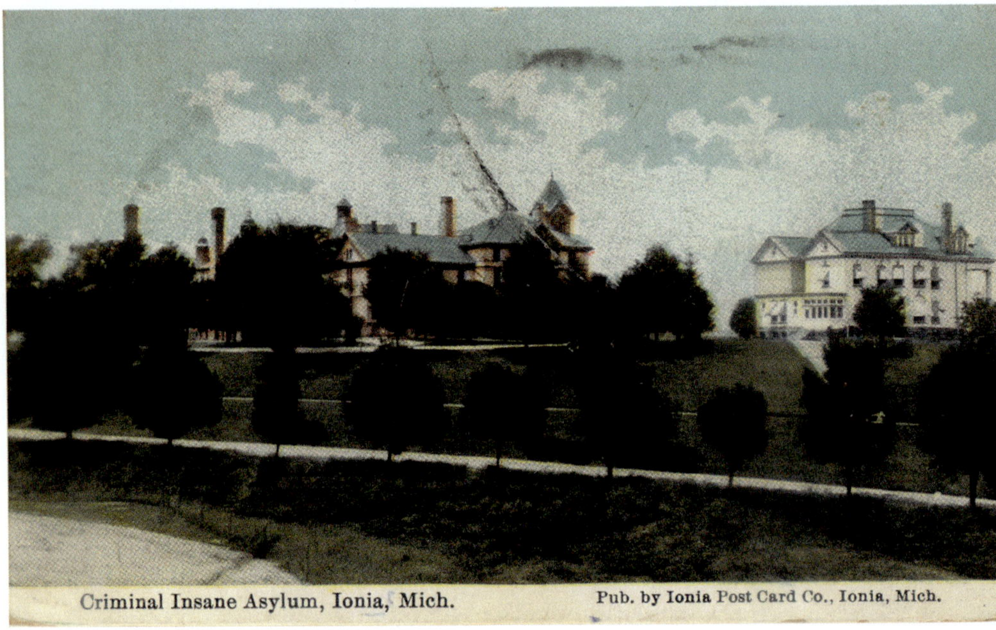
Criminal Insane Asylum, Ionia, Mich.
Pub. by Ionia Post Card Co., Ionia, Mich.

Figure 216

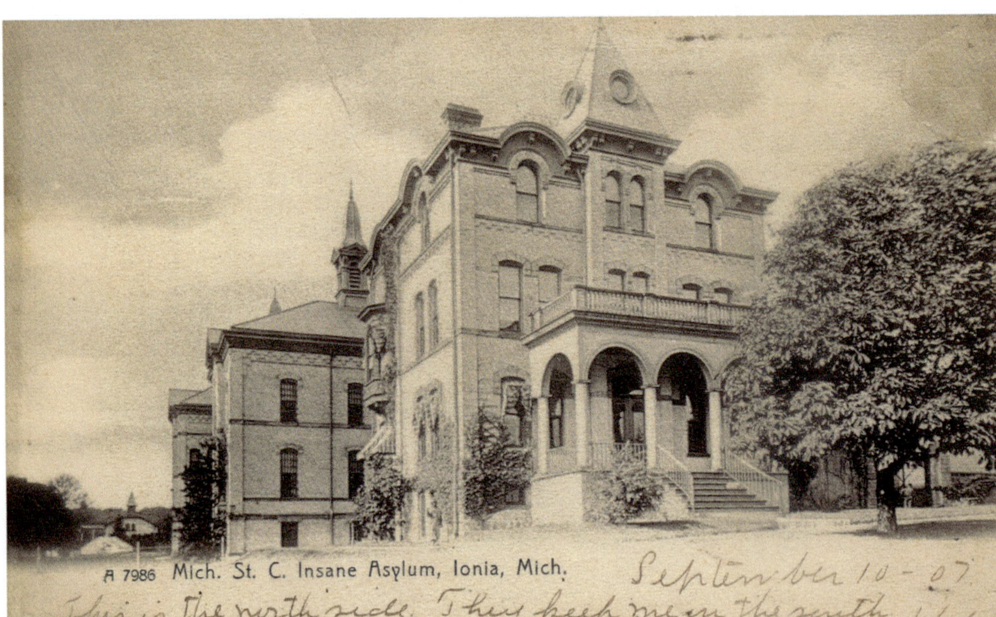
A 7986 Mich. St. C. Insane Asylum, Ionia, Mich.
September 10 - 07
This is the north side. They keep me in the south

Figure 217

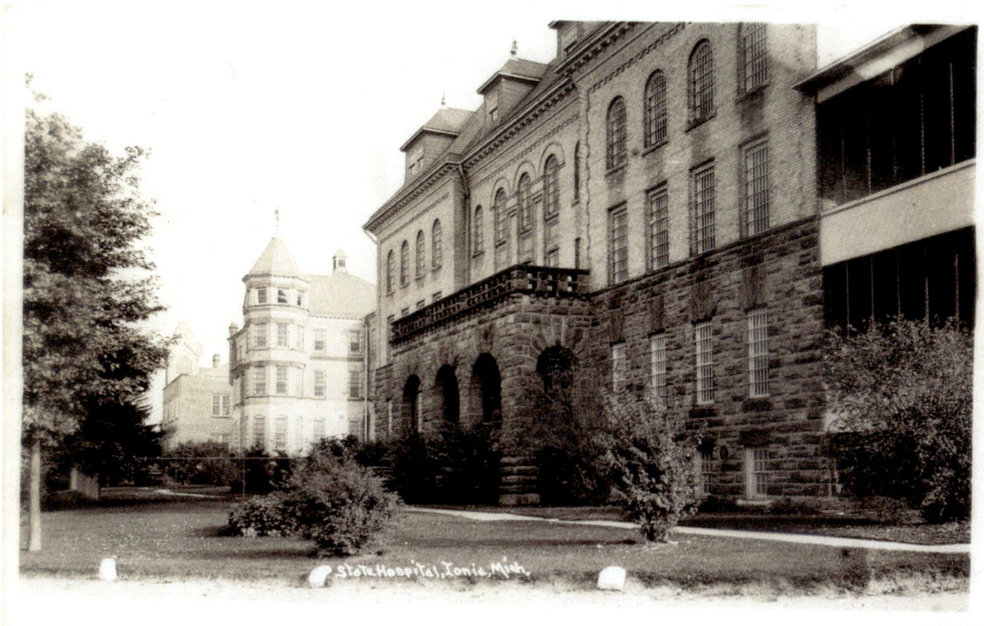
State Hospital, Ionia, Mich.

Figure 218

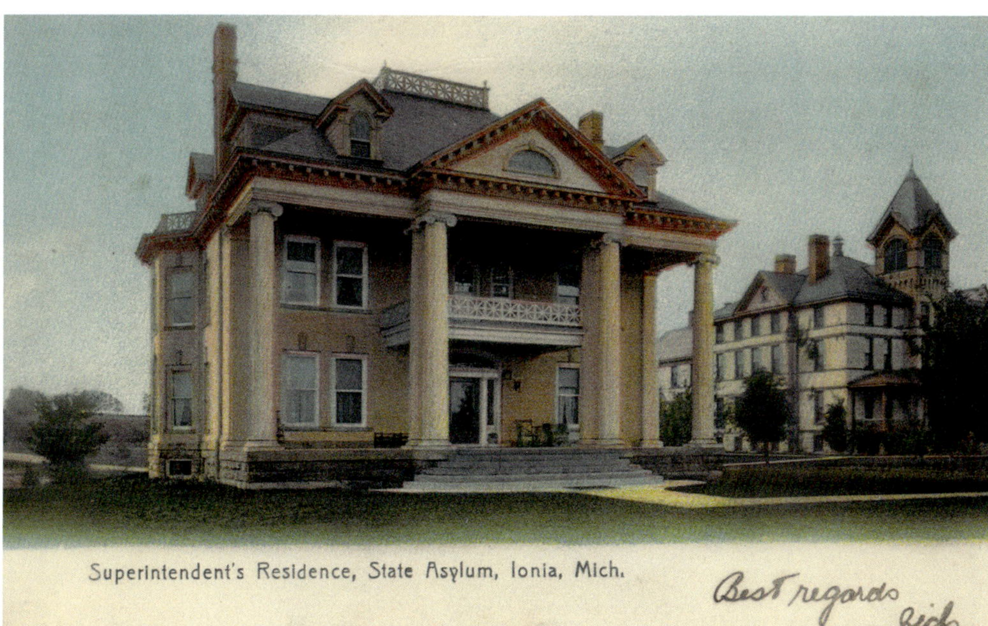
Superintendent's Residence, State Asylum, Ionia, Mich.
Best regards

Figure 219

North Dakota State Hospital for the Insane
Jamestown, North Dakota, 1885

The State Hospital for the Insane, authorized by the Dakota Territorial Legislature, opened in 1885 four miles from Jamestown. The buildings included an administration building, eight ward buildings containing three wards each, a hospital building, an assembly hall, an isolated building for female tuberculosis patients, a dining room, a kitchen, and other service and support buildings. By 1912, the capacity of the hospital was 650 patients but the institution was overcrowded with 797 patients.

Figure 220, postmarked 1908, shows the main building, along with a small greenhouse on the left.

The postcard in figure 221 is postmarked 1914.

A more recent view is provided on a postcard postmarked 1946 (figure 222).

An undated card (figure 223) provides a view of the grounds.

The State Hospital continues to operate in the same location. Many of the original buildings have been demolished, but some have been renovated to serve as part of a correctional facility.

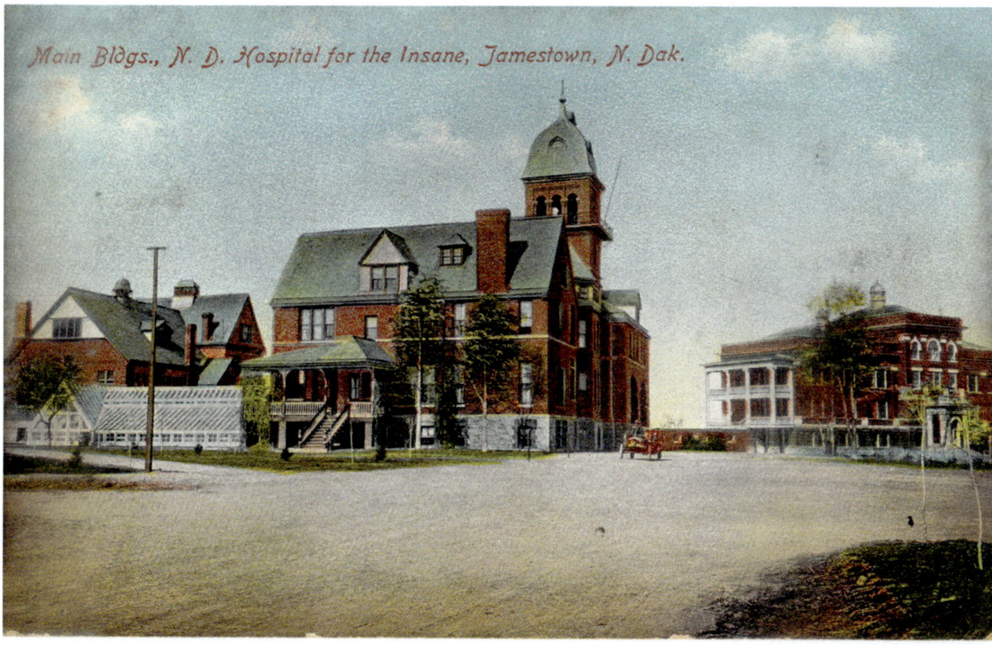

Figure 220

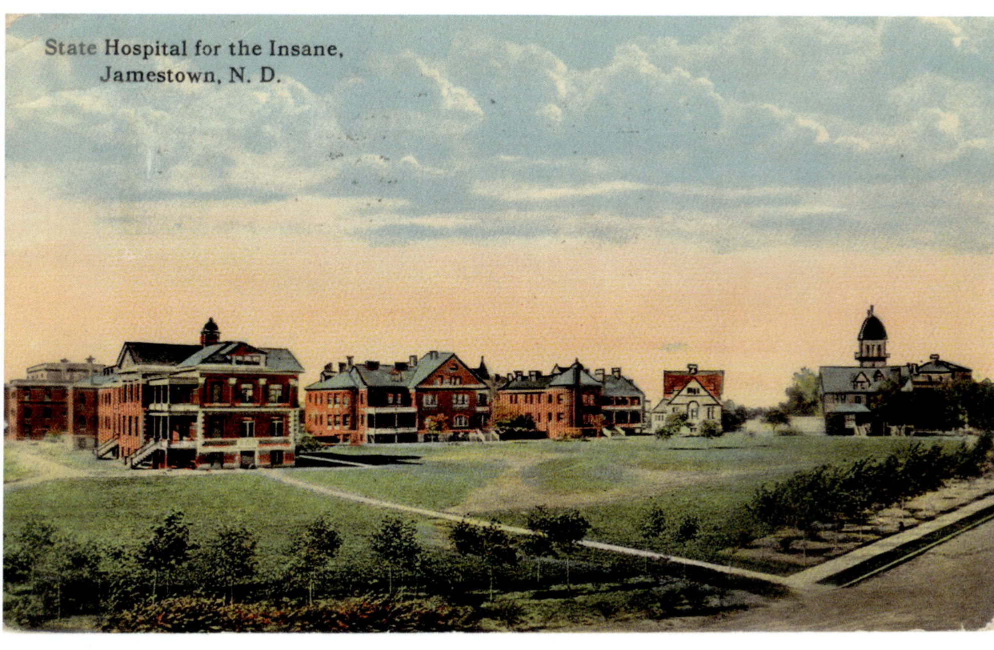

Figure 221

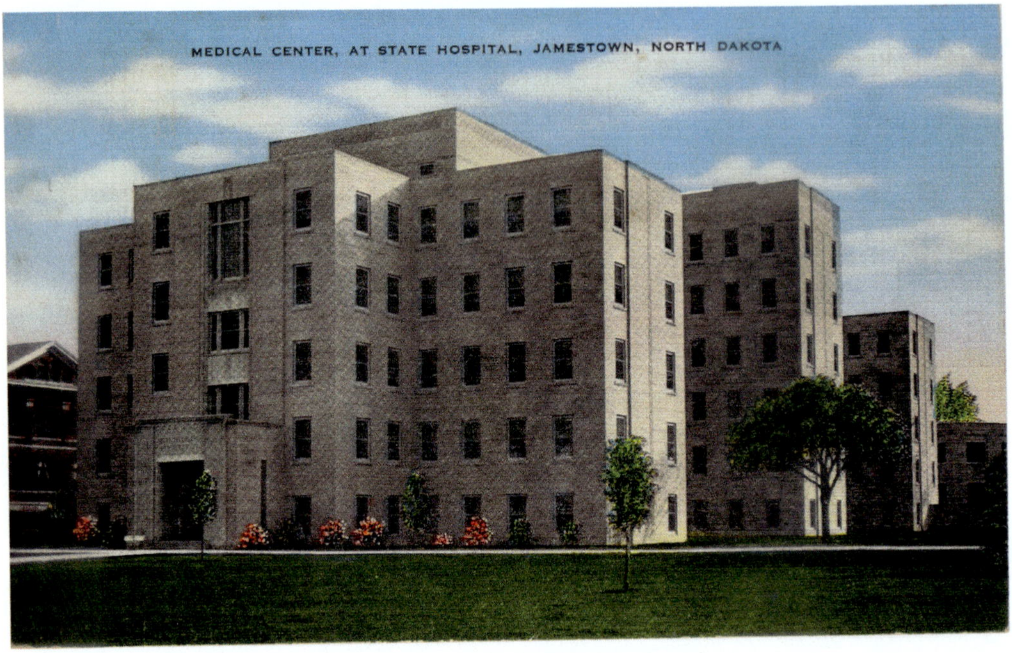
MEDICAL CENTER, AT STATE HOSPITAL, JAMESTOWN, NORTH DAKOTA

Figure 222

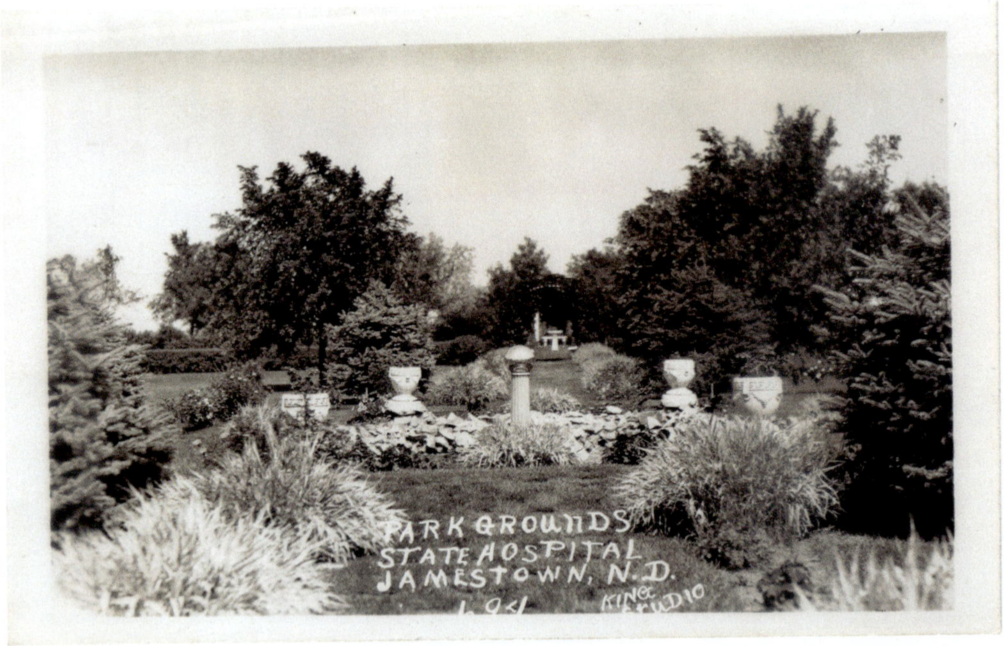
PARK GROUNDS
STATE HOSPITAL
JAMESTOWN, N.D.
KING STUDIO

Figure 223

North Texas Lunatic Asylum
Terrell, Texas, 1885

Originally named the North Texas Lunatic Asylum, this hospital was the second mental health facility in Texas. The original facility consisted of one building that housed 400 patients. By 1891, the wings were completed, increasing the capacity to 800. By 1914, the hospital had 1,912 patients.

This 1907 postcard (figure 224) shows the administrative building. The handwritten message reads, "Was dismissed a few days ago and trying to find the way home, expect to succeed Saturday, everything looks, makes a noise like water down here."

Like other state hospitals, Terrell had a band (figure 225) comprised of staff and patients that provided music for the patients.

The Terrell State Hospital (figure 226) continues to operate as a psychiatric inpatient facility. All of the original buildings have been demolished. A fountain from the original facility has been restored and remains on the grounds.

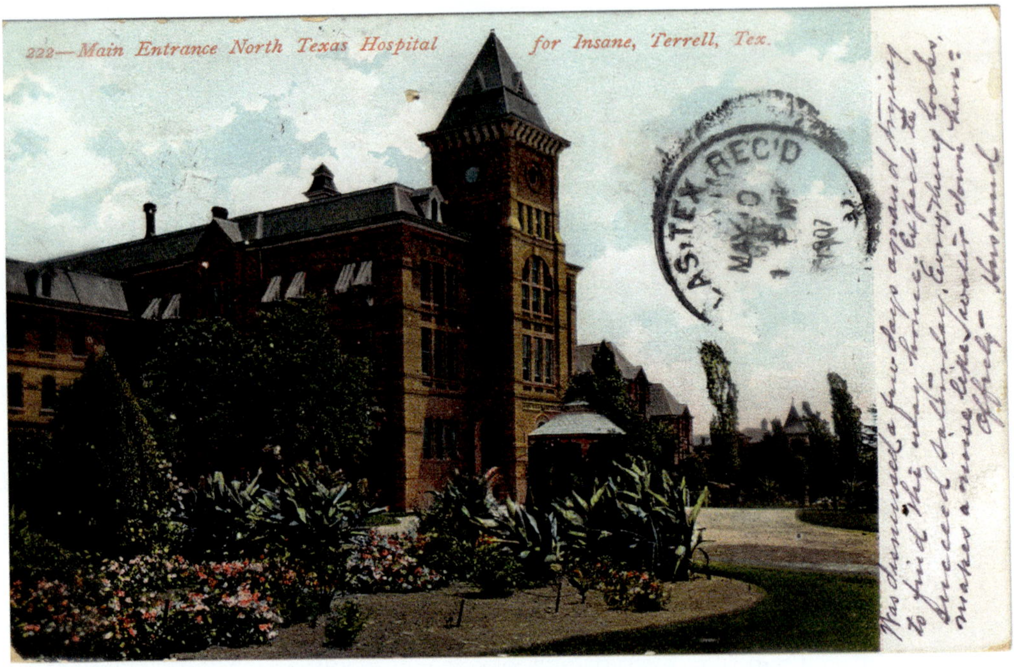
222—Main Entrance North Texas Hospital for Insane, Terrell, Tex.

Figure 224

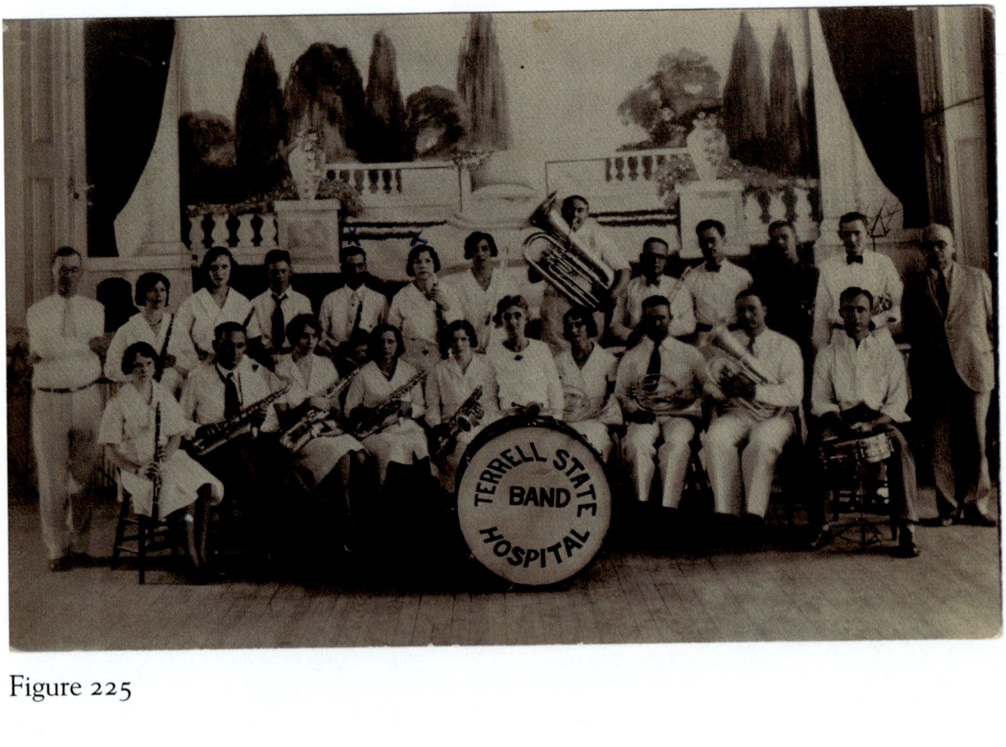
TERRELL STATE
BAND
HOSPITAL

Figure 225

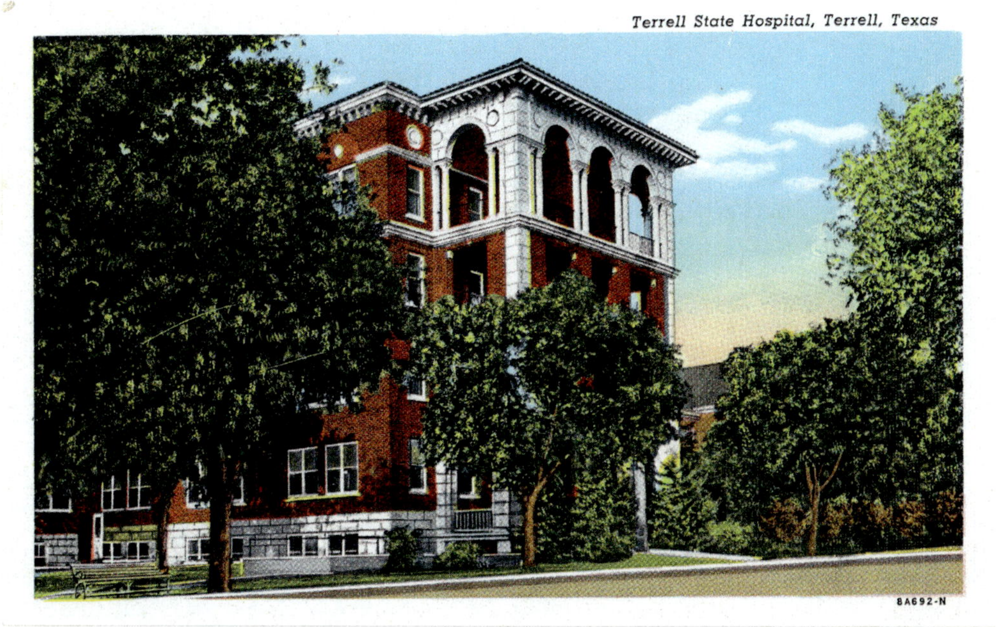
Terrell State Hospital, Terrell, Texas
8A692-N

Figure 226

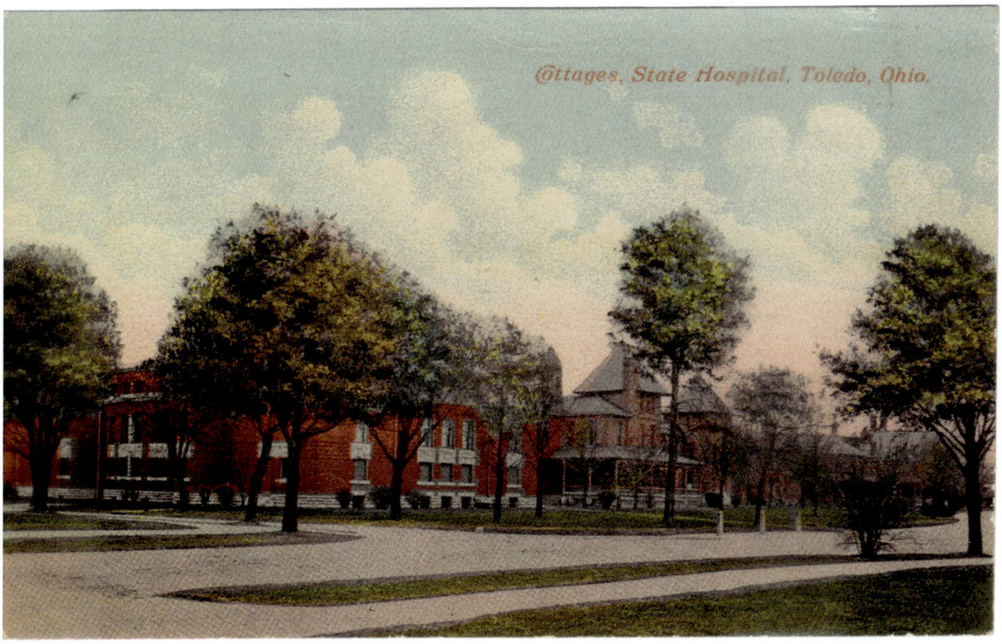
Cottages, State Hospital, Toledo, Ohio.

Figure 227

Toledo Asylum for the Insane
Toledo, Ohio, 1888

The Toledo Asylum for the Insane opened in 1888. This was the fifth state hospital built in Ohio. The building plans followed the cottage system, with detached buildings in the form of a parallelogram. The cottages could accommodate a total of 1,000 patients and, with the additional wards, the facility could house a total of 1,800 patients. Toledo's use of the cottage plan demonstrated the utility of the design and some suggested that it demonstrated the possibility of doing away with patient restraints.

The postcard in figure 227 was not sent through the mail, but the owner described the scene in figure 228.

The postcard in figure 229, postmarked 1907, shows the amusement hall used for recreational activities for patients.

Figure 230 shows the grounds at the Toledo State Hospital. About 160 additional acres were purchased and a farm and gardens were added in 1910.

The name has been changed to the Northwest Ohio Psychiatric Hospital, which provides psychiatric care in Toledo. All of the original buildings from the asylum have been destroyed.

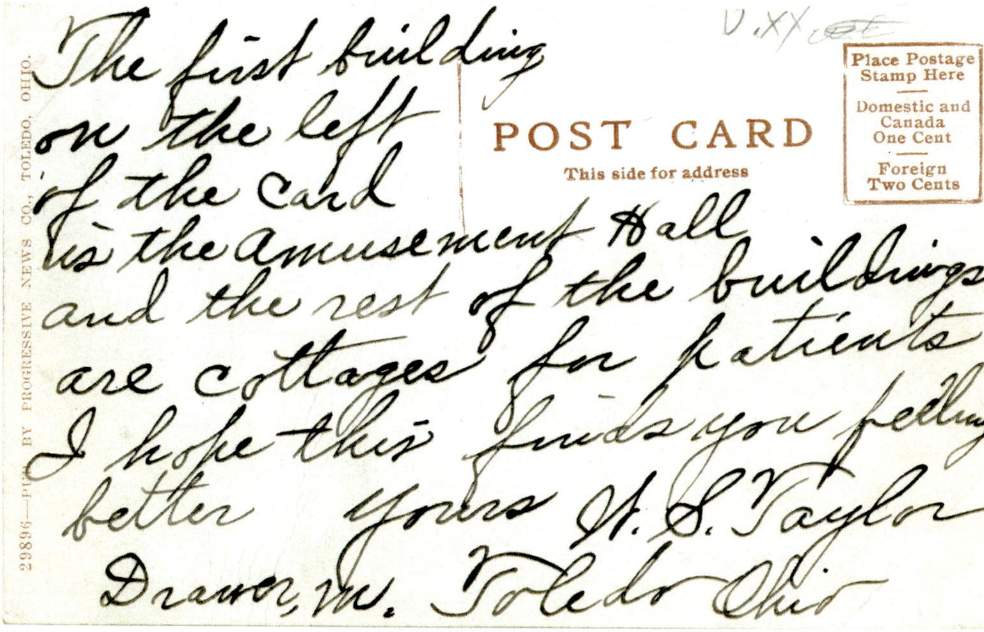

Figure 228

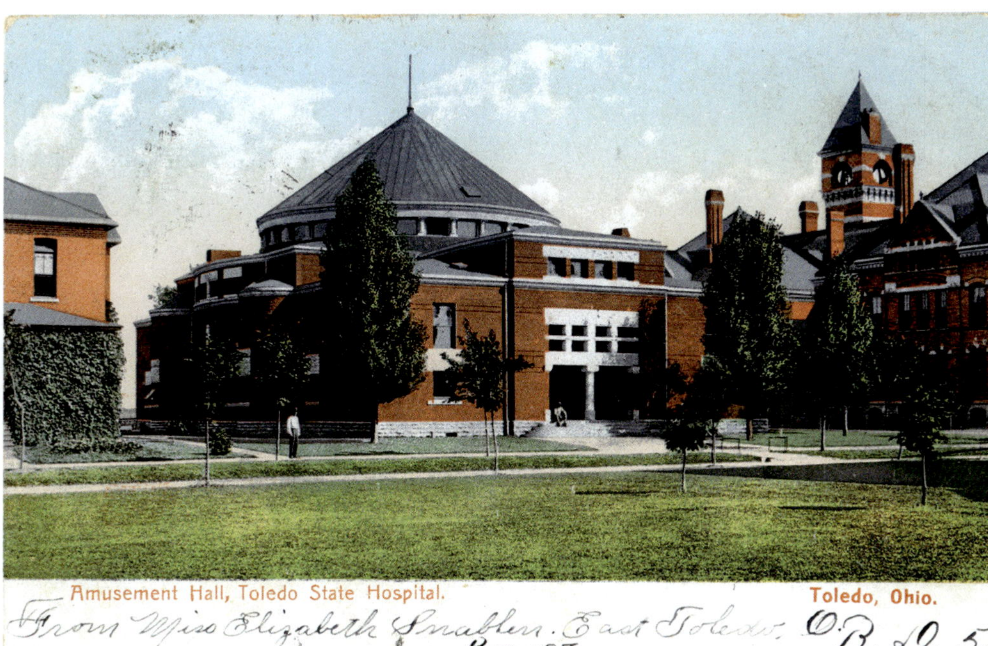
Amusement Hall, Toledo State Hospital.
Toledo, Ohio.
From Miss Elizabeth Snabley. East Toledo. O. R. D. 5.
Box 138.

Figure 229

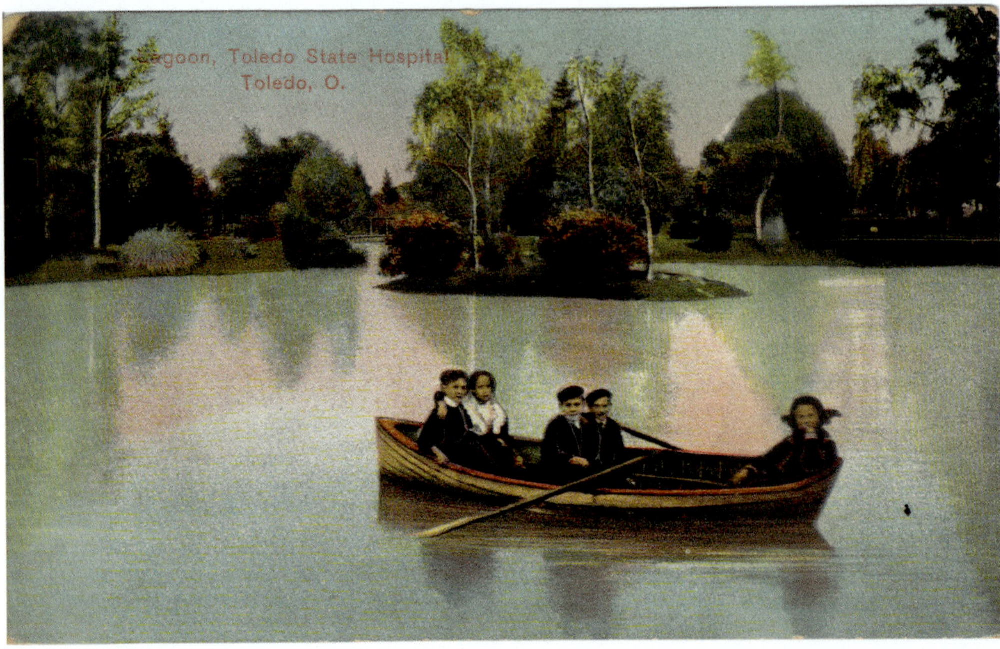
Toledo State Hospital
Toledo, O.

Figure 230

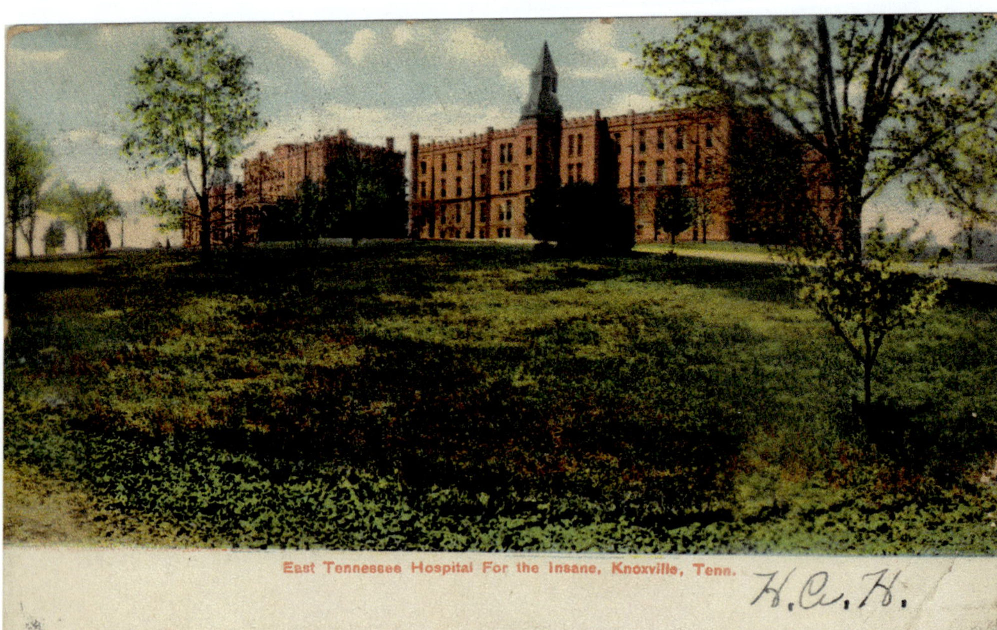
East Tennessee Hospital For the Insane, Knoxville, Tenn.
H.C.H.

Figure 231

East Tennessee Asylum for the Insane
Knoxville, Tennessee, 1886

Originally named the East Tennessee Asylum for the Insane, this facility was established on 305 acres of land on the Tennessee River about five miles from Knoxville. It was located within one mile of a railroad and had a large spring that could provide water for 1,000 patients. The institution was constructed on the Kirkbride plan with a capacity for 250 patients.

In 1895, a detached building was erected for black patients and two years later a building was erected for female patients. The original building was extended to double its original capacity increasing the census to 630 patients in care.

The postcard in figure 231 was postmarked 1907. The postcard of this facility in figure 232 is postmarked 1911. The postcard in figure 233 is postmarked 1913.

The hospital, renamed the Lakeshore Mental Health Institute in 1977, closed in 2012. Most of the original buildings have been demolished, but the central administration building has survived.

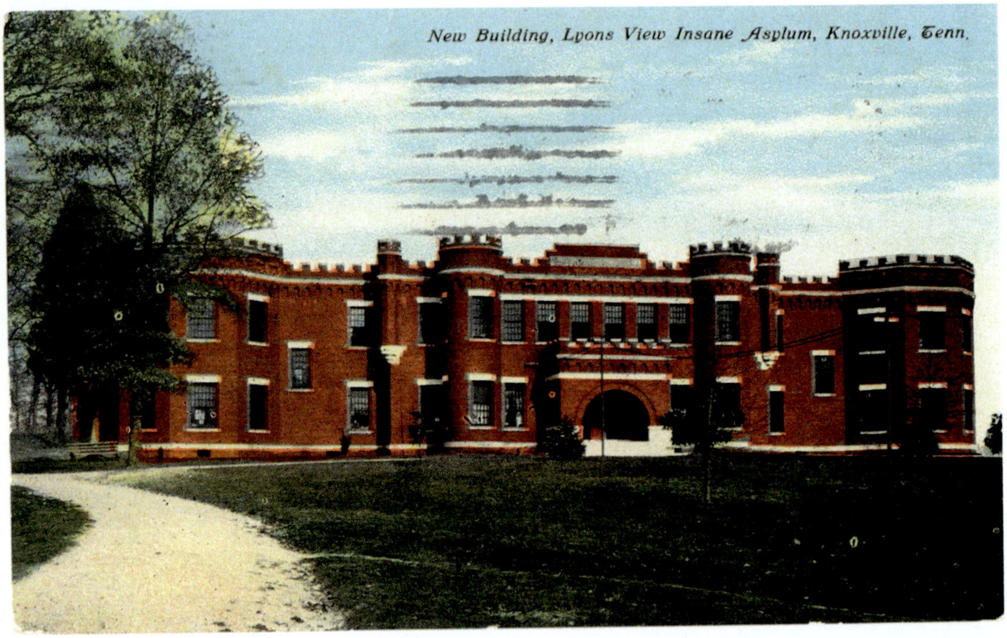
New Building, Lyons View Insane Asylum, Knoxville, Tenn.

Figure 232

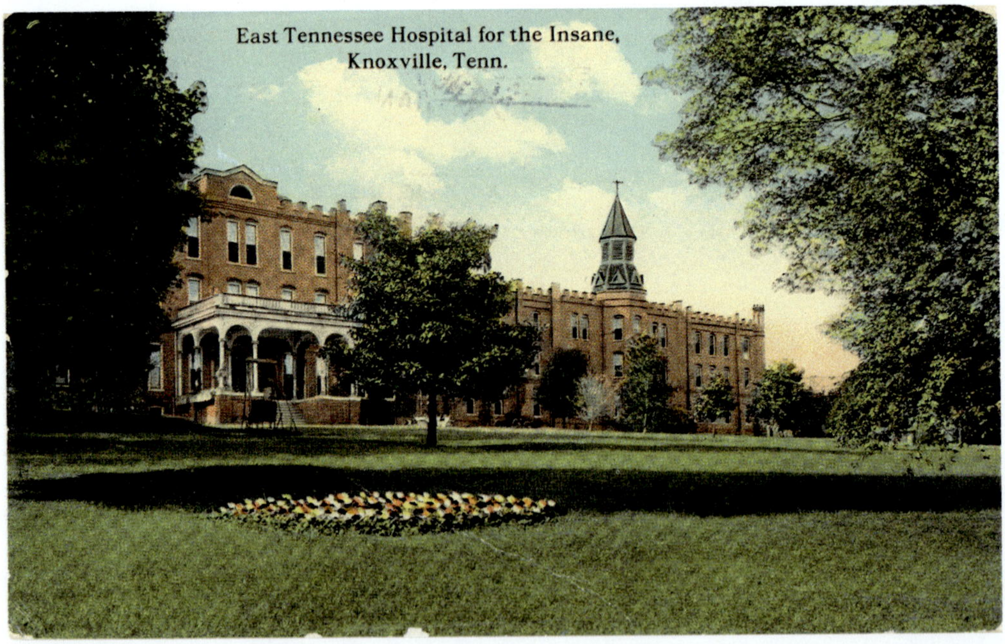
East Tennessee Hospital for the Insane,
Knoxville, Tenn.

Figure 233

Idaho Insane Asylum
South Blackfoot, Idaho, 1886

Originally named the Idaho Insane Asylum (figure 234), this hospital was established about one mile east of the village of Blackfoot. The asylum consisted of a three-story building and 73 acres of land.

In 1889, a fire completely destroyed the main buildings, resulting in at least two patient deaths and an additional five patients were never found. Patients were able to move into a new building that was nearly completed at the time. Several service and housing buildings were added slowly over the years and all future buildings were fireproofed.

Now known as State Hospital South, this facility continues to provide acute and long-term care for the mentally ill in Idaho.

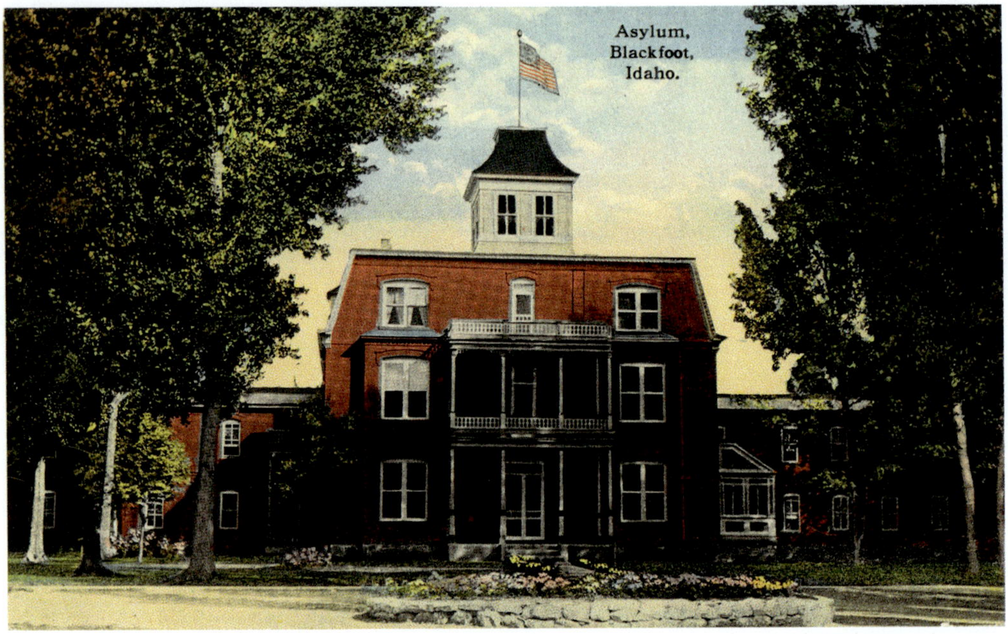
Asylum,
Blackfoot,
Idaho.

Figure 234

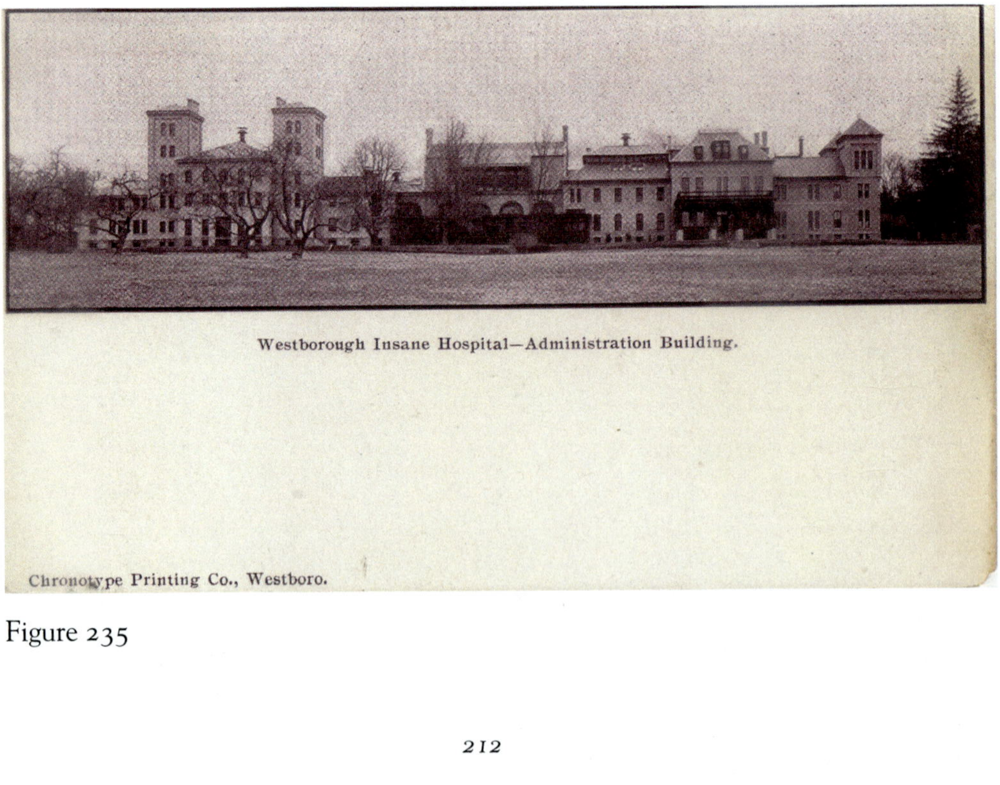
Westborough Insane Hospital—Administration Building.
Chronotype Printing Co., Westboro.

Figure 235

Westborough Insane Hospital
Westborough, Massachusetts, 1886

The Westborough Insane Hospital (figure 235) opened in 1886, using buildings and land previously occupied by the Massachusetts State Reform School for Boys. The hospital relied on homeopathic treatment, which involved rest, a special diet, massage, and hydrotherapy. The original reformatory building was remodeled to add a congregate dining room, a chapel, and patient wards.

In 1892, the hospital established its first satellite colony. A nearby farm, Stanley Farm, was purchased for $8,000. It included a farmhouse and a large barn (figure 236) that was used to store hay and corn. Other farm colonies were established in the early 1900s to house patients. By 1914, the hospital (figure 237) encompassed 768 acres of land with 60 buildings housing 1,213 patients.

Westborough State Hospital closed in 2010 and the site was purchased by the town of Westborough in 2014. Options for reuse of the site are being explored.

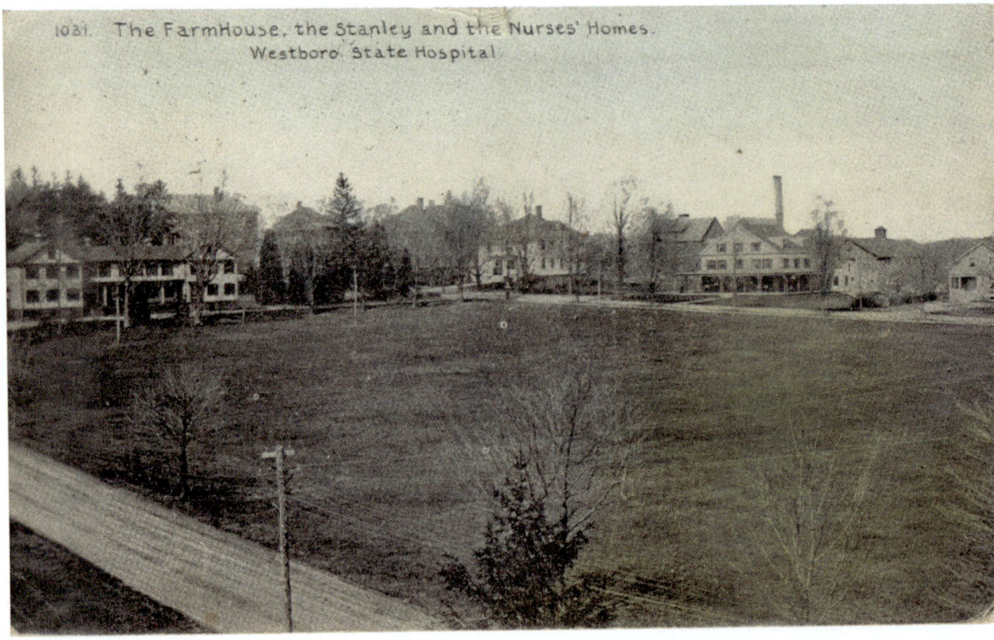
1031. The FarmHouse, the Stanley and the Nurses' Homes.
Westboro State Hospital

Figure 236

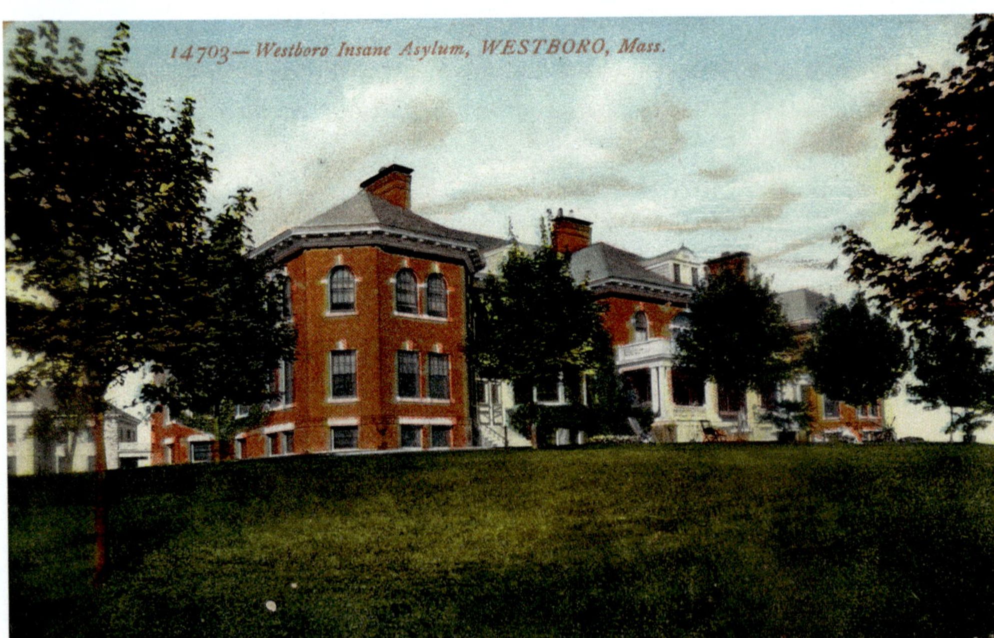
14703—Westboro Insane Asylum, WESTBORO, Mass.

Figure 237

Southwestern Lunatic Asylum
Marion, Virginia, 1887

Prior to the establishment of this facility, Virginia asylums, including those located at Williamsburg and Staunton, were crowded and the mentally ill were often housed in jails and almshouses. A new asylum, originally called the Southwestern Lunatic Asylum, was therefore opened in 1887. The facility had accommodations for 280 patients.

The central building of the hospital (figure 238) included six wards extending to the rear, three for male patients and three for female patients. A seventh ward was located on the upper floor of the central building. Physicians lived in the central building and attendants and nurses lived on the upper floors of the wards.

In 1902, the asylum was renamed Southwestern State Hospital (figure 239) and there were more than 440 patients living there. In 1910, two departments were added to care specifically for the "criminally insane," with Southwestern State Hospital caring for white patients while Central State Hospital in Petersburg, Virginia cared for black patients. The facility continued to grow, until by 1935, the hospital census reached 1,140.

In 1986, the original buildings were demolished and replaced with the Southwestern Virginia Mental Health Institute, which still operates today.

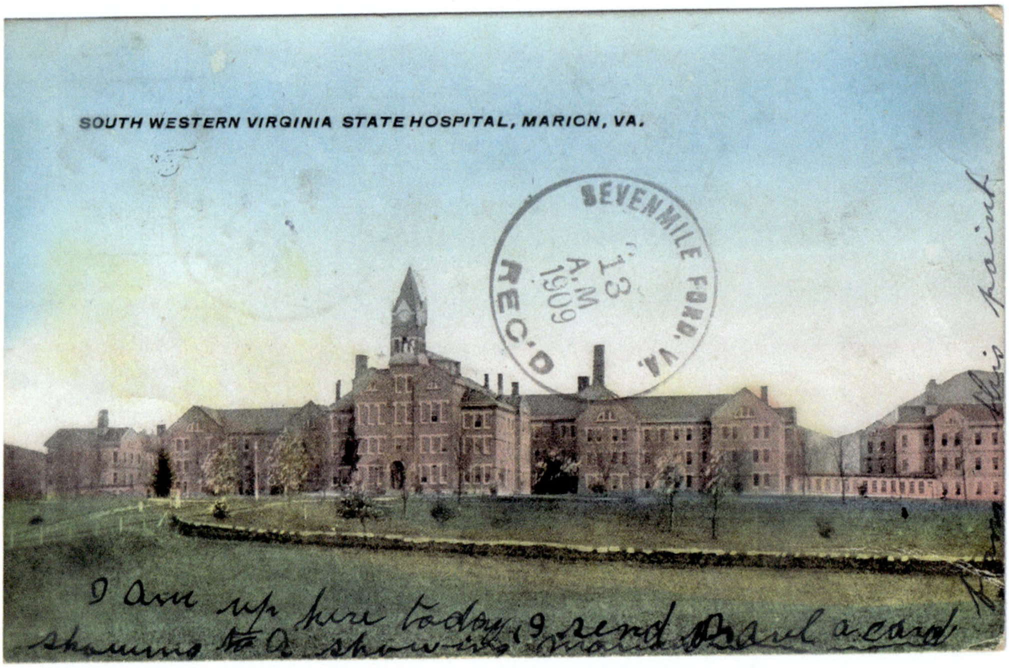

Figure 238

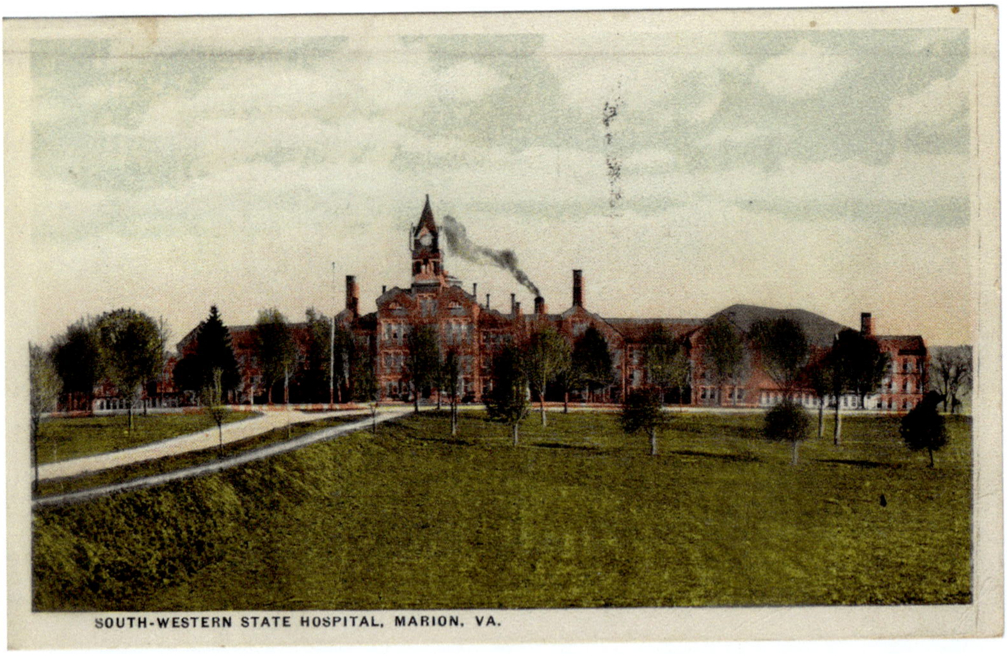

Figure 239

Lunatic Asylum No. 3
Nevada, Missouri, 1889

The crowded conditions of the other two state hospitals in Missouri made it necessary to open a third facility, originally called Lunatic Asylum No. 3, near the city of Nevada. Nevada was seen as an optimal location, due to its proximity to the Ozark Mountains; the altitude and pure air were considered an advantage for patient treatment and recovery. Within two years of opening, the hospital was home to 281 patients and 30 staff members.

The original building had two wings, a chapel, an electric light plant, a carpenter shop, storage rooms and shops, a training school for nurses and attendants, two buildings for tuberculosis patients, and a laundry house. The postcard in figure 240 was postmarked 1911.

An additional postcard (figure 241) appears to be from around the same time period.

By 1912, the total number of patients under treatment reached 1,791. Reports from the hospital indicate that 216 patients had died while 333 had been discharged as restored, improved, or stable.

State Hospital No. 3 closed in 1991 and the original Kirkbride building was demolished in 1999.

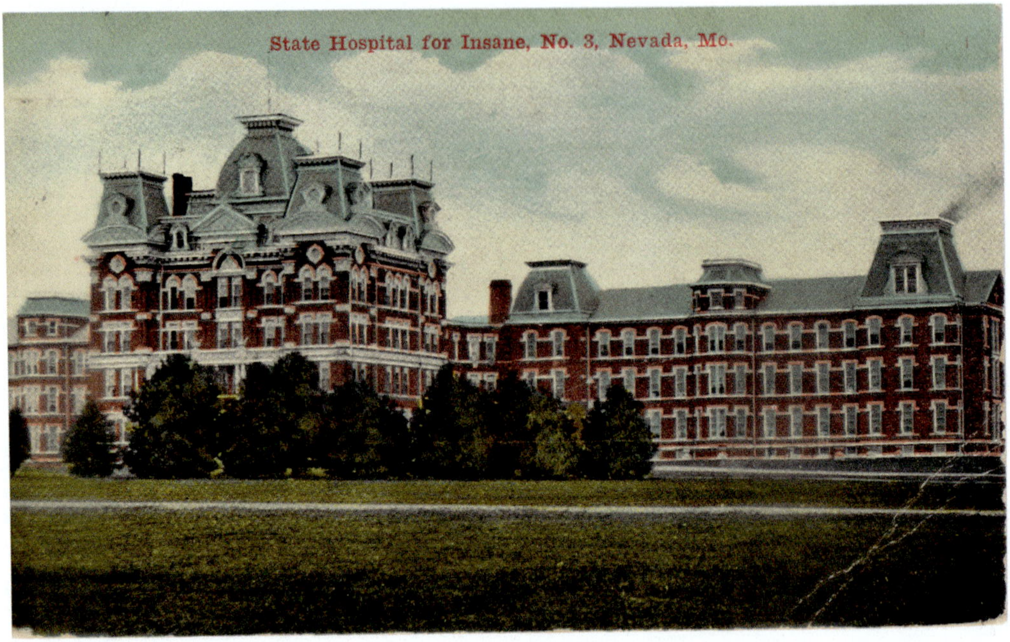

Figure 240

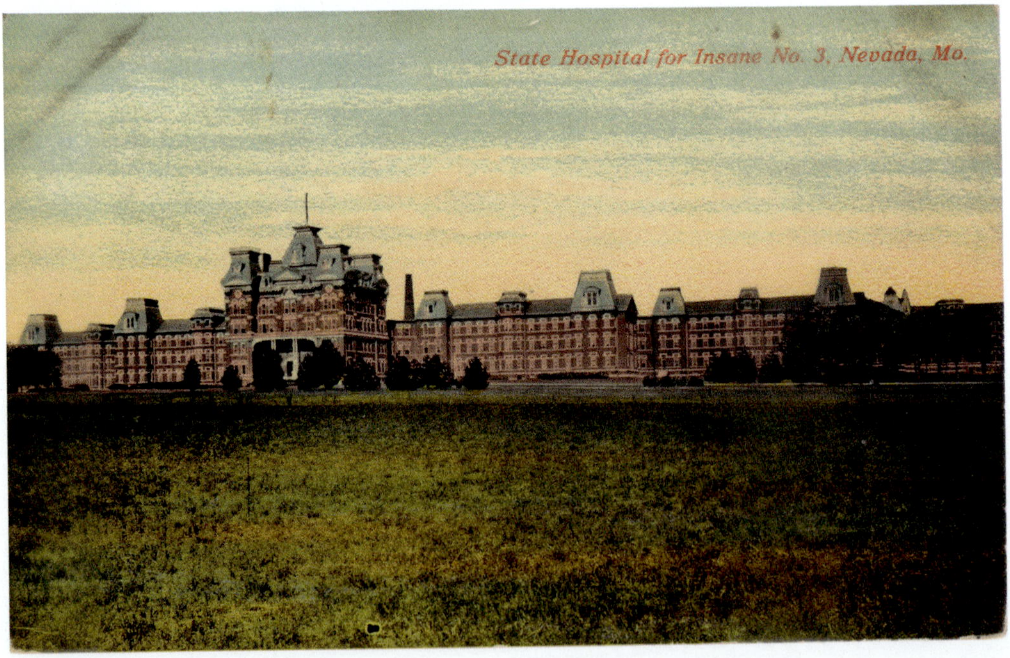

Figure 241

Territorial Insane Asylum
Phoenix, Arizona, 1887

The Territorial Insane Asylum opened in 1887. Prior to its opening, Arizona citizens suffering from mental illness were taken to a private asylum in Stockton, California. After this facility was opened for admission, 61 patients were transferred from the California facility.

The hospital, located less than 3 miles from Phoenix, included a central administration building, two patient wings, and 160 acres of land for cultivation.

The postcards in figures 242 and 243, postmarked 1907 and 1908, show the grounds and main building.

The original buildings were destroyed by a fire in 1911. After the facility was rebuilt in 1913, it was renamed the State Asylum for the Insane. By 1914, 442 patients were being treated.

This facility continues to operate as a State Hospital in Phoenix, Arizona. Only one of the original buildings, from when it was rebuilt in 1913, remains on the grounds.

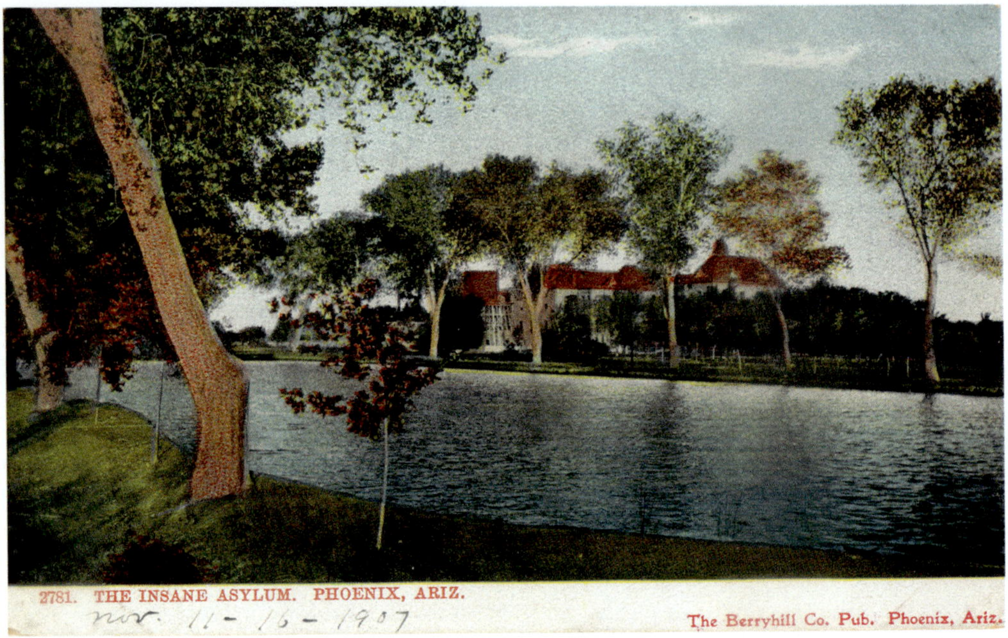

Figure 242

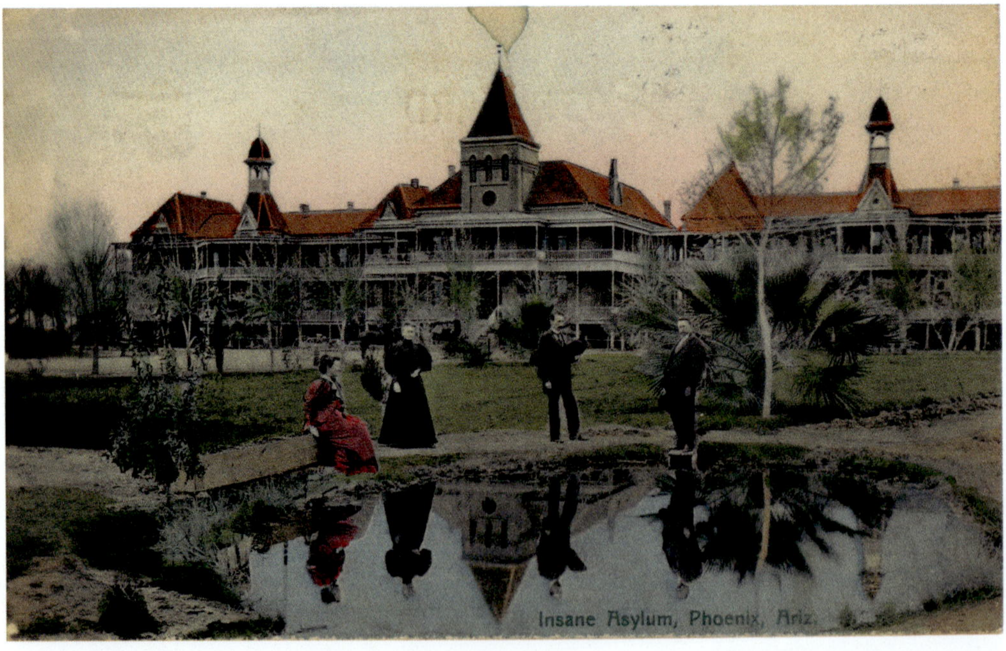

Figure 243

Northern Indiana Hospital for the Insane
Logansport, Indiana, 1888

The Northern Indiana Hospital for the Insane was the second facility for mental health care in the state. It consisted of an administration building, four wards for males and four for females, a rear center building, boiler house, and laundry. It was situated on the south bank of the Wabash River on a farm of 281 acres with picturesque views of the river. At the end of the first year, all beds were occupied and additional accommodations were being requested.

By 1899, two annexes and two additional buildings were built, providing space for nearly 300 more patients. By 1912, the capacity had reached 950, with 865 patients in residence.

The handwritten note in figure 244, dated 1906, reads, "Dear Nellie. Will write tomorrow. One of the homes for the insane. With love."

The postcard in figure 245, postmarked 1914, shows the facility in color. The entrance to the property appears in figure 246.

Loganspor State Hospital continues to operate as a psychiatric facility. Some of the original buildings still stand, including the administration building which houses a museum devoted to the history of the facility.

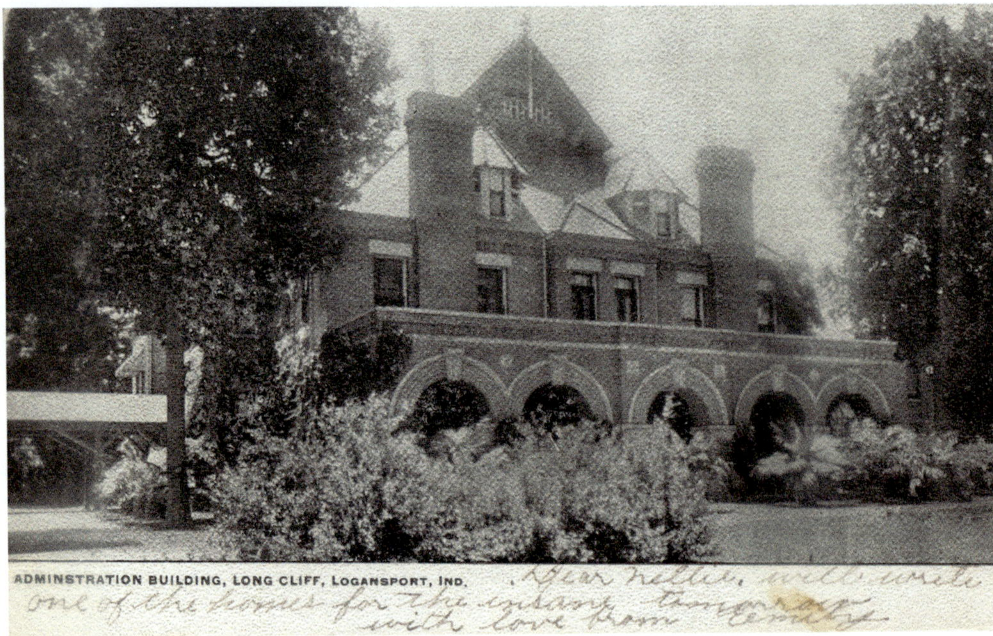

Figure 244

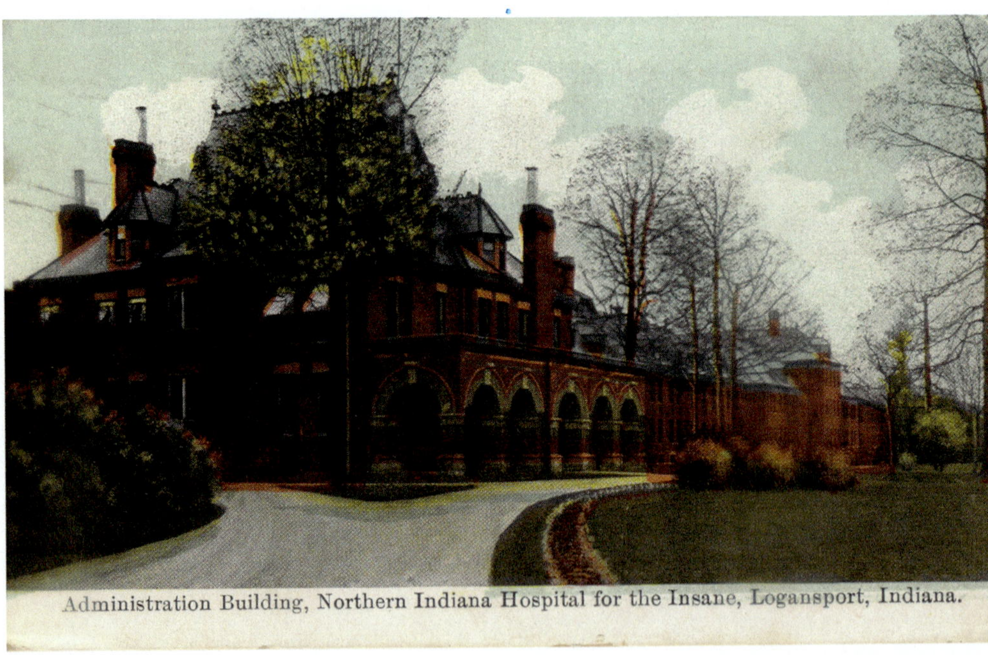

Figure 245

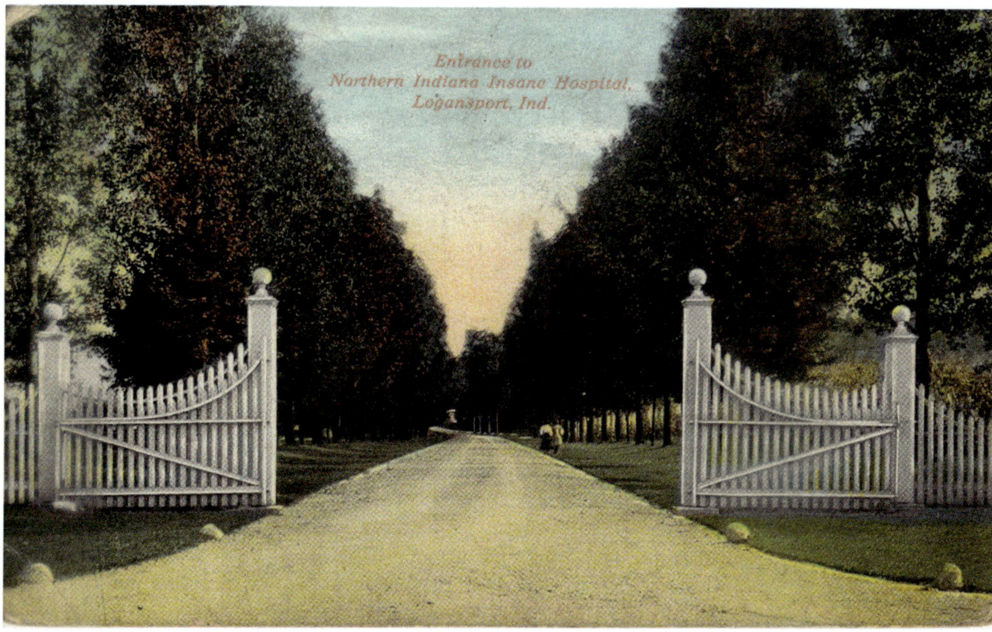

Figure 246

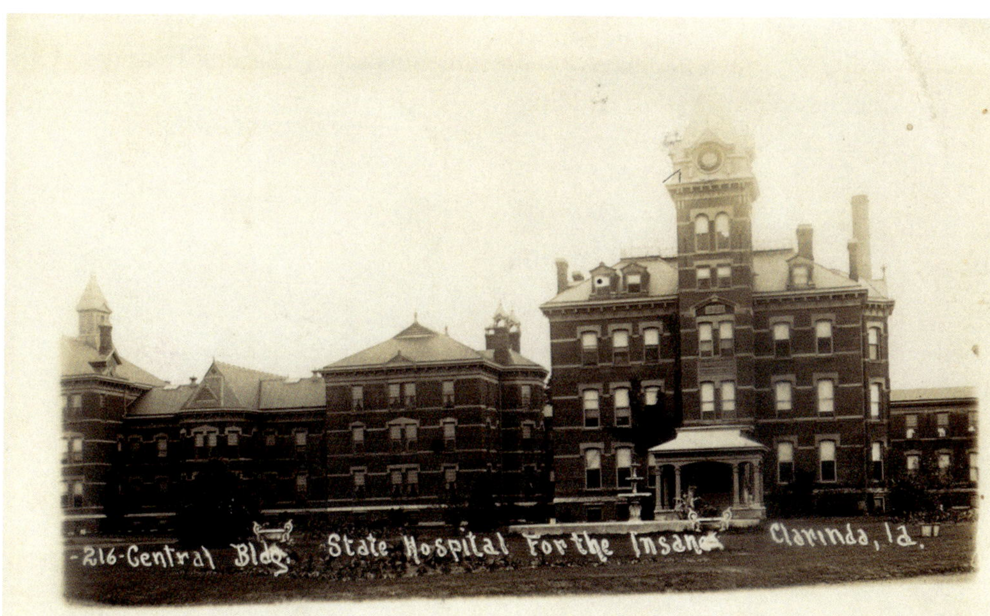

Figure 247

Iowa State Hospital for the Insane
Clarinda, Iowa, 1888

The Iowa State Hospital for the Insane in Clarinda opened in 1888 to care for the mentally ill in the southwest region of Iowa. The administration building and one wing were erected first, with additional buildings completed by 1897.

The picture in figure 247, postmarked 1913, shows the administration building which was four stories high with three-story wings. The buildings, implementing a modern Gothic design, were constructed of brick and stone with steep slated roofs.

The card in figure 248, postmarked 1907, provides an interior view.

The next card (figure 249), postmarked 1910, shows the interior of the amusement building, which was used for chapel services, theatrical performances, dances, and other activities.

This facility continues to operate on the same site as the Clarinda Treatment Center. The original administration building is still in use.

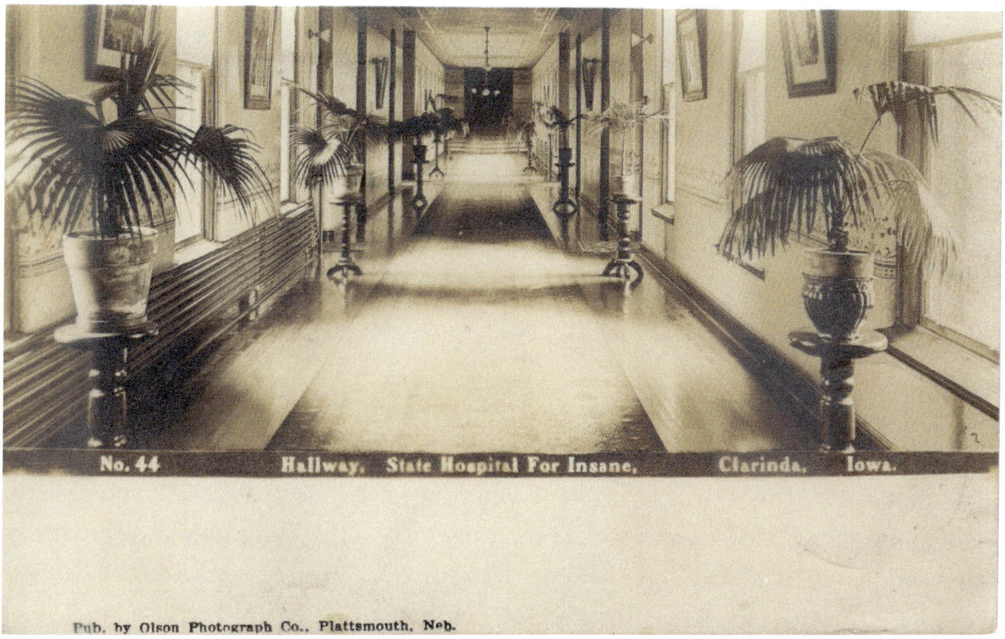
No. 44 Hallway, State Hospital For Insane, Clarinda, Iowa.
Pub. by Olson Photograph Co., Plattsmouth, Neb.

Figure 248

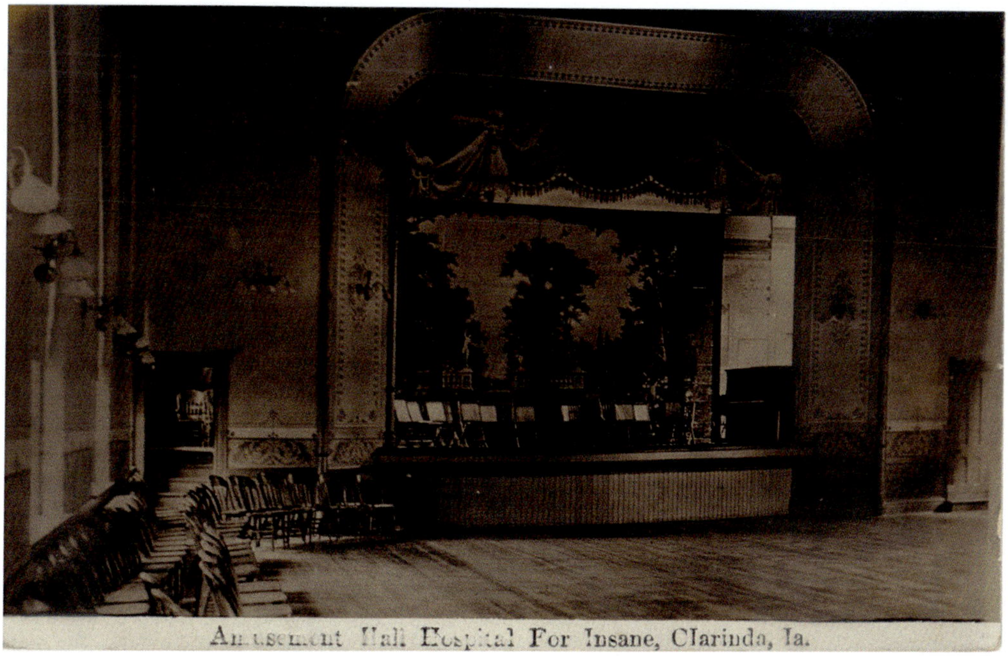
Amusement Hall Hospital For Insane, Clarinda, Ia.

Figure 249

California Hospital for the Chronically Insane
Agnews, California, 1888

This facility was opened to care for California citizens suffering chronic mental illness. It was located in the Santa Clara Valley partially because the area provided an abundant source of water. Prior to the California earthquake in 1906, 1,108 patients were in residence. More than 100 lost their lives when the building was destroyed by the earthquake. In addition, 99 patients were then transferred to Stockton. No new cases were admitted to the facility and the number of patients was reduced to 758 by 1909. After the earthquake, temporary quarters were used to house patients and the management began planning a new facility.

The new construction consisted of a modern cottage system, with patients being housed according to their diagnoses and degree of illness. Concrete one- and two-story buildings were erected, with the hope that such structures were better suited to an earthquake-prone area. A new hospital building was added with receiving wards and two infirmaries.

In 1926, a new site—which came to be known as the East Campus—was purchased just 1.5 miles from the original campus. In 1985, this became known as the Agnews Developmental Center and in 1996, the original West Campus was closed. In 2013, the Agnews Developmental Center also closed.

No postcards of this facility exist in the author's collection.

Insane Asylum
Norfolk, Nebraska, 1888

Founded as the Insane Asylum in Norfolk in 1885 and opened in 1888, this facility was established to care for patients in the northern part of Nebraska. Originally, the facility included an administration building and eight adjacent buildings. These were almost completely destroyed by fire in 1901. The facility was then rebuilt on the cottage plan. By 1910, the facility housed just over 300 patients.

While the postcard in figure 250 was undated, the back of the card is divided, which suggests that it dates from the period between 1907 and 1915. It shows the facility that was built after the 1901 fire.

Some of the buildings erected after the fire still stand, but are in a state of disrepair. The facility now operates as the Norfolk Regional Center.

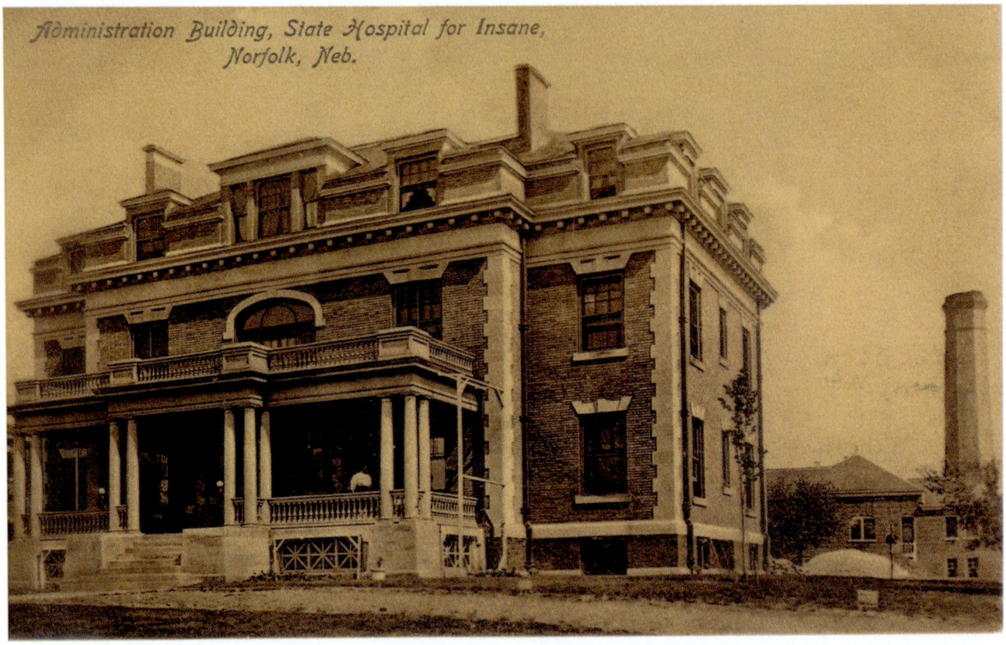
Administration Building, State Hospital for Insane,
Norfolk, Neb.

Figure 250

Department for Insane, Anamosa Penitentiary
Anamosa, Iowa, 1888

Anamosa Penitentiary was established in 1872, and in 1888 it added a department for the "criminal insane." Convicts with mental illnesses were housed separately from the other prison inmates, but the residents were governed by the prison warden along with the other convicts. Once their sentences were complete, those prisoners still considered suffering from mental illness were transferred to a state hospital. The three-story building contained small cells lining the outer north and south walls. A yard attached to the building was used for recreation and mandatory exercise. Due to cost constraints, patients were cared for by a regular physician who had no special training in caring for the mentally ill; because of this, the care was primarily custodial. One year after opening, the insane ward housed 32 inmates.

No postcards of this facility have been found. The facility continues to operate as a penitentiary.

West Tennessee Hospital for the Insane
Bolivar, Tennessee, 1889

This facility, later renamed the Western State Hospital, opened in 1889, taking 156 patients from another Tennessee asylum. The asylum, built to accommodate 300 patients, sat on a tract near a large lake. By 1892, the hospital census reached 319.

This hospital was built on the Kirkbride plan with an administration building and wings on each side, divided into six wards each. Each ward had a dining room and later additions included a ward for working patients, another for epileptic patients, a receiving ward, and a ward housing the infirmary and patients in the process of recovery.

The postcard in figure 251, postmarked 1909, provides a view of the hospital.

This facility continues to exist as the Western Mental Health Institute. The original administration building still stands and is in use, but the wings were removed in 1980.

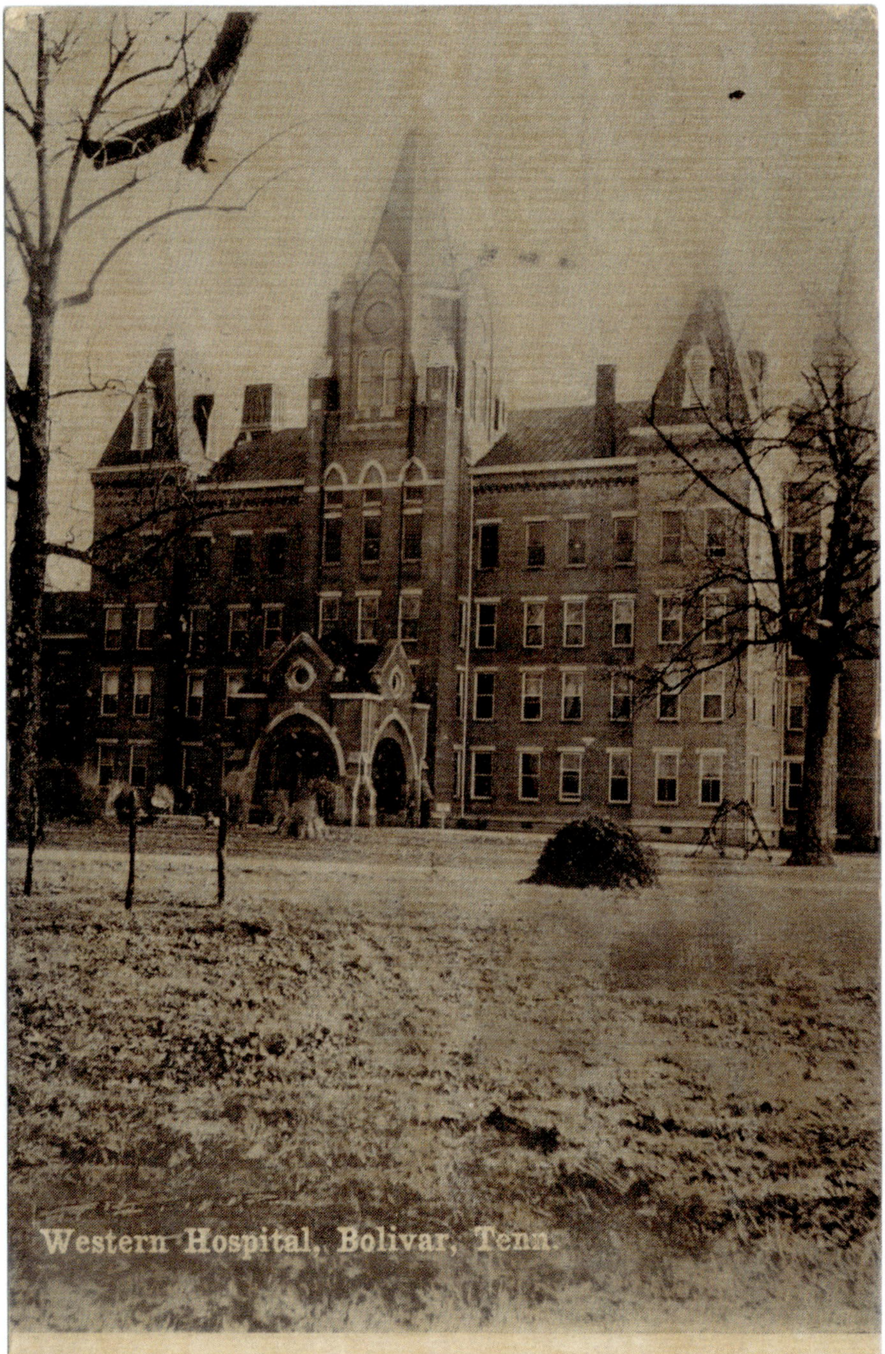

Figure 251

Hospital for the Incurably Insane
Hastings, Nebraska, 1889

The Hospital for the Incurably Insane opened in 1889 to care for patients deemed incurable or chronically ill. The original three-story building could house only 90 patients. Wings were added in 1891 and an additional annex was built the following year. Other additions included an amusement hall, a farm cottage, greenhouses, a dairy barn, a surgical building, a chapel, and a psychiatric hospital. By 1916, the hospital cared for 1,152 patients.

Three postcards provide images of this facility. The first two (figures 252–253) date sometime prior to 1907.

This third image (figure 254) dates between 1907 and 1914.

After several name changes, this facility now operates as the Hastings Regional Center, a center for treating adolescent substance abuse.

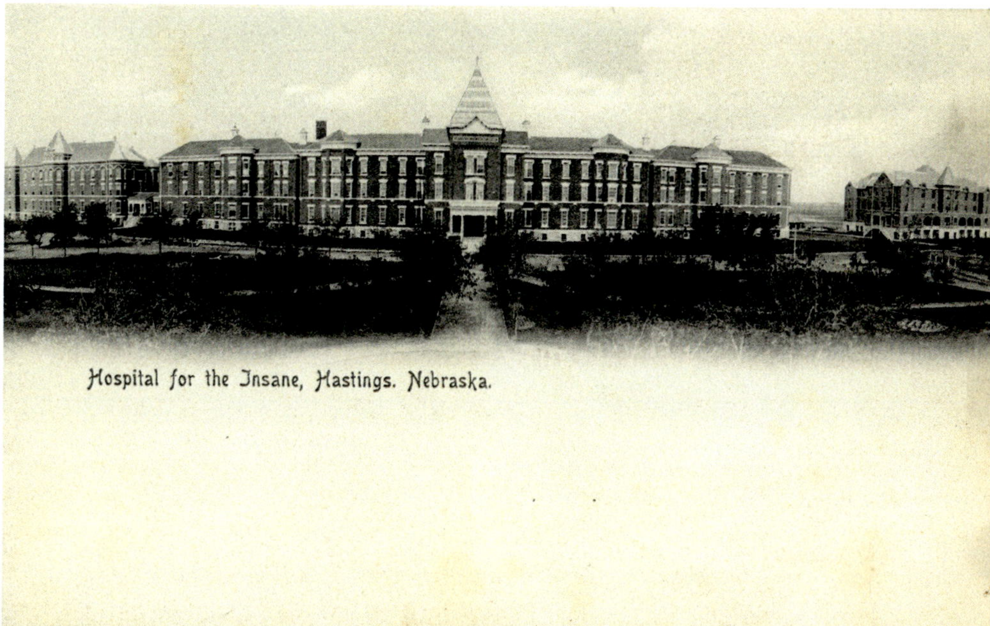

Figure 252

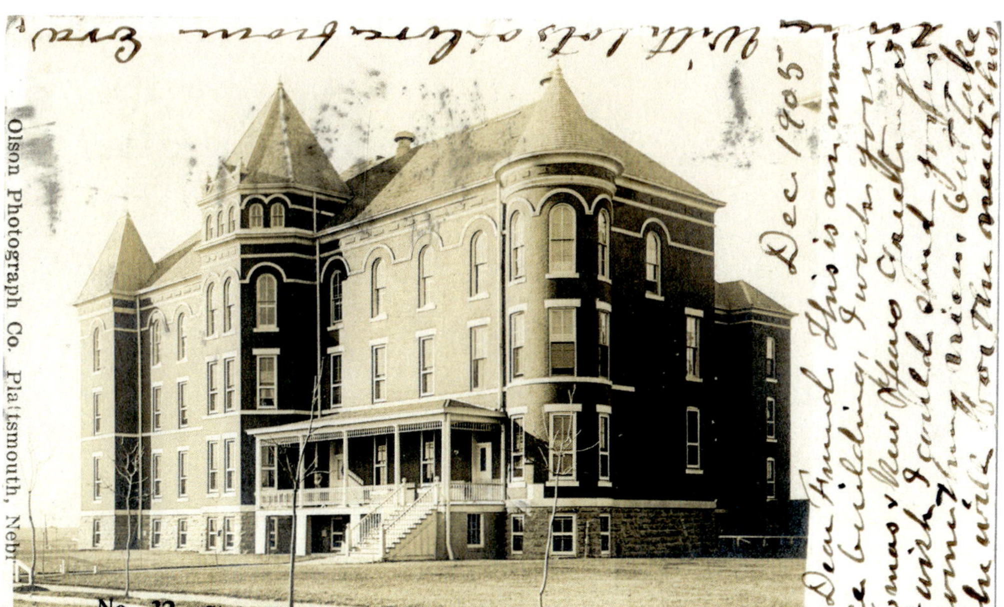

Figure 253

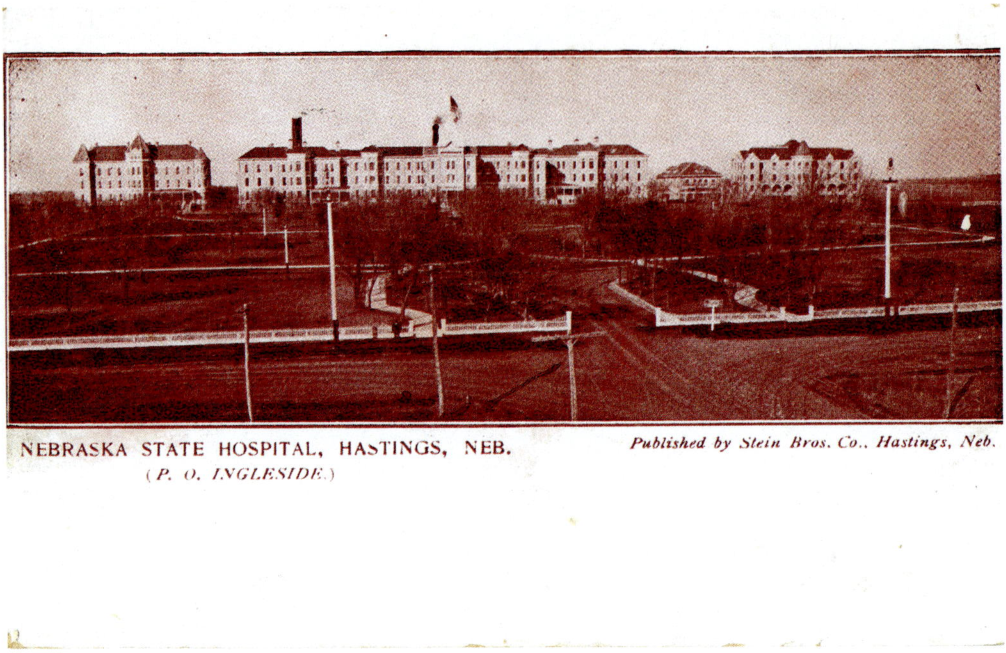
NEBRASKA STATE HOSPITAL, HASTINGS, NEB.
(P. O. INGLESIDE.)
Published by Stein Bros. Co., Hastings, Neb.

Figure 254

Wyoming Insane Asylum
Evanston, Wyoming, 1889

Established in 1886, the Wyoming Insane Asylum opened three years later to provide relief to other overcrowded facilities in Wyoming. When Wyoming was admitted to statehood in 1890, the State Board of Charities and Reform was created to manage the hospital. In 1891, the hospital was home to 31 patients, a number that rose to 129 just five years later.

The original building, a two-story brick structure, housed female patients on one floor and male patients on another. A building for the hospital superintendent was also added. A new wing was later added for male patients and an additional building was erected in 1910 to house female patients. The original building was destroyed by fire in 1917, but the wing for male patients survived.

The hospital farm flourished on more than 300 acres of land, producing vegetables, milk, livestock, and grains.

There were no postcards of this hospital in the author's collection. The facility continues to operate as the Wyoming State Hospital and many of the original buildings are still in use.

Insane Department and Hospital of New Castle County
Farnhurst, Delaware, 1889

The Insane Department and Hospital of New Castle County (figure 255), operated by the New Castle County Trustees of the Poor, was established in the late 1800s. Prior to this, the facility had operated as a poorhouse that also housed the mentally ill. In 1889, the facility's governance was transferred to the State Board of Trustees of the Insane and in 1891 it officially became known as the Delaware State Hospital.

The facility grew over the next few years. A superintendent's residence was added, along with a new laundry and an amusement hall, and 13 acres of grounds for greenspace, trees, grass, and walkways. At the close of 1894, the population had risen to 232. A new three-story building was added adjoining the existing structure to accommodate this growth.

In April of 1902, smallpox was discovered in one of the women's wards and the hospital was quarantined until the epidemic was suppressed. In 1904, a tuberculosis hospital was also opened to accommodate 20 patients. By 1907, the hospital population had steadily increased to 423 patients, despite the fact that it had been designed for 250.

The hospital has been administratively reorganized, becoming part of the Department of Health and Social Services. The original administration building is still in use.

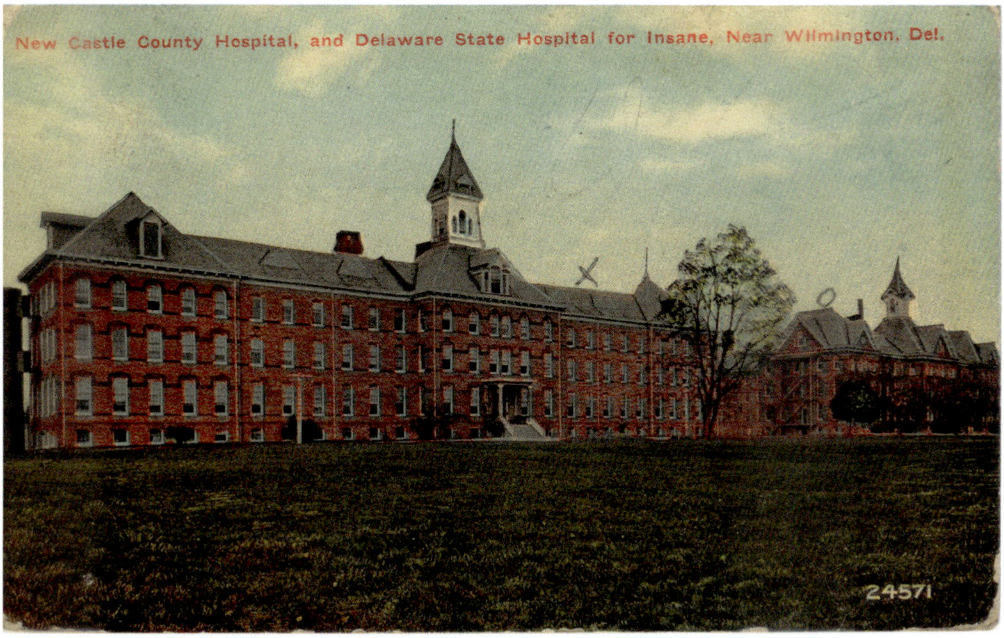

Figure 255

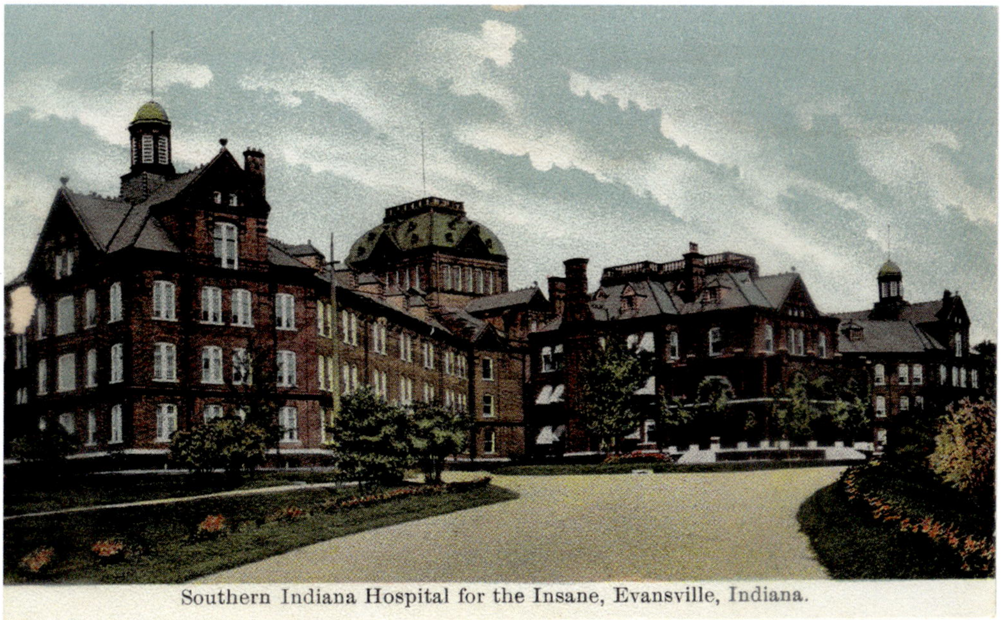

Figure 256

Southern Indiana Hospital for the Insane
Evansville, Indiana, 1890

This facility, frequently referred to as Woodmere, was established as the Southern Indiana Hospital for the Insane in 1890 on 879 acres of wooded land. The main buildings included a central block with two wings and an administration building. An additional patient wing was later added and although the original plan included separate dining rooms for men and women, two congregate dining rooms were instead created. Other detached buildings included a laundry, barn, stable, and coachman's house. The original capacity of the facility was 400, but the census reached 810 by 1911. A disastrous fire in 1943 destroyed the original building and forced the facility to close, but it reopened two years later in 1945.

Two 1907–1915 era postcards (figures 256–257) show the original buildings.

The original buildings were demolished in 2006, but the facility continues to operate as the Evansville State Hospital next to the original site.

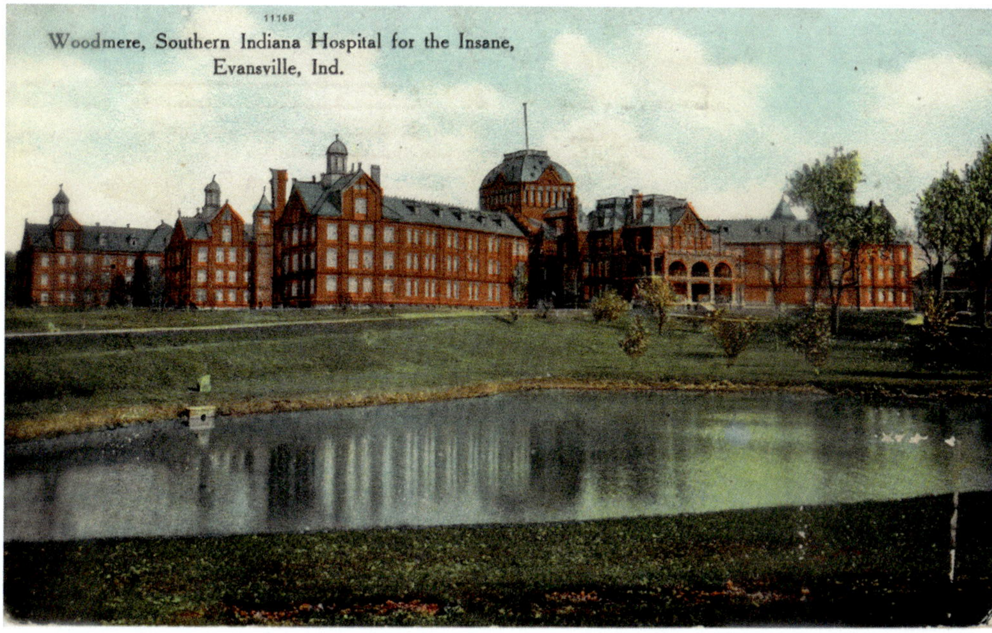

Figure 257

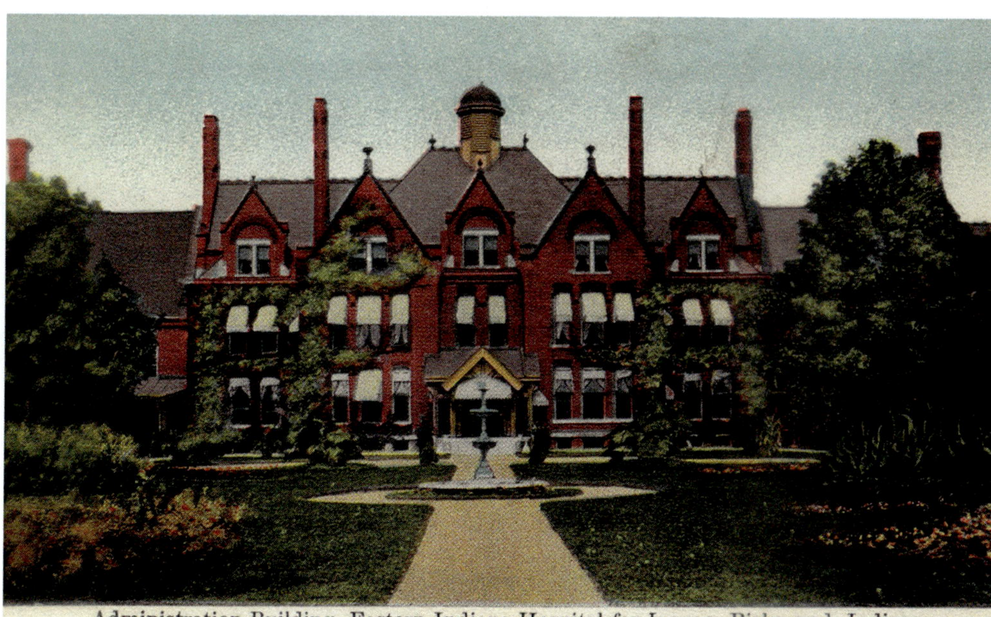

Administration Building, Eastern Indiana Hospital for Insane, Richmond, Indiana

Figure 258

Eastern Indiana Hospital for the Insane
Richmond, Indiana, 1890

The Eastern Indiana Hospital for the Insane, frequently referred to as "East Haven" and later renamed the Richmond State Hospital, opened in 1890. From 1887 to 1890, while the facility was still under construction, three of the buildings were used for the School for Feeble Minded Youth. These patients were transferred to another facility in 1890, and all of the buildings were then used for the hospital.

The hospital was constructed using the cottage plan, though a central administration building (figure 258) with wings strongly resembled other Kirkbride structures. By 1891, all beds were occupied. Over the next few years, a large general kitchen with two large dining halls was completed. A second floor assembly hall with seating capacity of 600 patients was also added along with more patient cottages and living quarters for male and female employees. In 1911, the facility was greatly enlarged when five farms were added. By 1912, the hospital consisted of 323 acres with 30 buildings. The capacity of the facility had reached 830, with an average of 794 patients in residence.

A 1907–1915 era postcard (figure 259) shows the expansive grounds.

The Richmond State Hospital continues to operate on the same site. The original administration building has been maintained and is still in use.

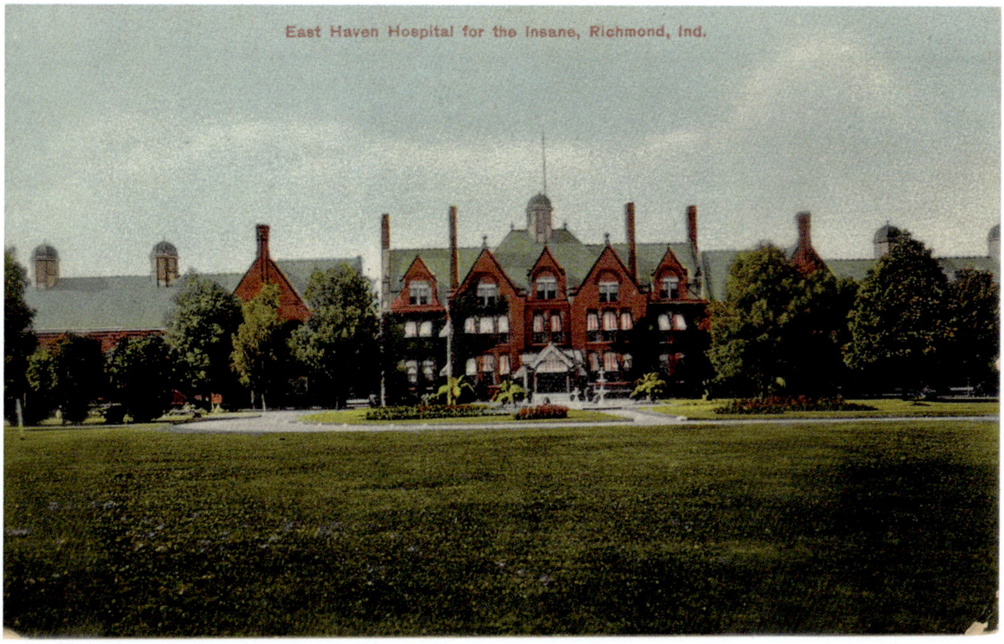

Figure 259

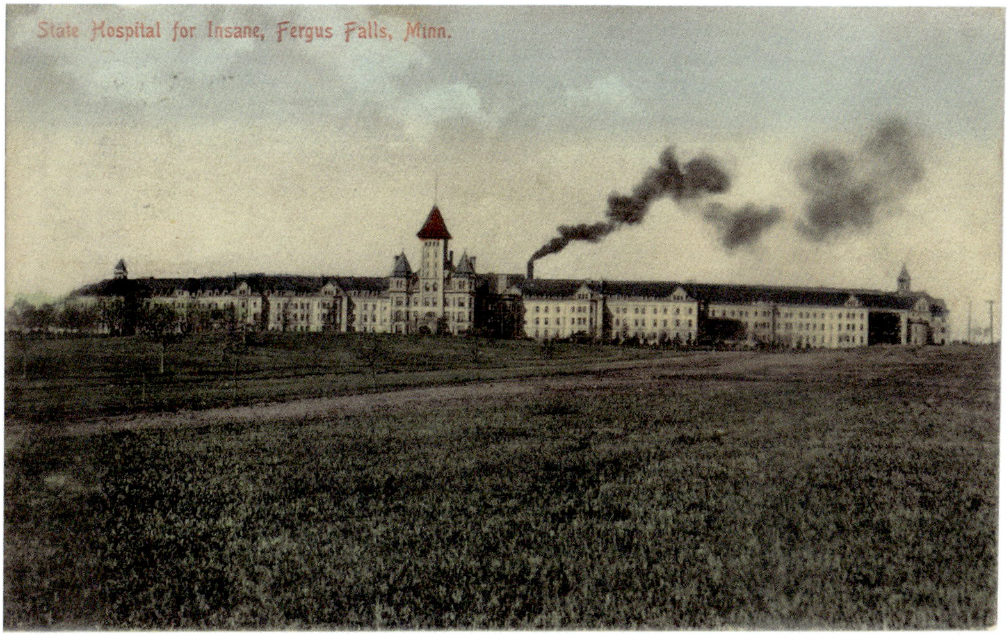

Figure 260

Fergus Falls State Hospital
Fergus Falls, Minnesota, 1890

This facility, the third in the state, was opened in 1890 to alleviate crowding at other institutions in Minnesota. It was located in Fergus Falls and was intended to be one of the few hospitals guided by homeopathic principles. Upon opening, 80 male patients were transferred from St. Peter State Hospital. Women were not admitted until 1893.

The ward buildings were based on the Kirkbride plan with a main wing and a detached wing. It was one of the last institutions built on the Kirkbride plan (figure 260) in the United States. The buildings were three stories high with a finished attic. The administration building, kitchen, nurses' home, amusement hall, and congregate dining rooms were all completed by the early 1900s. A training school for nurses was opened in 1894. By 1912, the patient population was 1,650, while the facility had a maximum capacity of 1,500.

The postcard in figure 261 is postmarked 1919.

The Fergus Falls State Hospital closed in 2005 and the original Kirkbride building has been sold to a private developer. It is being converted into a multipurpose residential and recreational facility.

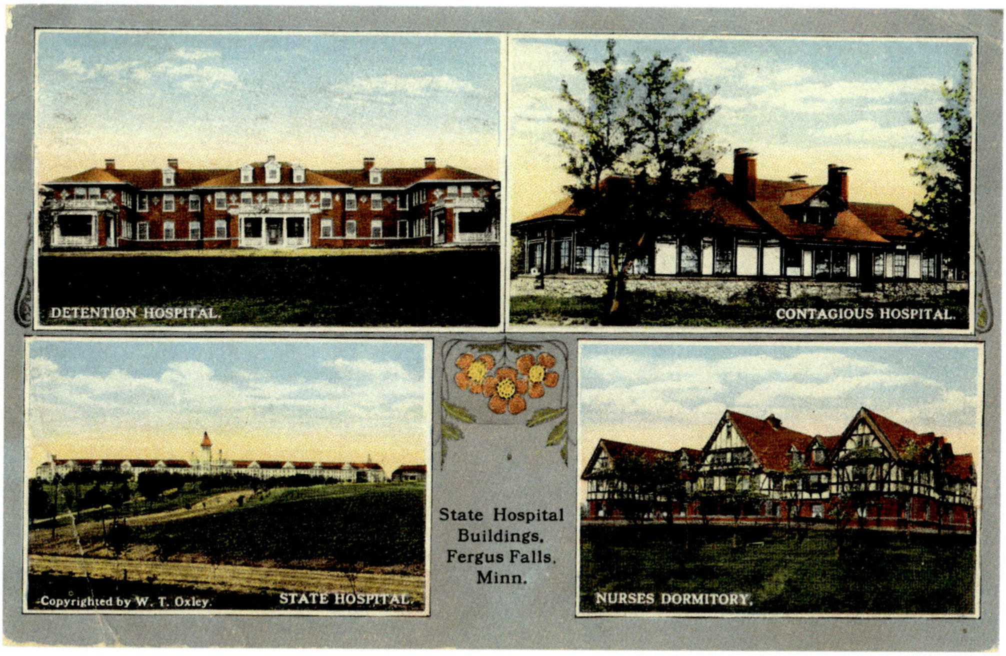
DETENTION HOSPITAL.
CONTAGIOUS HOSPITAL.
Copyrighted by W. T. Oxley.
STATE HOSPITAL.
State Hospital Buildings, Fergus Falls, Minn.
NURSES DORMITORY.

Figure 261

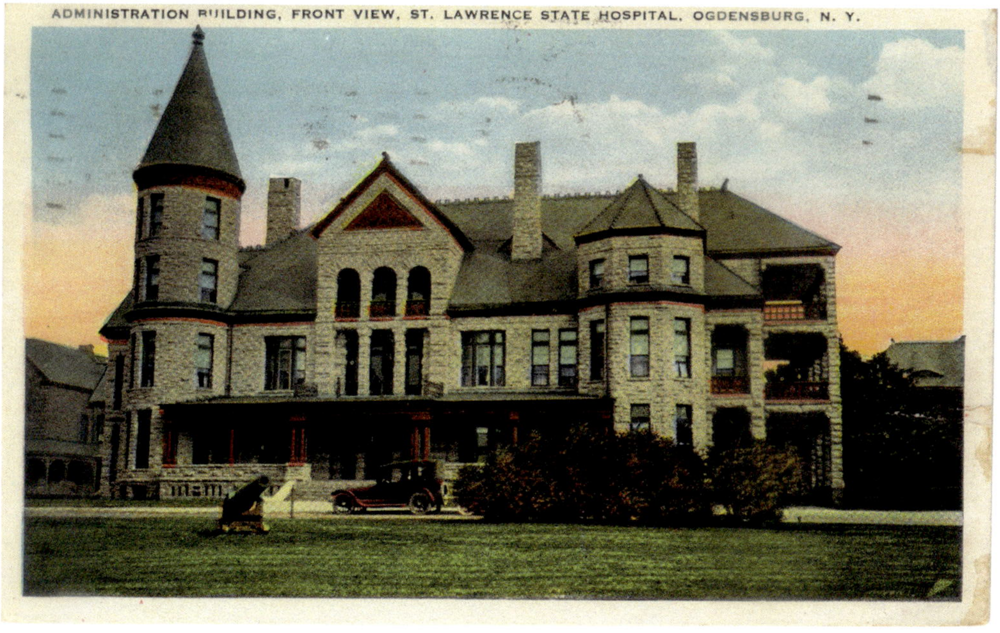
ADMINISTRATION BUILDING, FRONT VIEW, ST. LAWRENCE STATE HOSPITAL, OGDENSBURG, N. Y.

Figure 262

St. Lawrence State Asylum
Ogdensburg, New York, 1890

The St. Lawrence State Asylum opened in 1890, accepting the first 140 patients. Nestled on the banks of the St. Lawrence River, the facility grew over the next six decades, becoming a self-sustaining community with a police station, a fire station, a hospital, a nursing school, a patient library, and five-hundred acres of farmland. By 1905, a pavilion for tuberculosis was constructed, providing for 100 patients. Over the next ten years, a general operating room was installed and dining rooms were built to connect with cottages where patients were received.

Two early postcards show the facility. The first (figure 262) shows the administration building.

The image in the card in figure 263 appears to be of the Letchworth Complex, completed in 1899 to house the "chronic insane."

The facility has been renamed the St. Lawrence Psychiatric Center operating on the same grounds. Many of the original buildings have survived but are in a state of disrepair.

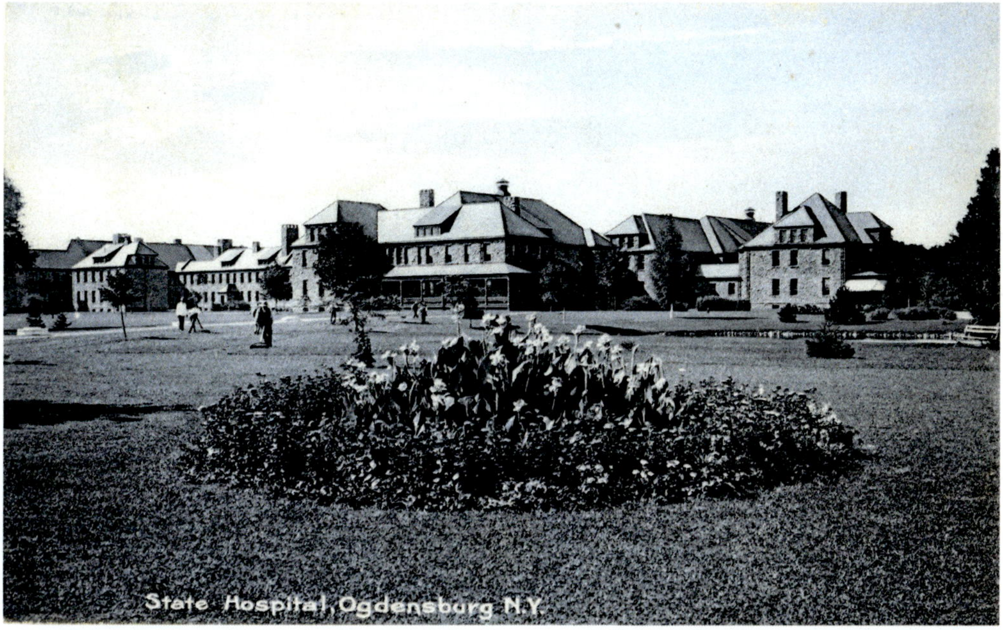
State Hospital, Ogdensburg N.Y.

Figure 263

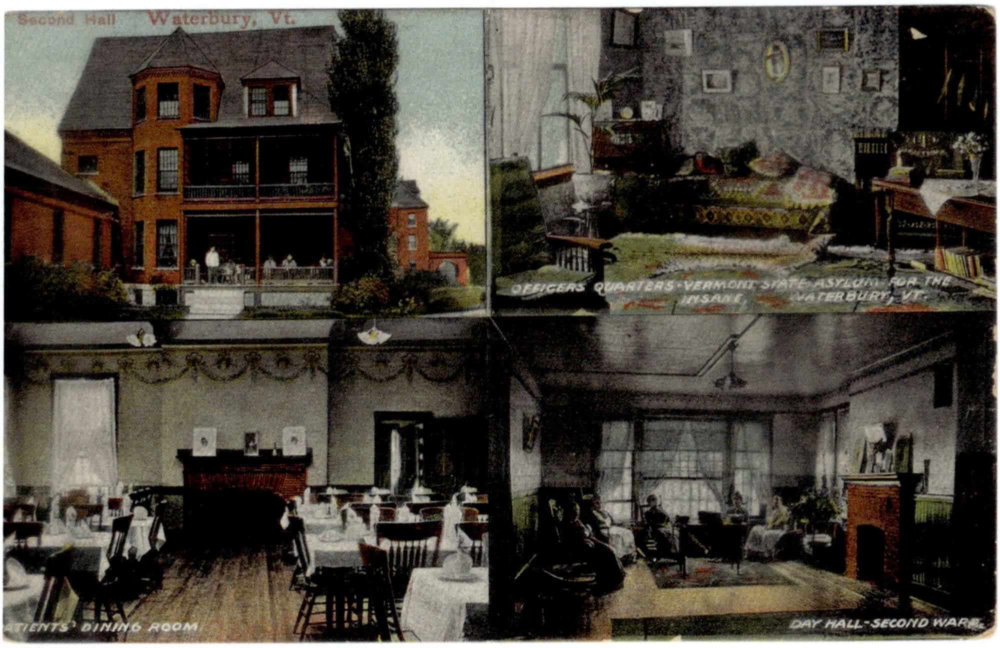
Second Hall
Waterbury, Vt.
OFFICERS QUARTERS-VERMONT STATE ASYLUM FOR THE INSANE, WATERBURY, VT.
DINING ROOM
DAY HALL-SECOND WARD

Figure 264

Vermont State Hospital for the Insane
Waterbury, Vermont, 1891

This Vermont Hospital for the Insane in Waterbury, Vermont was opened in 1891 with an expected capacity of 350 patients. It had been established to relieve the overcrowding of the asylum at Brattleboro. Only one-third of the institution had been completed in 1892. By 1914, the capacity of the hospital had been increased to 675.

The original buildings (figure 265) consisted of two wings and a central building for the administrative offices and kitchen. The wings had three floors containing two wards for patients with the dining rooms and bath rooms on each floor (figure 264).

The rare photograph in figure 266 shows a cabin built by one of the patients. It was taken by an amateur photographer and preserved.

The Vermont State Hospital at Waterbury closed in 2011 due to damages inflicted by Tropical Storm Irene. Some of the original buildings have been renovated and are part of a larger office complex that has been built on the site. A new psychiatric facility has been established in nearby Berlin, Vermont.

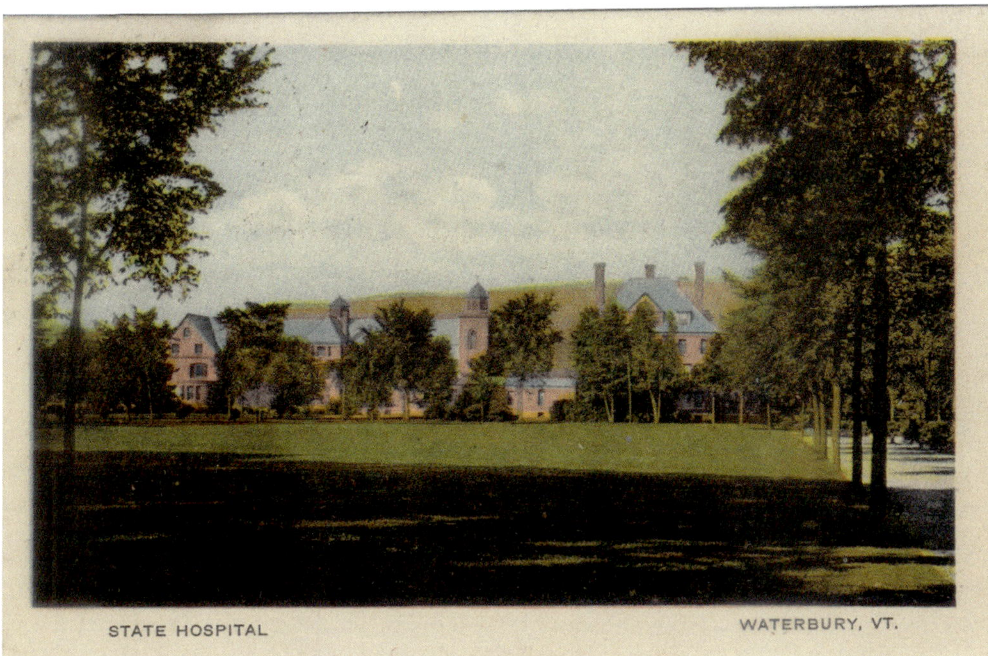

Figure 265

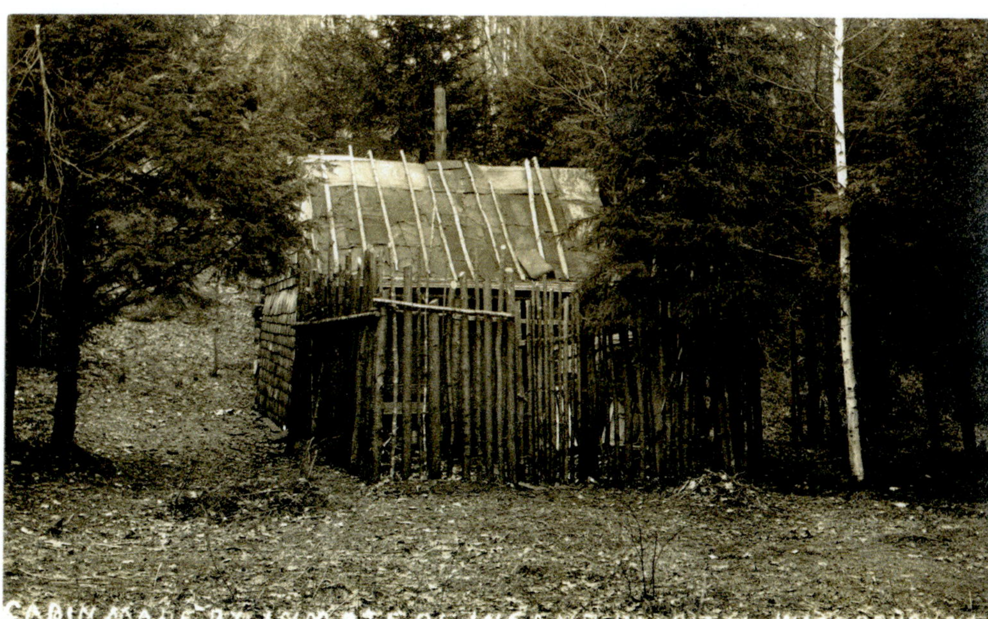

Figure 266

Asylum for Insane Criminals
Menard, Illinois, 1891

This facility, formerly the Asylum for Insane Criminals, opened in 1891 in Menard. All convicts deemed insane were transferred from state penitentiaries to this facility. Patients who were deemed homicidal or dangerous were also transferred from other hospitals in the state. By 1914, the number of patients reached 228 while the capacity of the institution was 150.

The main building was T-shaped with administrative offices, the superintendent's and employees' quarters, four wards for the patients, employee and patients dining rooms, and a general kitchen. The facility also consisted of the usual outlying buildings such as laundry, stables, dairy, and a barn. A site consisting of 17 acres owned by the state was rented for the farm and garden.

There were no images of this facility in this collection. The facility continues to operate as the Chester Mental Health Center, but the original building has been torn down.

Eastern State Hospital for the Insane
Medical Lake, Washington, 1891

Eastern State Hospital for the Insane was the second asylum built in the state of Washington. The facility originally consisted of a central administrative building with a wing on each side and a rear wing for the kitchen, engine room, and laundry. The entire facility was constructed of brick and each wing was three stories. Some claimed Eastern State Hospital was the largest building in the entire state. Designed using the Kirkbride plan, the hospital accommodated 150 patients in each wing.

The growth of the hospital population made it necessary to erect additional wards. By 1903, a three-story wing was built for 105 women and in 1907, another wing was built to accommodate 150 men. A fourth wing was added to care for patients deemed criminally insane. By 1914, the hospital cared for 1,056 patients.

Two postcards (figures 267–268), dated between 1907 and 1915, provide images of the hospital.

Eastern State Hospital continues to operate on the same site. The original Kirkbride building no longer exists.

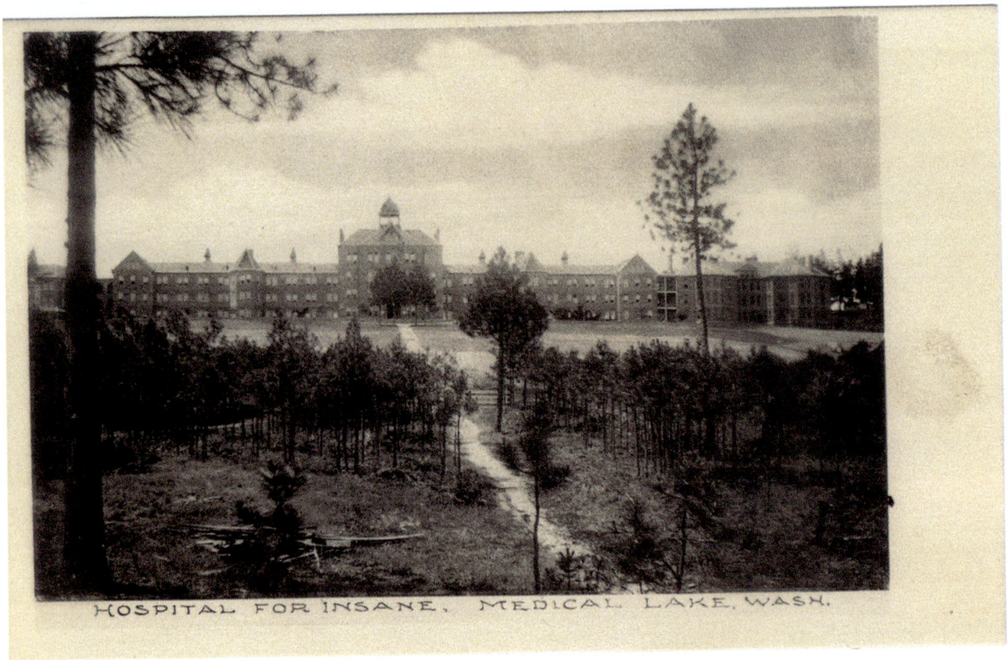

Figure 267

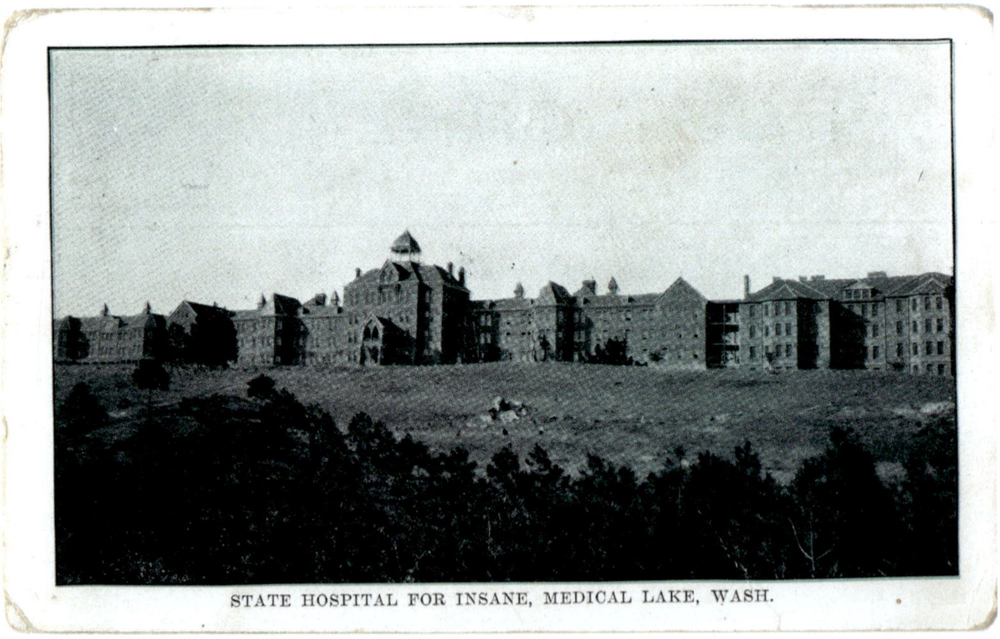

Figure 268

New Mexico Insane Asylum
Las Vegas, New Mexico, 1893

The New Mexico Insane Asylum was built on five acres of land one mile northwest of Las Vegas. The original facility was a four-story structure built of white sandstone. The basement contained a kitchen and laundry while the first floor included a dining hall, twelve rooms for patients, and staff offices. The upper floors each had 13 patient rooms.

By 1895, funds had been secured for a new three-story building and by 1902, the average census of the hospital had reached 100 patients. A third building was added the following year. The postcard in figure 269, produced some time before 1907, shows the three-story addition. It provided space for 110 additional patient rooms.

In 1968, the asylum was renamed New Mexico State Hospital and continues to operate as the New Mexico Behavioral Health Institute.

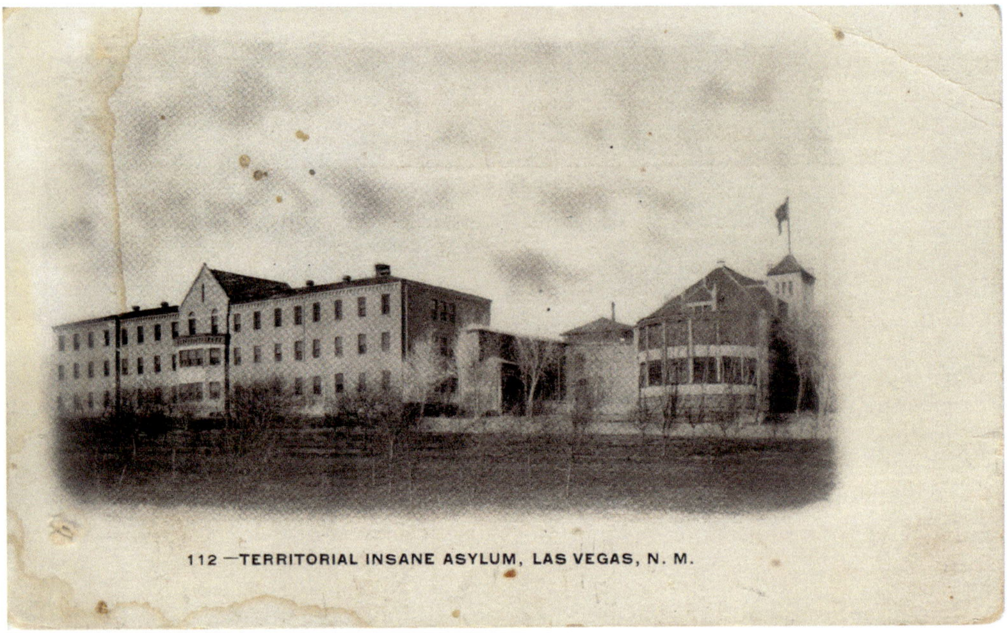

Figure 269

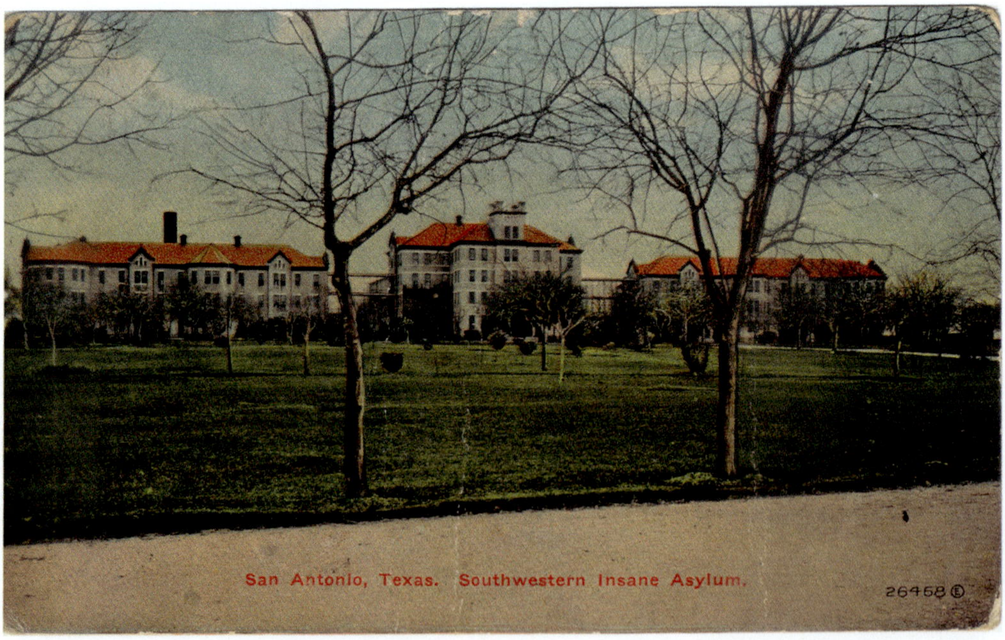

Figure 270

Southwestern Insane Asylum
San Antonio, Texas, 1892

The Southwestern Insane Asylum (figure 270) opened in San Antonio, Texas in 1892, becoming the third asylum in Texas. It was built to house 200 patients and within eight months, it housed 142.

Two more buildings were added, providing room for 200 more patients. There were also two cottages for tuberculosis patients, one for men and one for women; each accommodated 24 patients. These improvements were completed in 1910 and the population quickly increased to 1,000.

The back of the postcard (figure 271), published during the period 1907–1915, describes the facility.

The postcard in figure 272 is postmarked 1907.

This facility continues to operate as the San Antonio State Hospital.

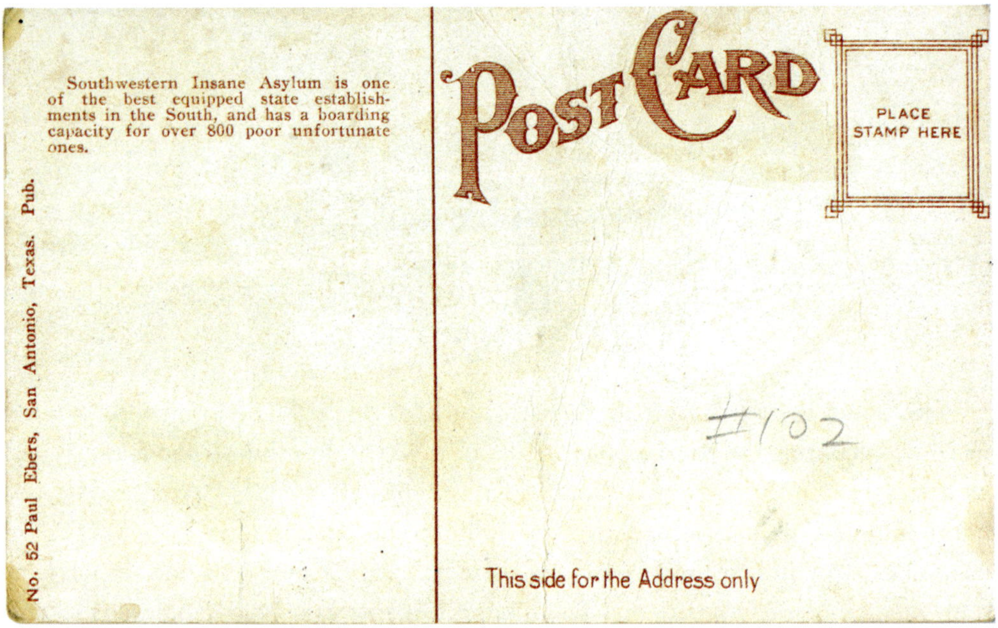

Figure 271

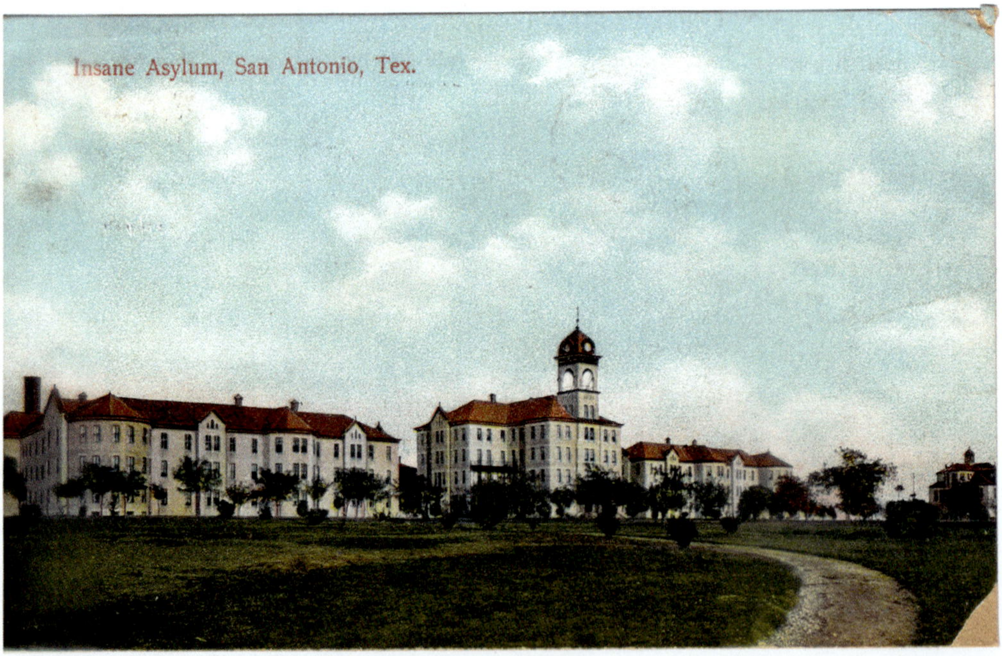

Figure 272

Second Hospital for the Insane
Spencer, West Virginia, 1893

Crowding at the First Hospital for the Insane at Weston prompted the Virginia Legislature to establish another facility. When the Second Hospital for the Insane opened, it received 54 patients with 26 patients arriving from Weston. Two more ward buildings were added to the original administration building and another wing was added within three years. The second floor of the administration building was used for the living quarters of the superintendent and family while the third floor housed the assistant physician and stenographers. There was a chapel and sleeping rooms for kitchen employees on the fourth floor.

A dining room was located in a three-story building to the rear of the administration building. The first floor consisted of a kitchen and the second floor had two large dining rooms. A third floor held rooms for employees.

By 1899, the hospital housed 389 patients and by 1910, this number had risen to 696.

The postcard in figure 273 provides an early view of the state hospital.

Later renamed the Spencer State Hospital, this facility was closed in 1989. The original buildings have been demolished.

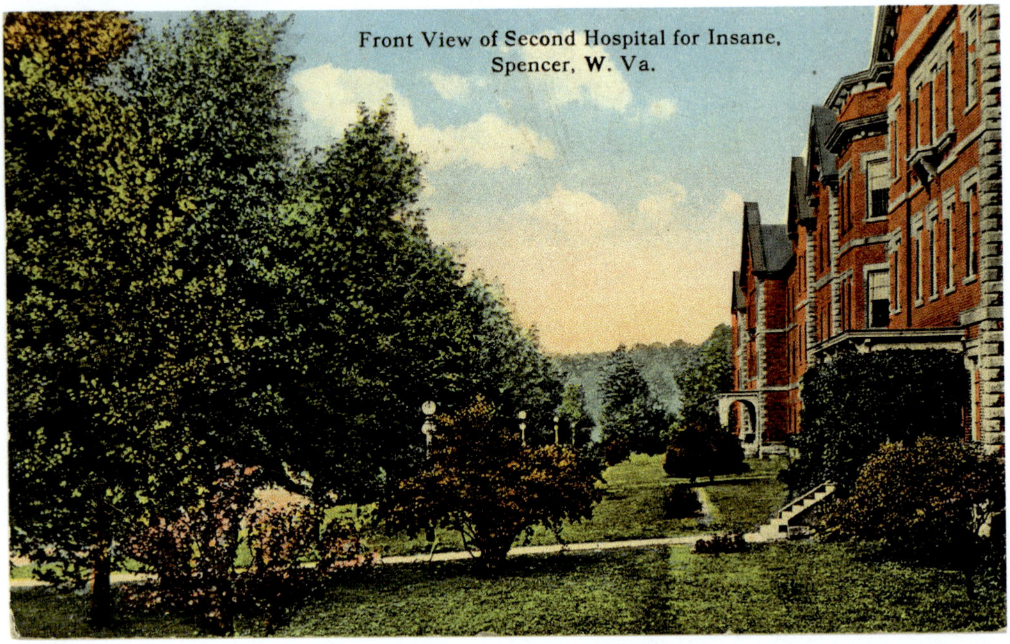
Front View of Second Hospital for Insane,
Spencer, W. Va.

Figure 273

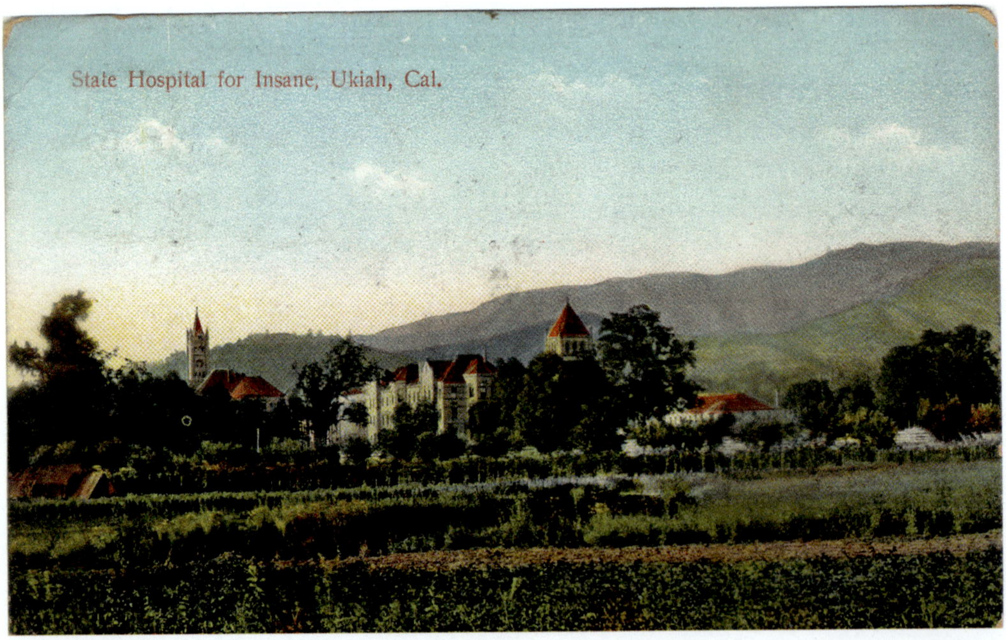
State Hospital for Insane, Ukiah, Cal.

Figure 274

Mendocino State Asylum for the Insane
Talmage, California, 1893

The Mendocino State Asylum for the Insane in Talmage, near the city of Ukiah, opened in July of 1893. The first patients, all male, arrived from state asylums at Napa and Stockton. The ward for female patients was still under construction and the first female patients were received after its completion in 1894.

By 1901, 270 acres had been added to the hospital for growing fruits and vegetables and raising cows. In the early 1900s, tents were also erected for treating tuberculosis patients, with the idea that open air encouraged a speedy recovery.

The 1906 earthquake caused damage to the buildings, but no major injuries were reported. The administration building was badly damaged and patients were transferred to other buildings. Two additional wards were added in 1910 and 1918.

By 1932, the hospital (figure 274) had more than 1,900 patients and 30 employees.

The original building was razed in 1952 and the Mendocino State Hospital was closed in 1972.

Southern California State Asylum for the Insane and Inebriates

Patton, California, 1893

This hospital was located on a tract of land lying along the foot hills in the shadow of the Arrowhead, six miles northeast of the city of San Bernardino. The original plan followed the cottage system and numerous buildings, some brick and others concrete, were added over the years. By 1904, the hospital had room for 800 patients.

The grounds included lawns, flower gardens, and scenic views. Moving pictures, band concerts and dancing were provided for patient recreation, along with outdoor walks and hayrides.

By 1915, the hospital cared for 1,369 men and 811 women and housed 239 employees.

This postcard in figure 275 was postmarked 1917.

An earlier postcard postmarked 1908 (figure 276) provides a view of the buildings.

An earthquake in 1923 badly damaged the original buildings and they were demolished. This facility continues to operate as Patton State Hospital.

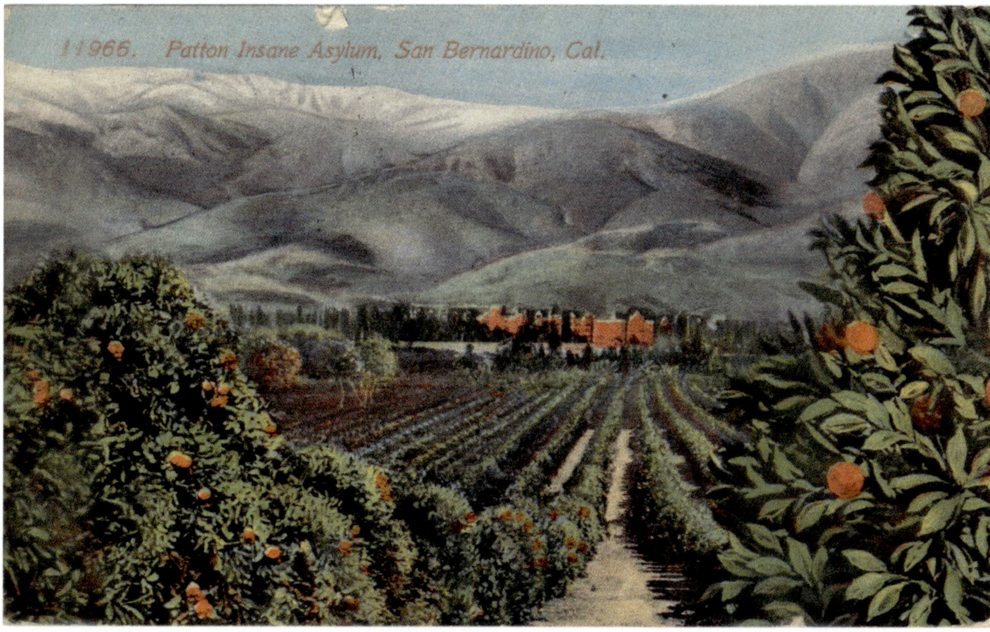
11966. Patton Insane Asylum, San Bernardino, Cal.

Figure 275

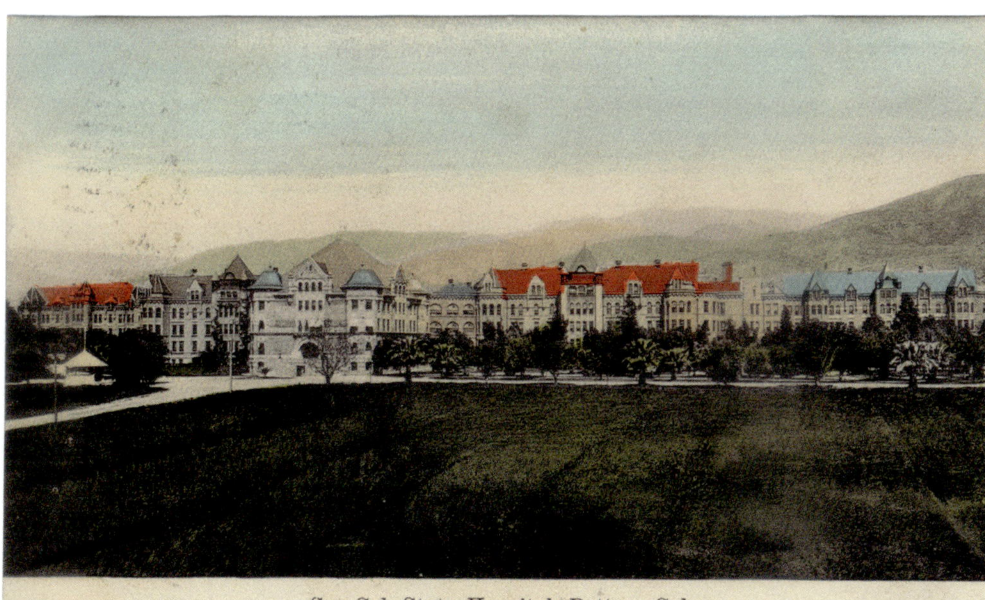
So. Cal. State Hospital, Patton, Cal.
LEE.

Figure 276

Asylum for the Chronic Insane of Pennsylvania
Wernersville, Pennsylvania, 1893

The Asylum for the Chronic Insane of Pennsylvania opened in 1893 on 540 acres of farmland. The three-story administration building was modeled after Independence Hall. The eight dormitories and a larger building used for dining and assembly rooms were two stories with half a basement. The facility had three farms, a mill, a chapel, a bakery, a boiler house, and a filtration plant.

By 1893, there were 147 patients in the facility. The next year an additional 147 patients were transferred from nearby asylums that had become overcrowded. Records from the facility indicate that in 1894, there were 662 patients. Reports from the hospital show that five patients had died during 1893. The average cost of caring for a patient for one week was $2.50.

The postcard in figure 277 provides a view of the administration building.

The men's infirmary is depicted in figure 278.

Figure 279 provides an image of the recreation quadrangle, presumably a place for patients to walk and enjoy the outdoors.

This facility continues to operate as the Wernersville State Hospital. A museum detailing the history of the hospital operates in the original buildings.

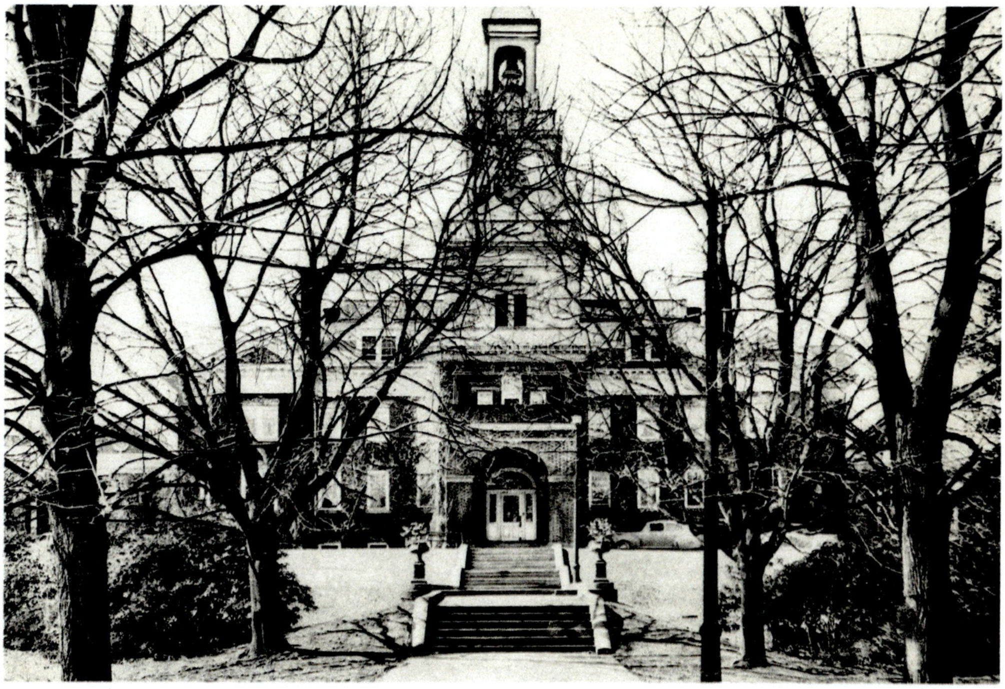

Figure 277

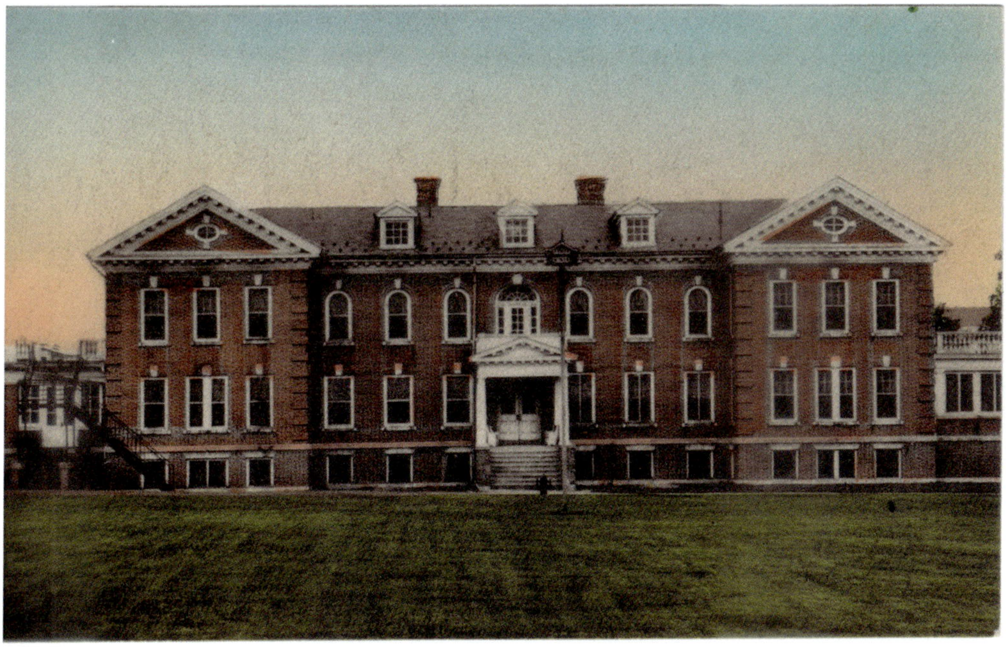

Figure 278

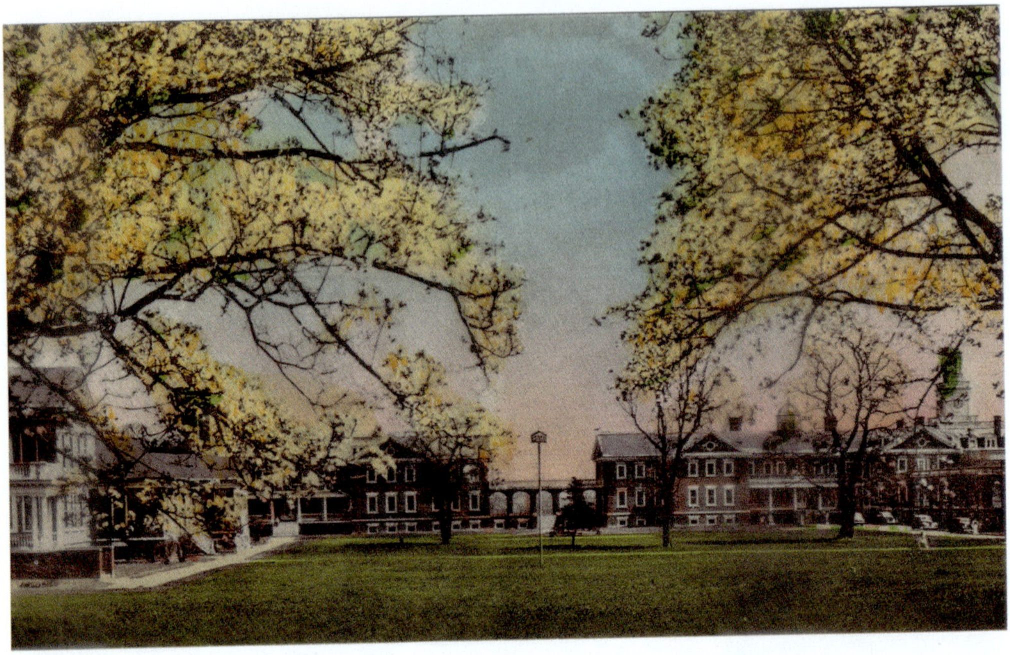

Figure 279

Asylum for Insane Criminals
Bridgewater, Massachusetts, 1895

Opened in 1852 as an almshouse for the poor, this facility also served as the State Workhouse in 1866 for the poor who had been convicted of petty crimes, for juvenile delinquents, and later—for "insane paupers" and "insane criminals." In 1887, the name of the facility was changed to Massachusetts State Farm when 50 patients from other state hospitals were transferred. In 1895, a division called the Asylum for Insane Criminals was officially established. Originally constructed primarily of wood, the facility was almost entirely destroyed by fire in 1883 and the workhouse was transferred to a new location.

The institution was rebuilt using brick and concrete. The facility was again rebuilt in 1974 and continues to operate as Bridgewater State Hospital in Bridgewater, MA.

There were no postcards of this facility in the author's collection.

Upper Peninsula Hospital for the Insane
Newberry, Michigan, 1895

The Upper Peninsula Hospital for the Insane consisted of 20 cottages arranged in the form of a quadrangle, connected by covered walkways. The general kitchen and dining rooms were included in the quadrangle while the heating plant, laundry, storerooms, and other industrial buildings were situated at the rear. A hospital with separate receiving wards for men and women also included a laboratory, operating rooms, and hydrotherapy treatment room. In 1905, the hospital cared for 880 patients and had 147 employees.

The postcard in figure 280 is a rare photograph of the facility prior to 1907.

The commercially produced postcard in figure 281, dated sometime before 1907, shows the whole facility.

This hospital, later named the Newberry State Hospital, closed in 1992.

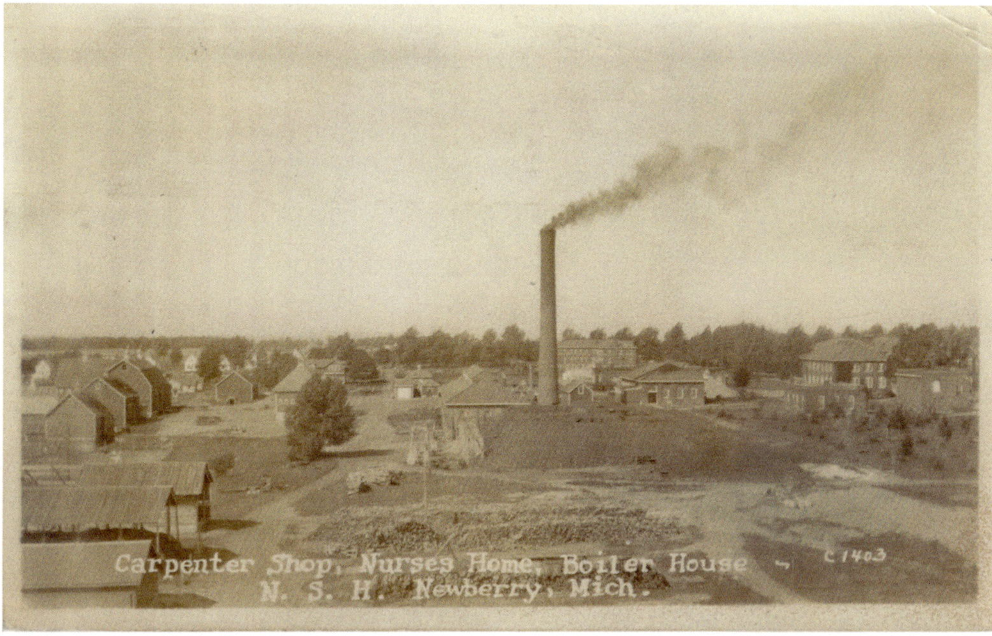
Carpenter Shop, Nurses Home, Boiler House
N. S. H. Newberry, Mich.
C 1403

Figure 280

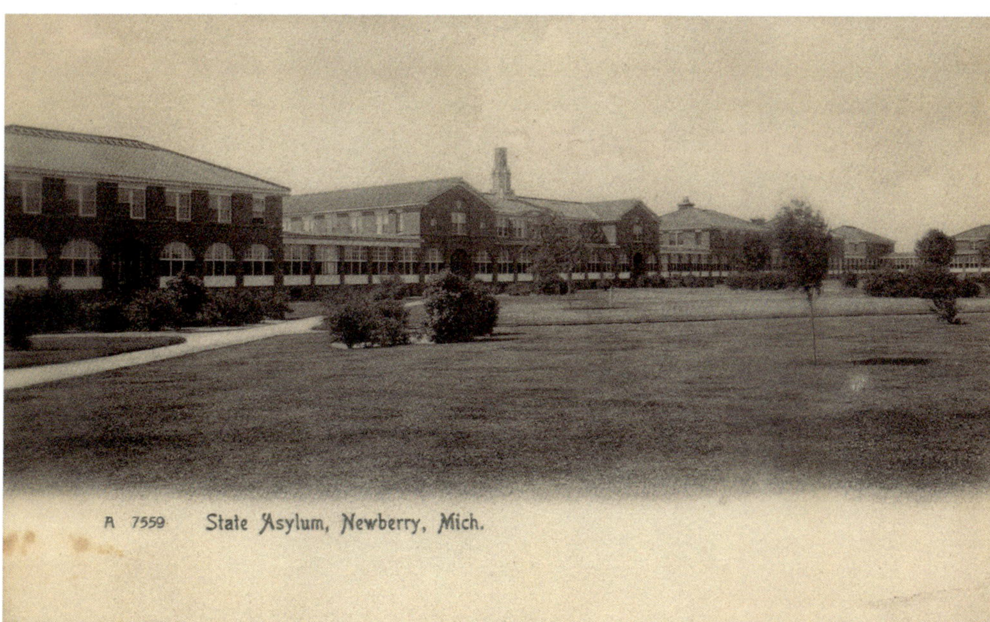
A 7559 State Asylum, Newberry, Mich.

Figure 281

Medfield Insane Asylum
Medfield, Massachusetts, 1896

The Medfield Insane Asylum was the first asylum in Massachusetts to be built on the cottage plan. It consisted of a kitchen, two general dining rooms, a power plant, a laundry room, an administration building, and twelve buildings for patients. When it opened in 1896 there were 120 patients, half men and half women, received from the Taunton State Hospital. By the end of the year, there were 563 patients. A chapel, stable, and six more buildings were completed the next year. During the succeeding years additions were built and renovations were made and the capacity was increased from 1,000 to 1,800 patients.

A nurses' home for 75 female attendants was completed in 1902 and the following year, a large building for 150 "excited" female patients was built. Three years later, a similar building was built for male patients.

The postcard in figure 282, postmarked 1908, shows the chapel. On the reverse (figure 283), the sender describes the chapel.

In 1909, the name of the institution was changed to Medfield State Asylum and in 1914 it was again changed to Medfield State Hospital. The hospital closed in 2003, but many of the original buildings have survived. The site was contaminated by a 1978 oil spill and in 2013, plans were approved for clean-up and reuse of the site and the buildings.

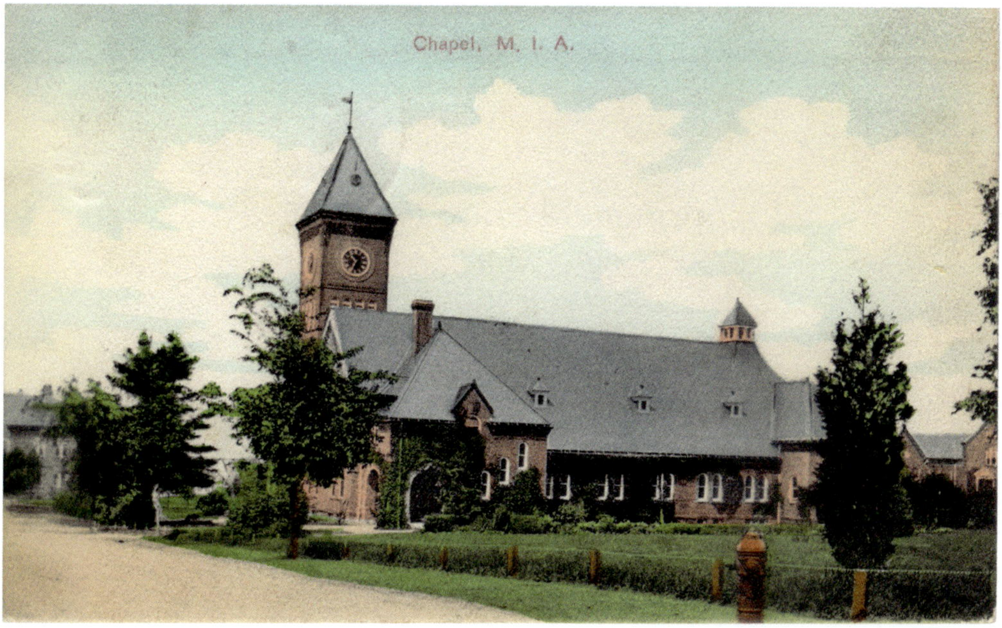

Figure 282

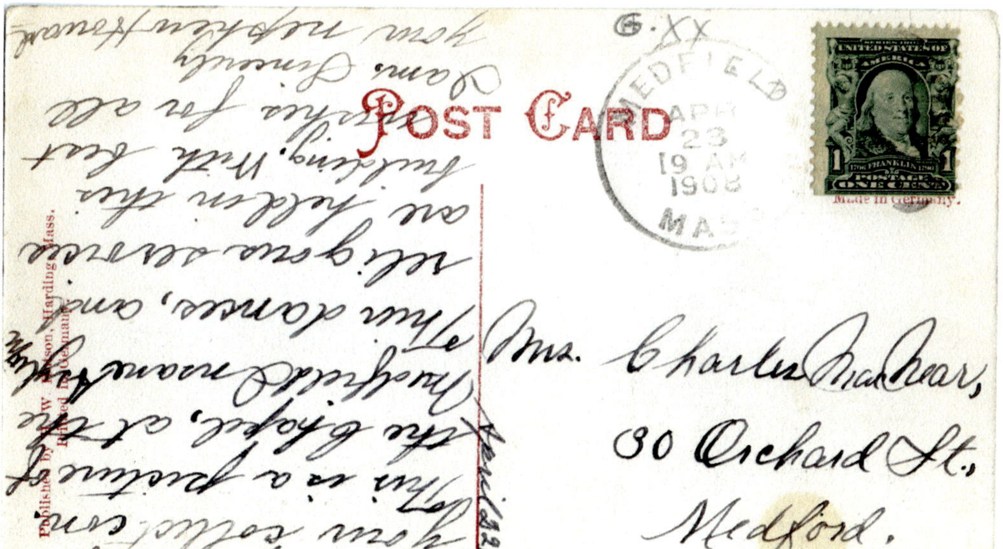

Figure 283

Springfield State Hospital
Sykesville, Maryland, 1896

This facility was located on a farm with over 700 acres near the town of Sykesville, in Carroll County, Maryland. When the first patients were accepted in 1896, the facility was still under construction and patients were housed in existing renovated farm houses. The men's and women's facilities were completed by 1900. The demand for admission was so great that additional buildings were added over the years.

By 1912, there were 20 detached cottages with 1,425 patients, 7 physicians, and 127 nurses. Other added buildings included two isolated cottages for tuberculosis patients, each with a capacity of 40 patients, and a receiving hospital.

This facility continues to operate as Springfield Hospital Center. The women's facility still stands and was placed on the National Register of Historic Places in 2000.

No images of this facility exist in the author's collection.

Eastern Ohio Asylum for the Insane
Massillon, Ohio, 1898

The Eastern Ohio Asylum for the Insane opened in 1898 as the sixth asylum in Ohio. Built on the cottage plan, the facility (figure 284) was comprised of a number of buildings including a kitchen and bakery, a store house, a carpenter shop, a hospital, an infirmary, and seven cottages. A school for patients was opened in the early 1900s. Constructed by patients, the two-story school included classrooms, a library, and a gymnasium.

By 1918, there were 1,650 patients and the facility occupied 1,100 acres of land containing a farm and gardens cultivated by the patients (figure 285). Therapy included recreation in the form of motion pictures and dances.

Postcards of the Massillon facility are plentiful.

The activity center was called McKinley Hall (figure 286).

Another postcard (figure 287) shows the outside of McKinley Hall and the cottages.

The practice of providing separate housing for superintendents, nurses and/or other officials became common by the early 1900s. The postcard in figure 288 shows a view of the superintendent's residence.

This facility is now called Heartland Behavioral Center. Some of the original buildings have survived.

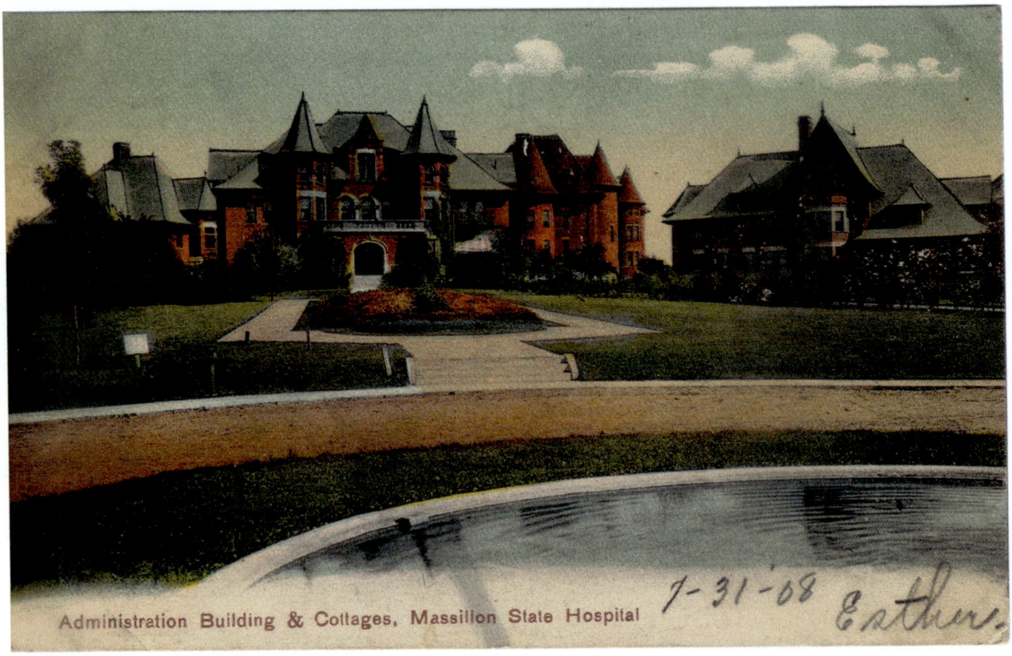
Administration Building & Cottages, Massillon State Hospital
1-31-08 Esther.

Figure 284

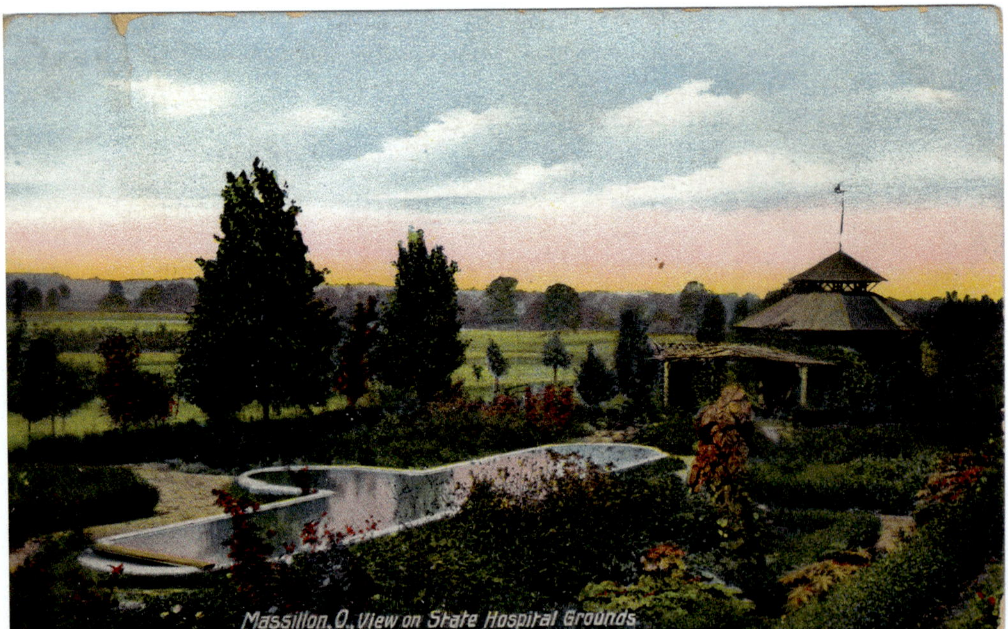
Massillon, O., View on State Hospital Grounds.

Figure 285

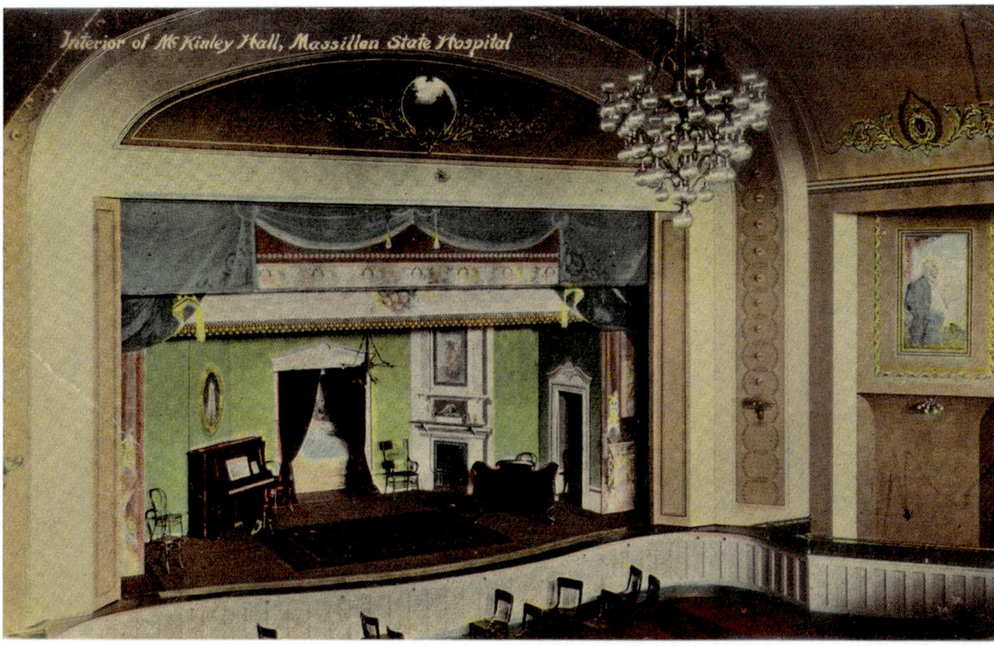
Interior of McKinley Hall, Massillon State Hospital

Figure 286

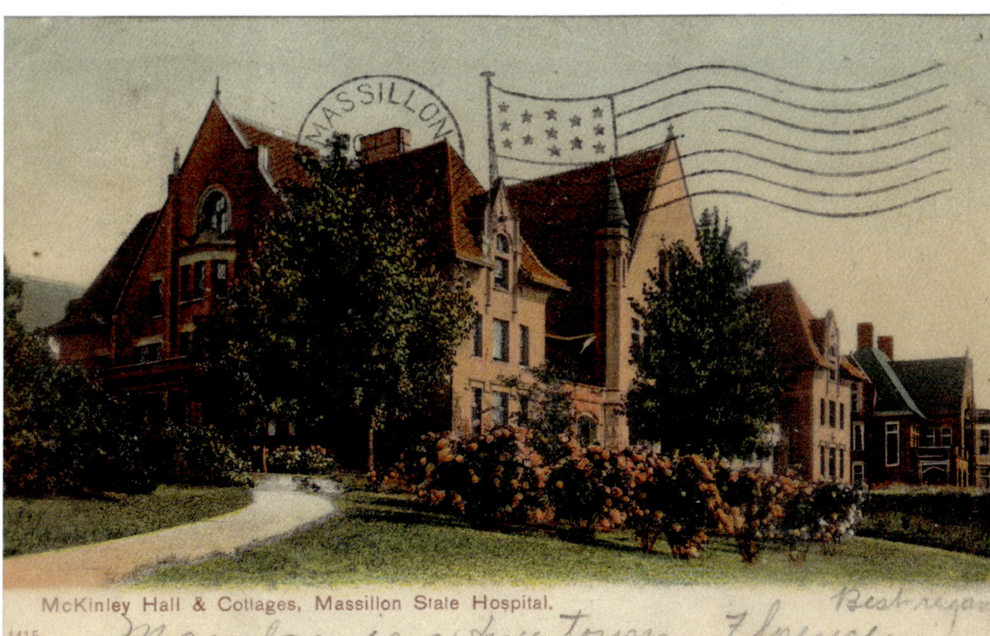
MASSILLON
McKinley Hall & Cottages, Massillon State Hospital.
4415

Figure 287

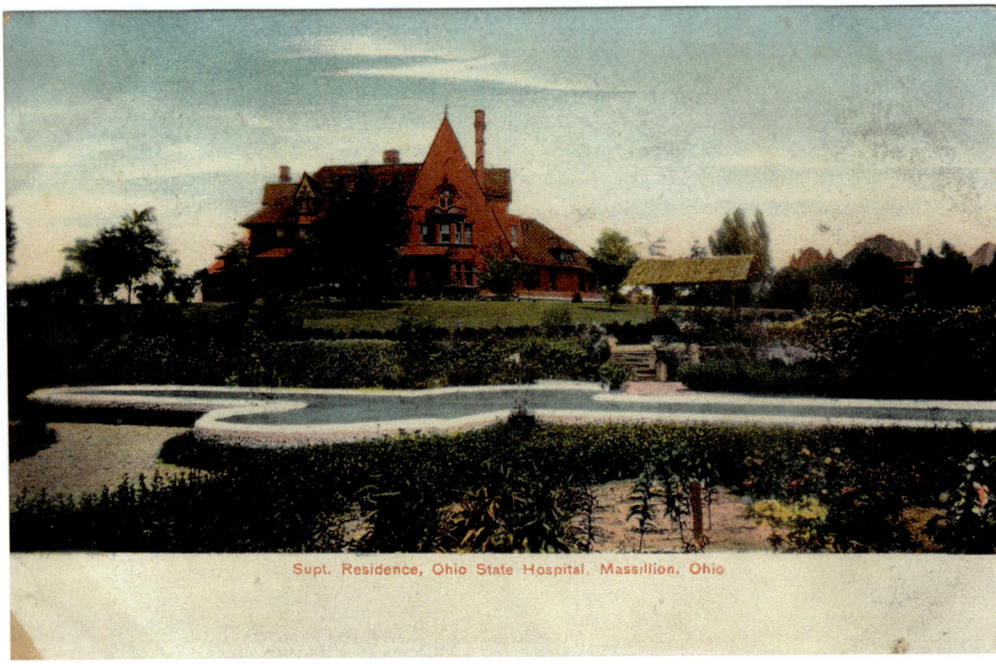
Supt. Residence, Ohio State Hospital, Massillion, Ohio

Figure 288

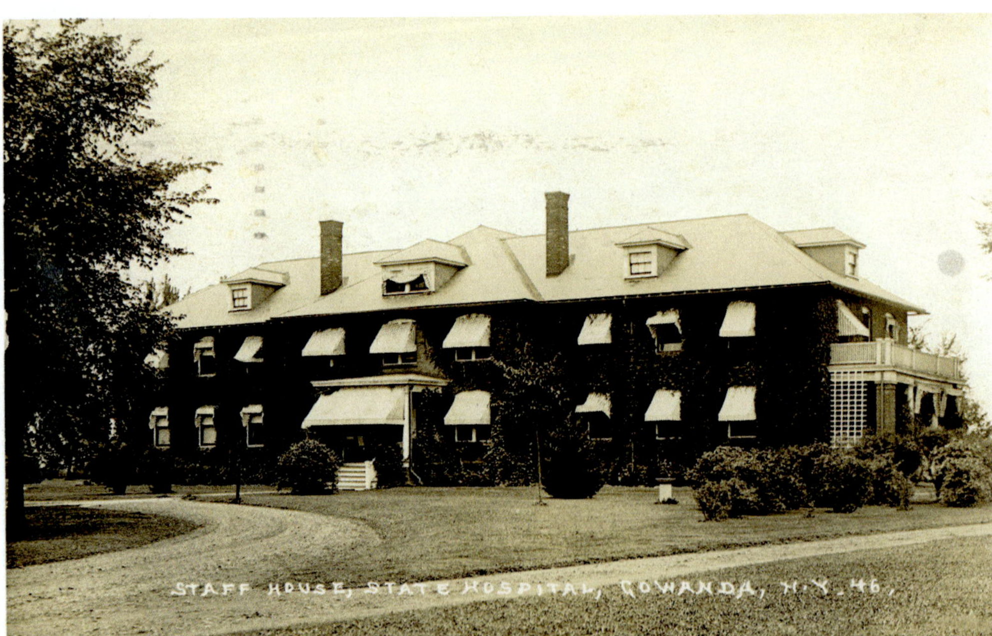
STAFF HOUSE, STATE HOSPITAL, GOWANDA, N.Y. 46.

Figure 289

Gowanda State Homeopathic Hospital
Helmuth, New York, 1898

The Gowanda State Homeopathic Hospital opened in 1898 to provide homeopathic care for the mentally ill in New York. A 500-acre farm near the town of Collins was purchased and the original buildings—including an administration building, an annex, and one wing—were constructed. Additions were made and the hospital (figures 290–291) became a self-sufficient facility, equipped with laundry, a power house, an electrical plant, dining rooms, and a kitchen.

By 1904, a superintendent's residence, staff housing for 150 nurses (figure 289), and an amusement hall with seating for 750 patients were completed. Shortly after, the hospital received a transfer of 100 more patients from the Kings Park State Hospital. By 1913, the census had reached 1,129 while the official capacity was 978.

The Gowanda State Homeopathic Hospital closed in the 1990s and the site is now home to a correctional facility.

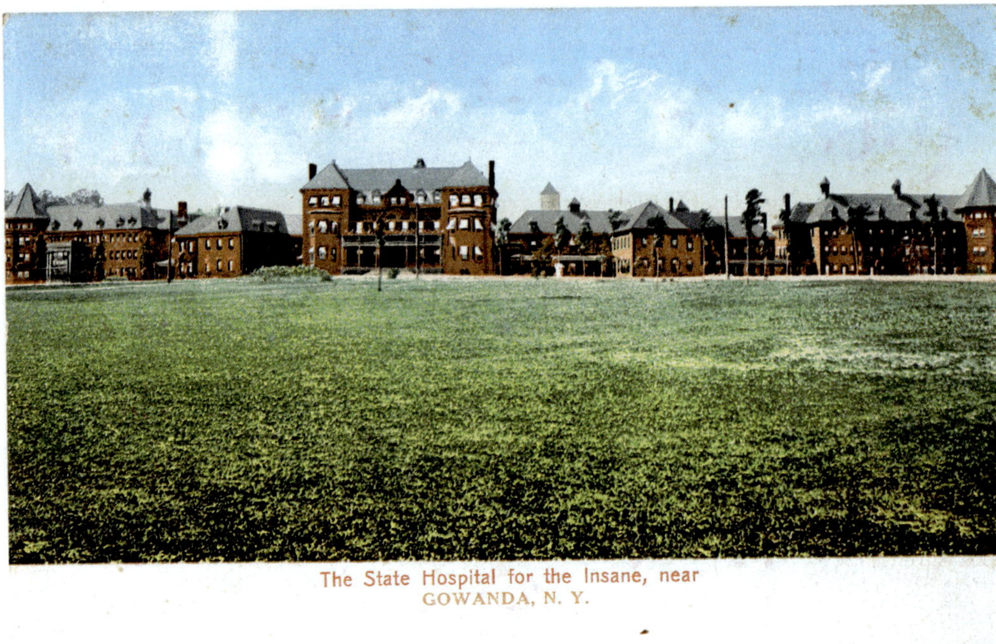
The State Hospital for the Insane, near
GOWANDA, N. Y.

Figure 290

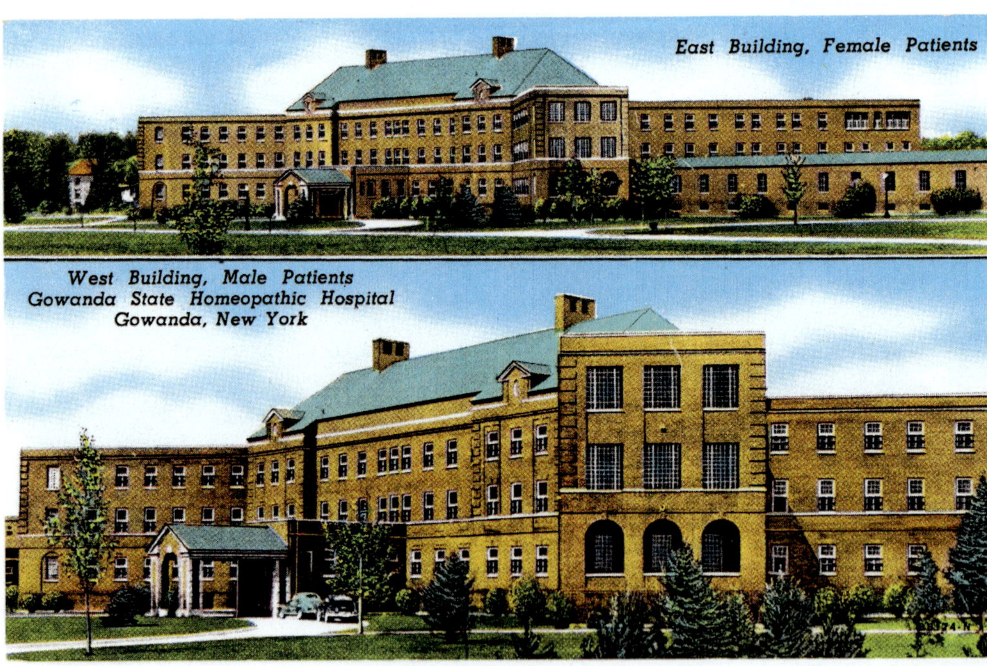
East Building, Female Patients
West Building, Male Patients
Gowanda State Homeopathic Hospital
Gowanda, New York

Figure 291

Part II:

Private, County, and Government Hospitals

Pennsylvania Hospital
Philadelphia, Pennsylvania, 1752

In 1751, the Pennsylvania Hospital was founded on Market Street in Philadelphia. It opened in 1752. By 1841, the general hospital, which included departments for the mentally ill, was located at Eighth and Spruce Streets in West Philadelphia. Benjamin Rush, considered by many to be the father of American psychiatry, was part of the medical staff at this hospital from 1783 until 1813. Thomas Kirkbride, the father of the Kirkbride asylum design, also worked at this facility for about 40 years.

A postcard (figure 292) from around 1910 shows the facility during the early 1900s.

This facility continues to operate as the Pennsylvania Hospital (figure 293) and several of the original buildings have been maintained. It is the oldest hospital in the United States.

Pennsylvania had a number of other county and private asylums by the early 1900s, most caring for between 100 and 200 patients each. The County Alms and Asylum at Lancaster, Pennsylvania is shown on a 1910 postcard in figure 294.

Most Pennsylvania county asylums were phased out by the middle 1900s.

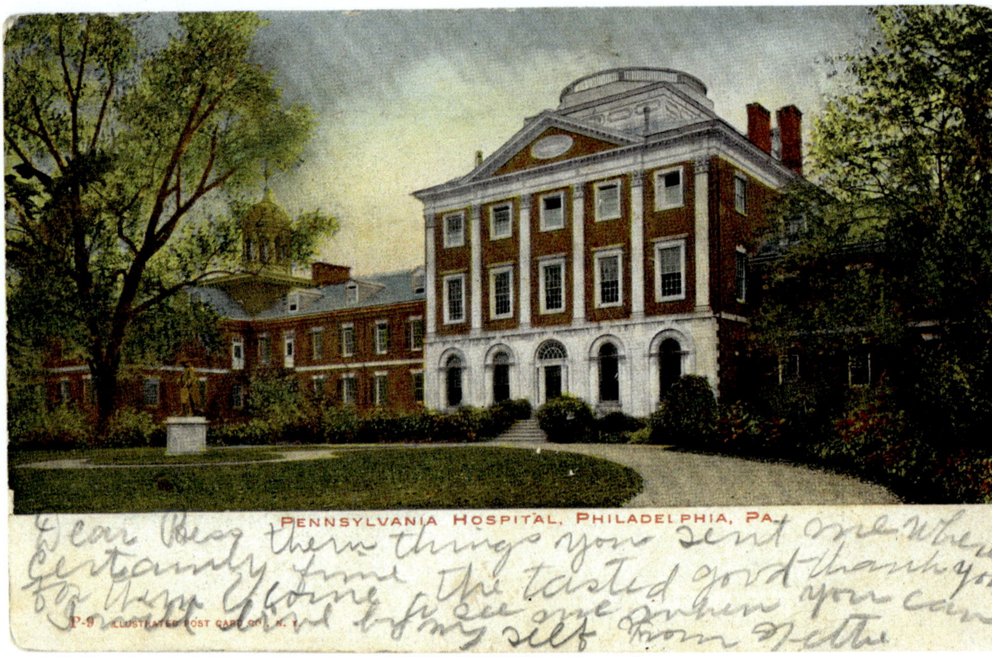

Figure 292

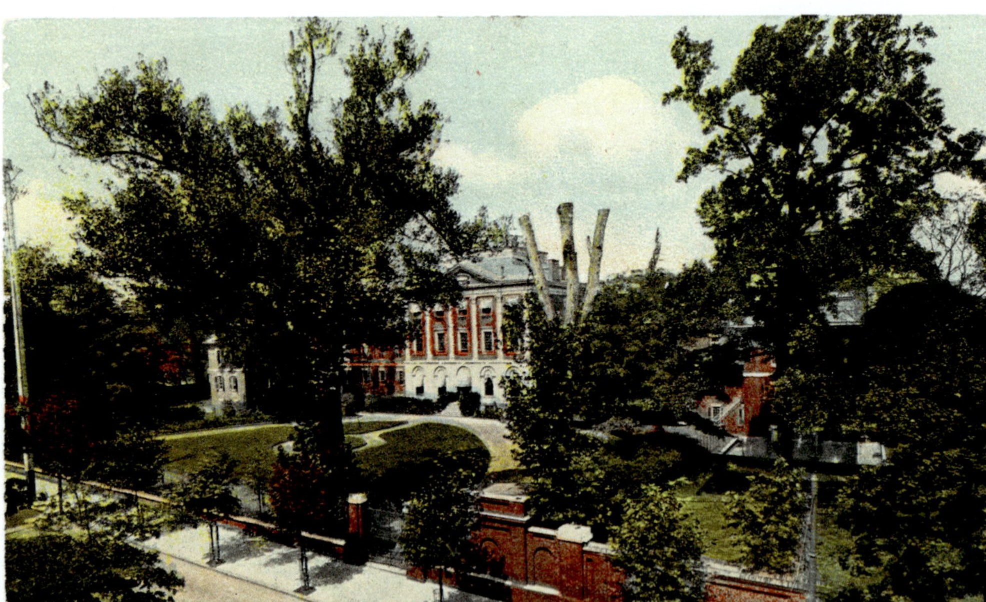

Figure 293

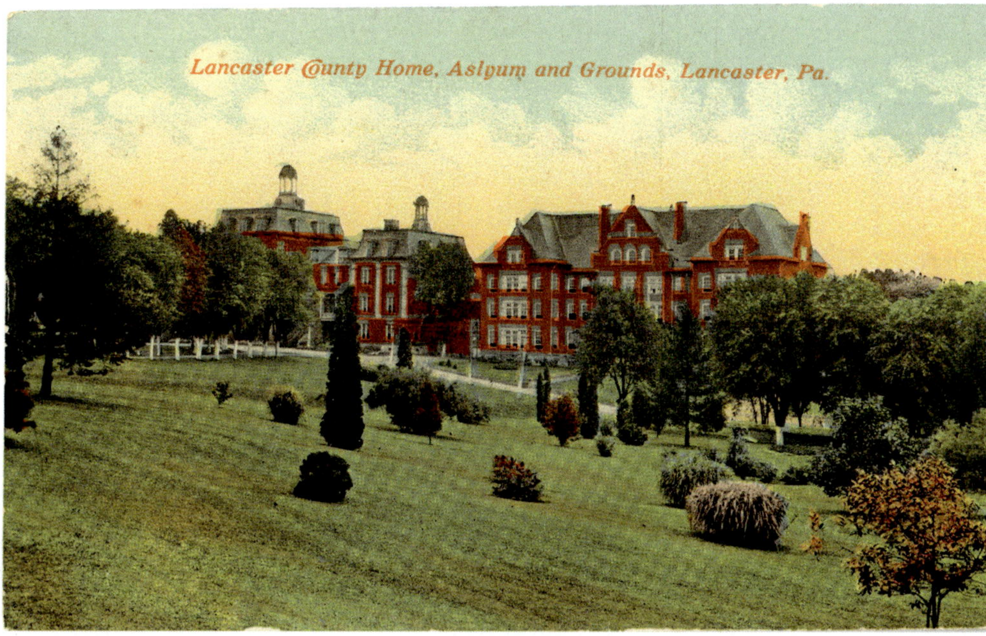
Lancaster County Home, Aslyum and Grounds, Lancaster, Pa.

Figure 294

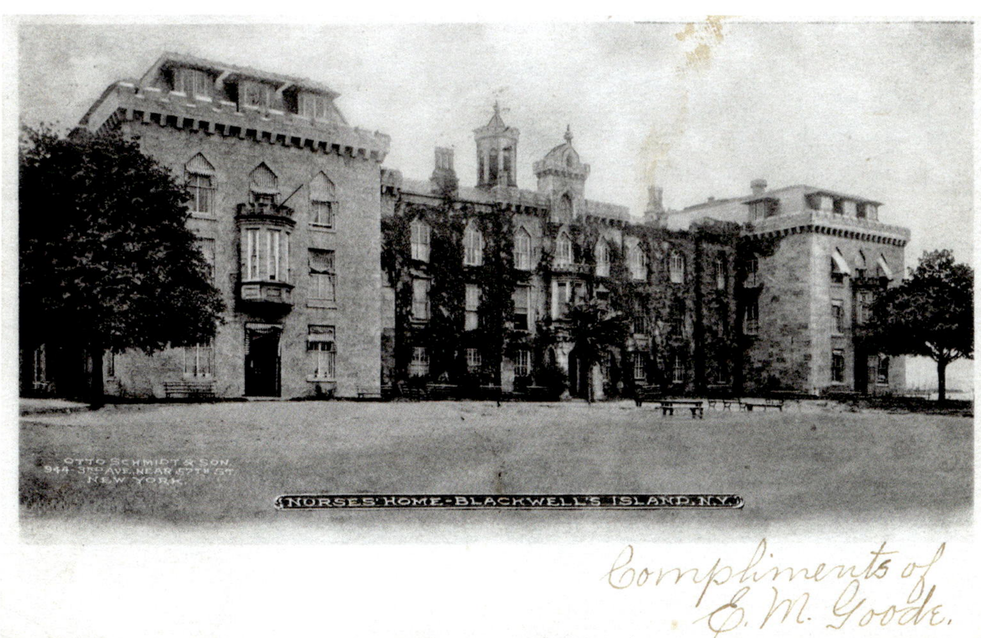
OTTO SCHMIDT & SON
944-3RD AVE. NEAR 57TH ST.
NEW YORK.
NURSES' HOME-BLACKWELL'S ISLAND, N.Y.
Compliments of
E. M. Goode.

Figure 295

Asylum on Blackwell Island
New York, 1839

In 1839, an institution for the mentally ill was established on Blackwell Island, now known as Roosevelt Island. The island was also home to an almshouse and a prison. One year after it opened, the asylum held 278 patients. Just 30 years later, the population had risen to 1,300 and the facility was severely overcrowded. This overcrowding was only slightly alleviated by the opening of asylums on Ward's Island and Hart Island, along with a facility on Long Island.

In 1887, the *New York World* newspaper had journalist Elizabeth Jane Cochrane feign mental illness to gain admission to Blackwell. Under the pseudonym "Nellie Bly," Cochrane spent ten days at the asylum and later detailed her experience and exposed the poor conditions of asylum life.

The postcard in figure 295, postmarked 1905, shows the Nurses Home on Blackwell Island.

All patients had been transferred off of Blackwell Island by 1894, when the facility became part of the Metropolitan Hospital. In 1955, the hospital abandoned the buildings. An octagon tower building from the original facility has been preserved.

Another county asylum was also established in the mid-1800s in New York. Initially called Kings County Insane Asylum, it was eventually purchased by the state and became part of Long Island State Hospital. The postcards in figures 296–297 show the same image, but also show the facility's name change.

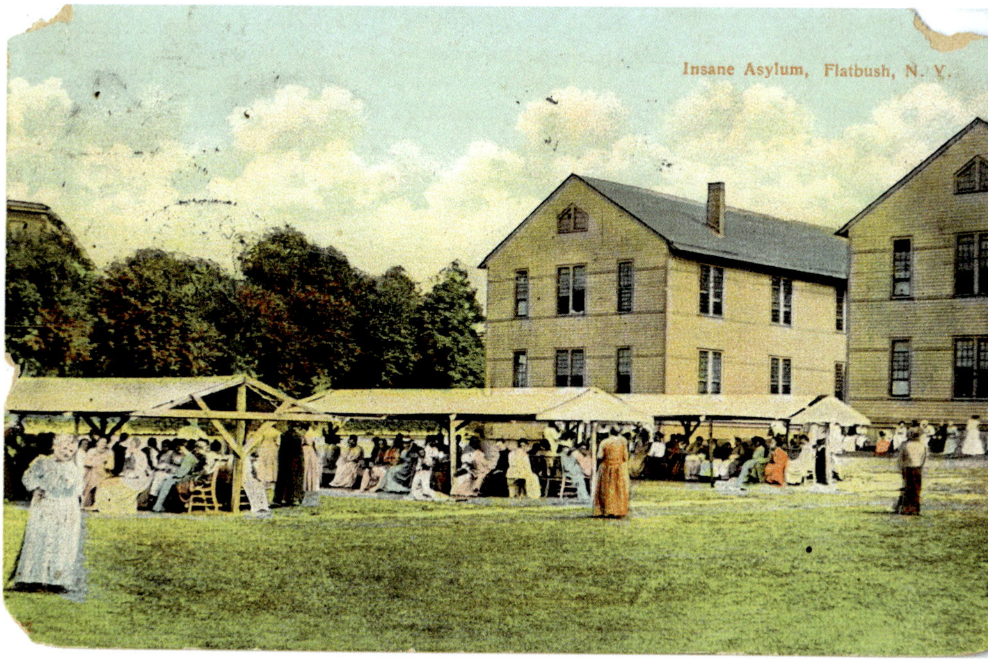
Insane Asylum, Flatbush, N. Y.

Figure 296

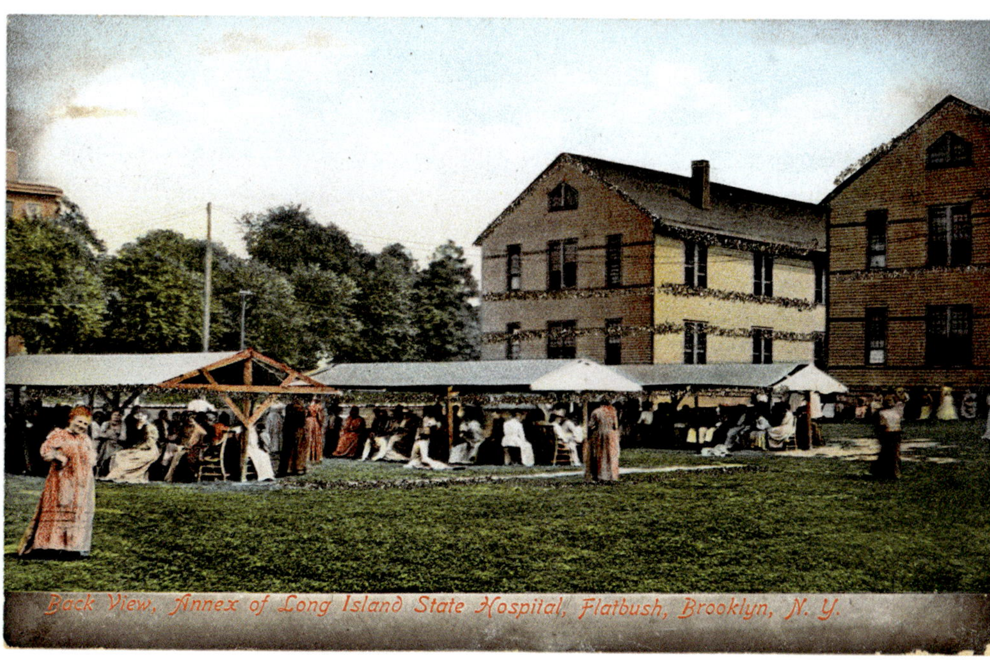
Back View, Annex of Long Island State Hospital, Flatbush, Brooklyn, N. Y.

Figure 297

County Asylums in Wisconsin, 1880

In 1854, a legislative act approved the establishment of the Wisconsin State Lunatic Asylum near Madison, Wisconsin. The first patient was admitted in 1860. However by 1870, the asylum did not have the capacity to care for all of the mentally ill in the state of Wisconsin. A county facility, the Milwaukee County Asylum, was therefore opened in 1880. The facility, which cared for 244 patients, was open only to residents of that county. The appointed trustees controlled the general operations of the asylum, but the state oversaw administration of the asylum. By 1910, there were 35 county asylums in Wisconsin.

The Milwaukee County Asylum (figure 298) was established in Wauwatosa, Wisconsin. This facility was closed in 1914.

Another county asylum, called Rock County Insane Asylum, is pictured in the postcard in figure 299, which has a postmark date of 1907.

This facility was opened in 1881 and demolished in the 1960s. Several buildings were added during its time as a poor house and county hospital. By 2007, newer buildings had been built for the housing of county government services.

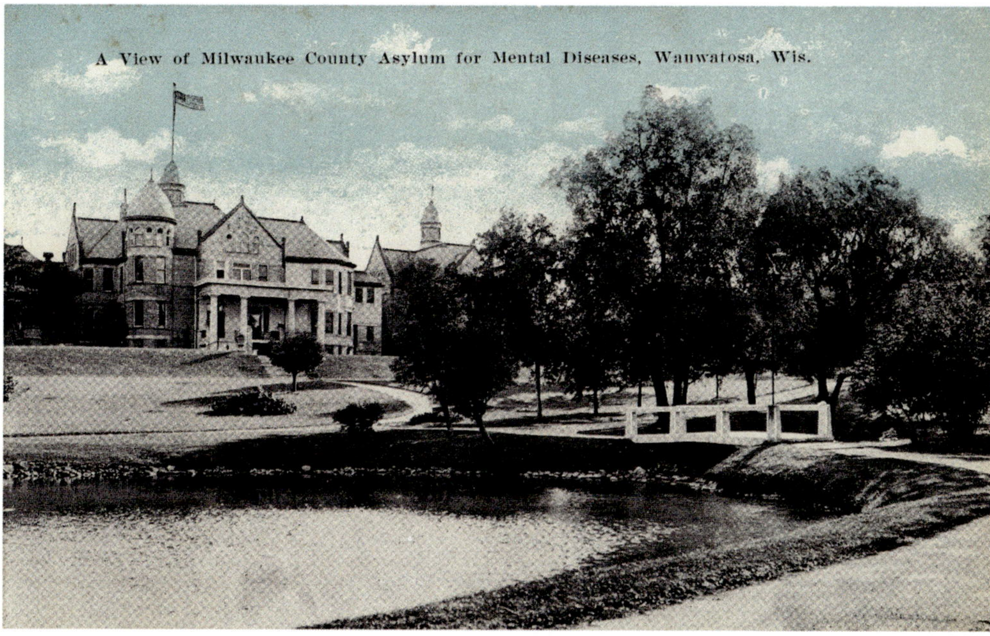
A View of Milwaukee County Asylum for Mental Diseases, Wauwatosa, Wis.

Figure 298

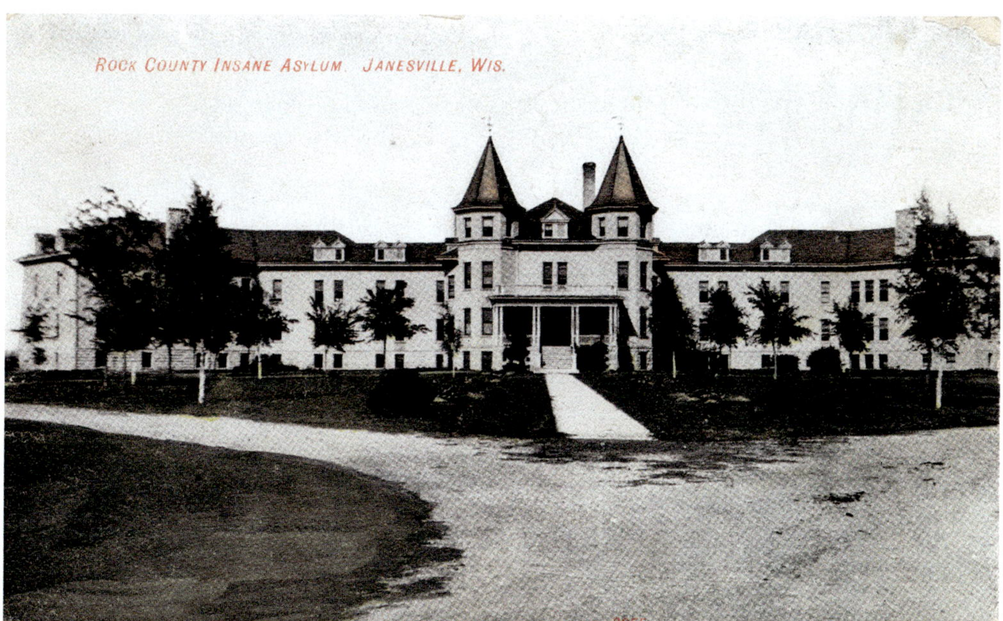
ROCK COUNTY INSANE ASYLUM. JANESVILLE, WIS.

Figure 299

Asylum for Insane Indians
Canton, South Dakota, 1898

This asylum, also called the Canton Indian Insane Asylum or the Hiawatha Insane Asylum, opened in 1903 on 100 acres of land in Canton, South Dakota. The facility, which consisted of 21 buildings, was the first and only federal asylum created specifically for American Indians. During its 31 years of operations, American Indians from a wide variety of tribes were committed to the asylum.

The buildings included pathological, bacteriological, and chemical laboratories and an operating room, dispensary, and mortuary. The basement contained a room for hydrotherapy treatments and a gymnasium.

Very little federal money was allotted to the asylum and several investigations revealed that many of the people confined to the asylum did not suffer from mental illness.

The asylum is pictured in the postcard in figure 300, sent in 1907.

The asylum was closed in 1934. Nothing remains of the original buildings.

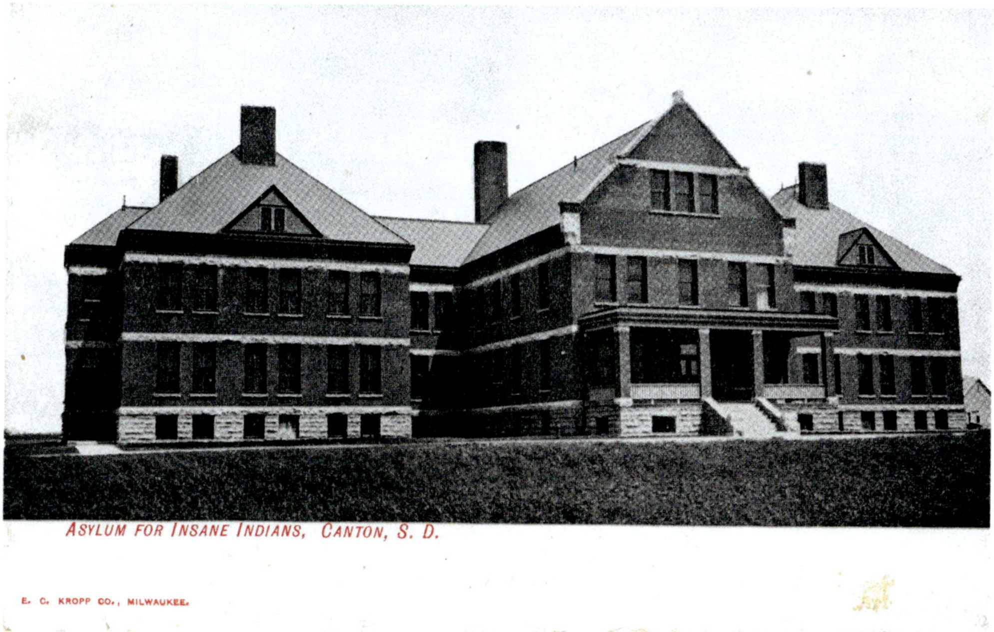
ASYLUM FOR INSANE INDIANS, CANTON, S. D.
E. C. KROPP CO., MILWAUKEE.

Figure 300

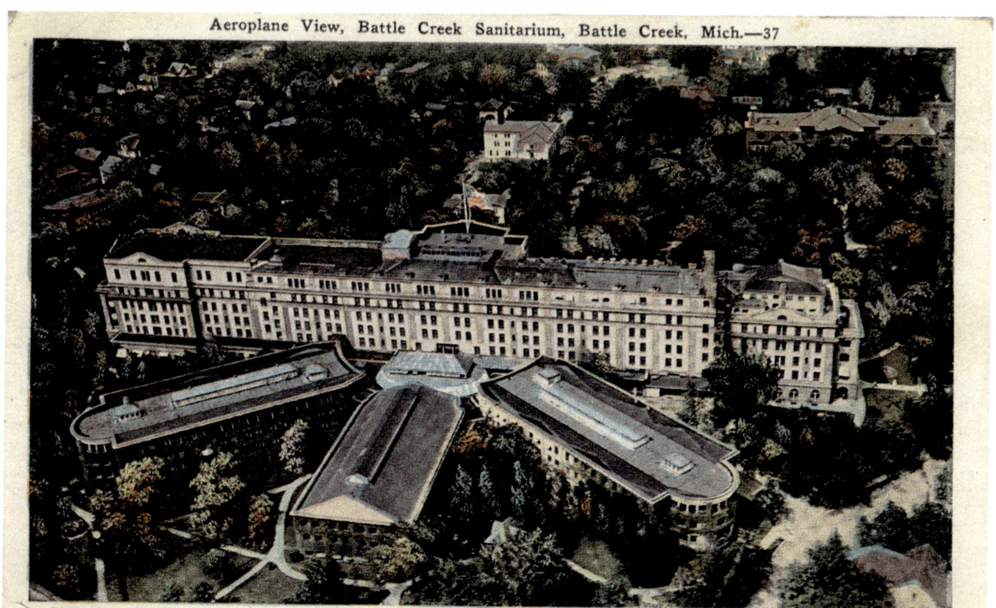
Aeroplane View, Battle Creek Sanitarium, Battle Creek, Mich.—37
Showing Rear of Main Bldg., Women's Bath House, Gymnasium, Men's Bath House, in Foreground.

Figure 301

Battle Creek Sanitarium
Battle Creek, Michigan, 1866

One of the most advertised private mental health facilities was the Western Health Reform Institute, opened in 1866 and based on the health principles advocated by the Seventh-day Adventist church. The name was changed to Battle Creek Sanitarium in 1876. The facility originally operated out of a small farmhouse.

In 1878, new buildings were erected to house the growing number of patients. These buildings were destroyed by fire in 1902, and a larger structure was erected the next year. It included a 550-foot building with wings that extended from the rear.

The divided back of the postcard in figure 301 indicates that it was produced between 1907 and 1915.

Treatment at the facility emphasized the importance of mind and body in health and included a low-fat diet, daily intake of fresh air, and exercise. Breathing exercises were also included. The card in figure 302 includes writing on the back that states, "You can't see me for I'm under the trees. F."

When the sanitarium first opened, many of the staff had no medical training. Eventually, the facility became a training site for student nurses, physicians, dieticians, and others. Nursing courses began at the sanitarium in 1877 and the first nurses' training school was established in 1883 (figure 303).

Another postcard (figure 304) shows some of the recreational facilities. The first image shows the swimming pool in the men's outdoor gymnasium. The second shows the gymnasium, which included "movement machines" for exercise.

The next postcard image (figure 305), taken in the early 1900s, shows Dr. J. H. Kellogg, who became the director of the Battle Creek Sanitarium in 1876 and frequently gave lectures there. Kellogg followed a strict health regime that excluded meat, stimulants, and alcohol and required plenty of fresh air and exercise.

The kitchen and dining room were located on the top floor to avoid having cooking odors penetrating other spaces. The dining room ceiling (figure 306) included a dome that rose 22 feet above the floor. Kellogg's and Post breakfast cereals originated at the sanitarium, when Dr. Kellogg and others began experimenting with healthful alternatives for patients who could not chew tougher grains.

Staying at the Battle Creek Sanitarium was expensive and after the stock market crash in 1929, few could afford it. In 1942, it was purchased by the US Army and converted into the Percy Jones General Hospital, serving as a place for treating wounded soldiers. The hospital closed in 1953 and in 1954 became the Battle Creek Federal Center, which houses federal agencies.

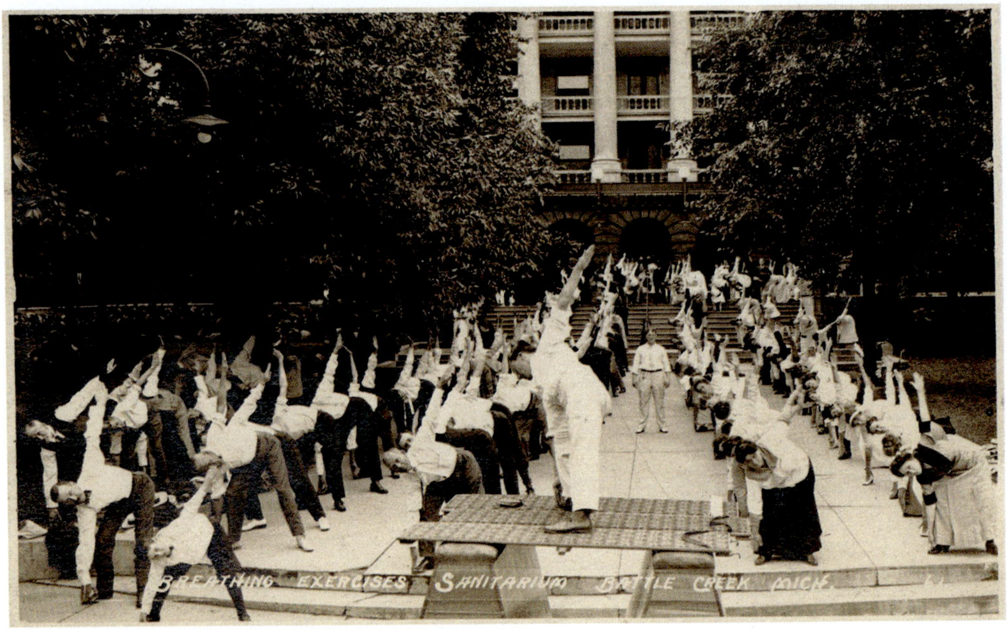
BREATHING EXERCISES SANITARIUM BATTLE CREEK MICH.

Figure 302

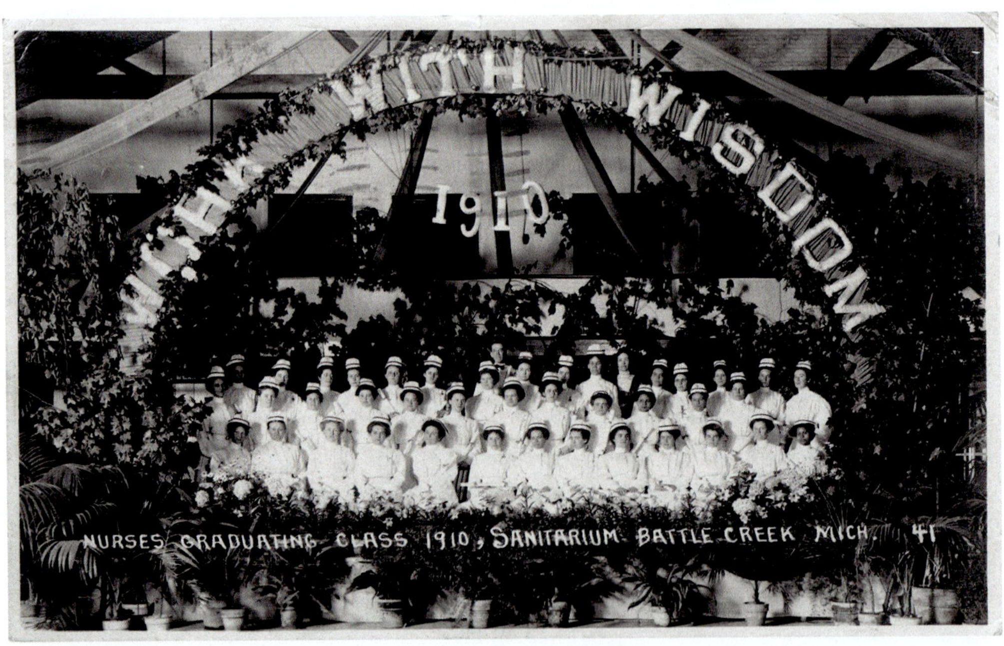
WITH WISDOM
1910
NURSES GRADUATING CLASS 1910, SANITARIUM BATTLE CREEK MICH. 41

Figure 303

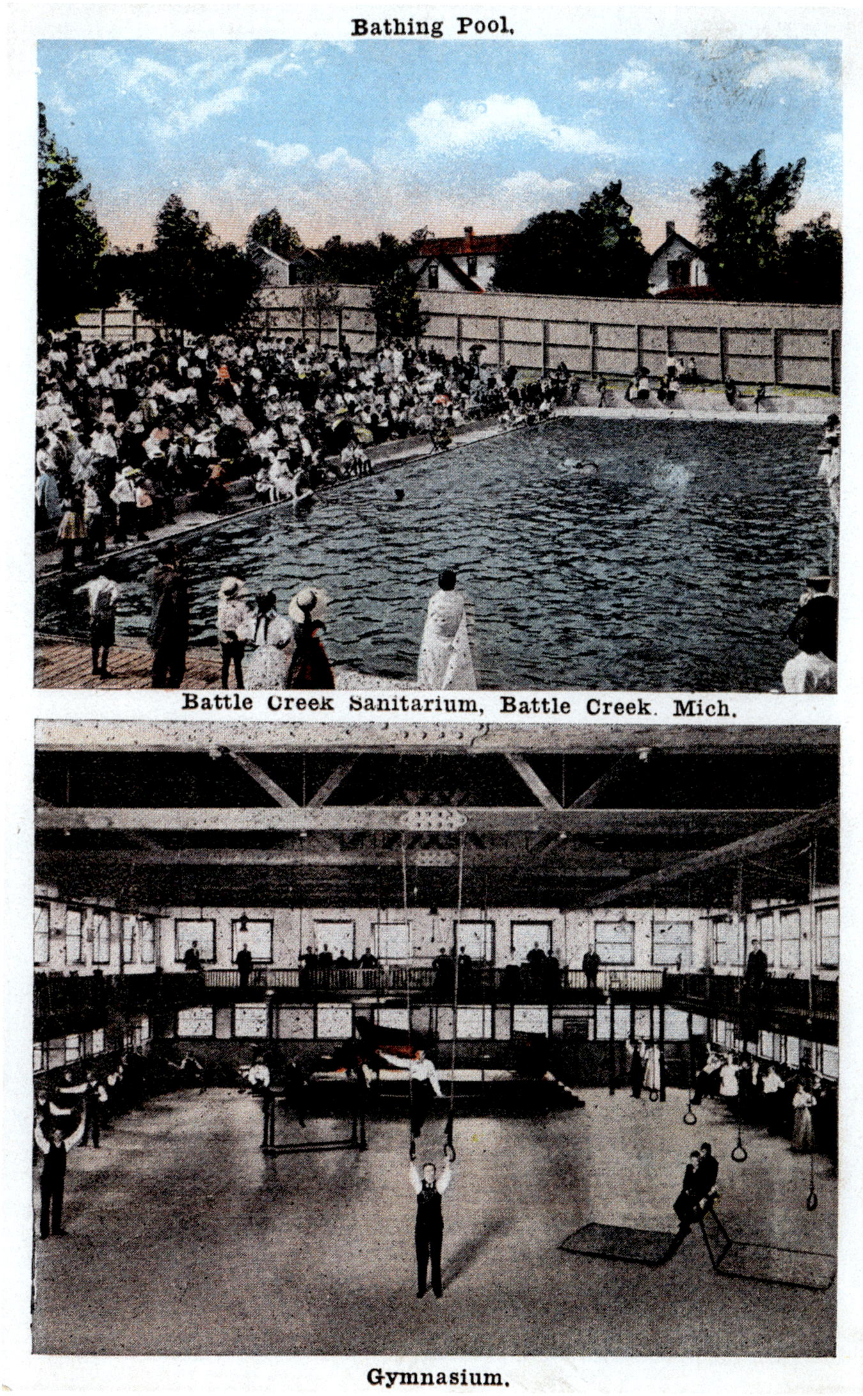
Bathing Pool.
Battle Creek Sanitarium, Battle Creek. Mich.
Gymnasium.

Figure 304

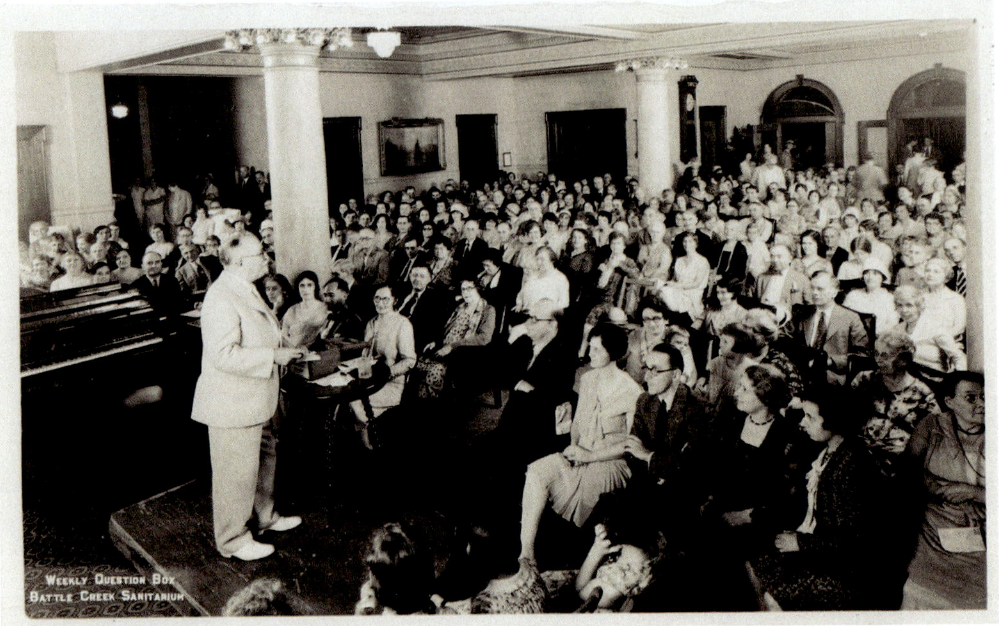

Figure 305

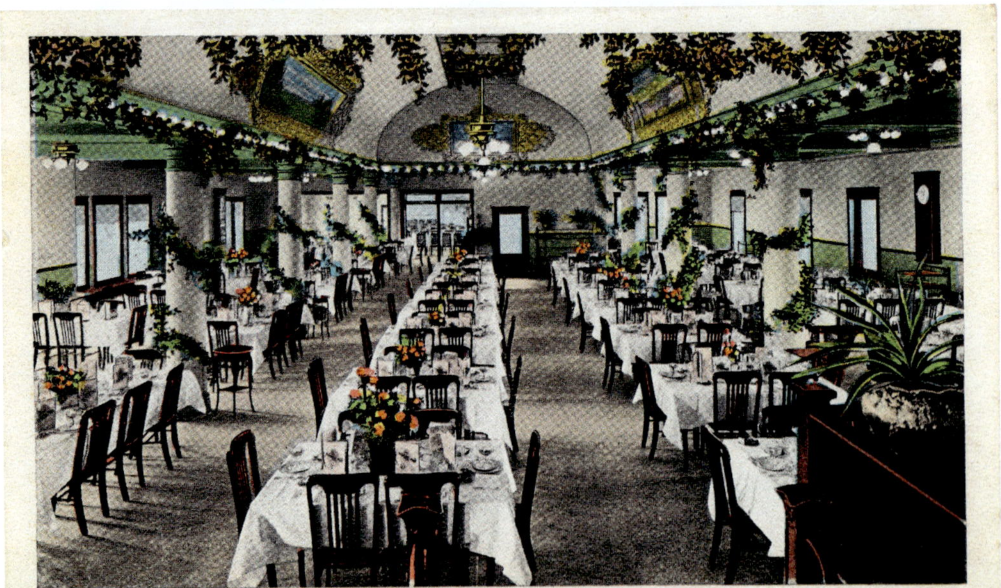

Main Dining Room, Sanitarium, Battle Creek, Mich.

Figure 306

Asylums in Attleboro, Massachusetts

The Attleboro Sanitarium was established in 1902. It is shown in figure 307, postmarked 1910. Advertisements for the facility invited guests who were ill, nervous, or tired to come for rest and treatment.

Another small sanitarium was opened in the late 1800s by a female physician. The Attleboro Home Sanitarium (figure 308) operated in a small home that cared for about ten patients at a time.

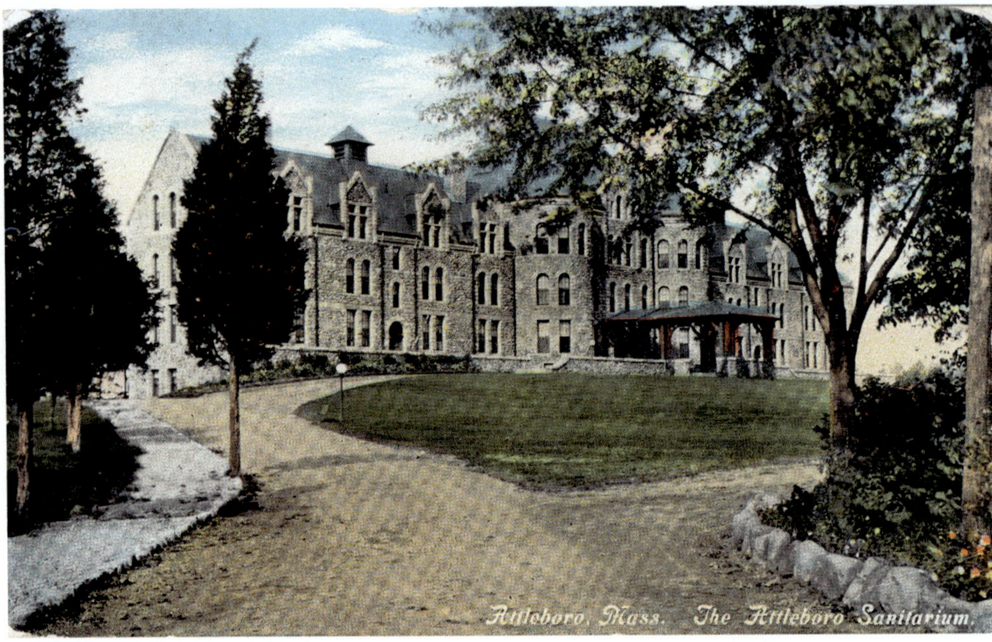

Figure 307

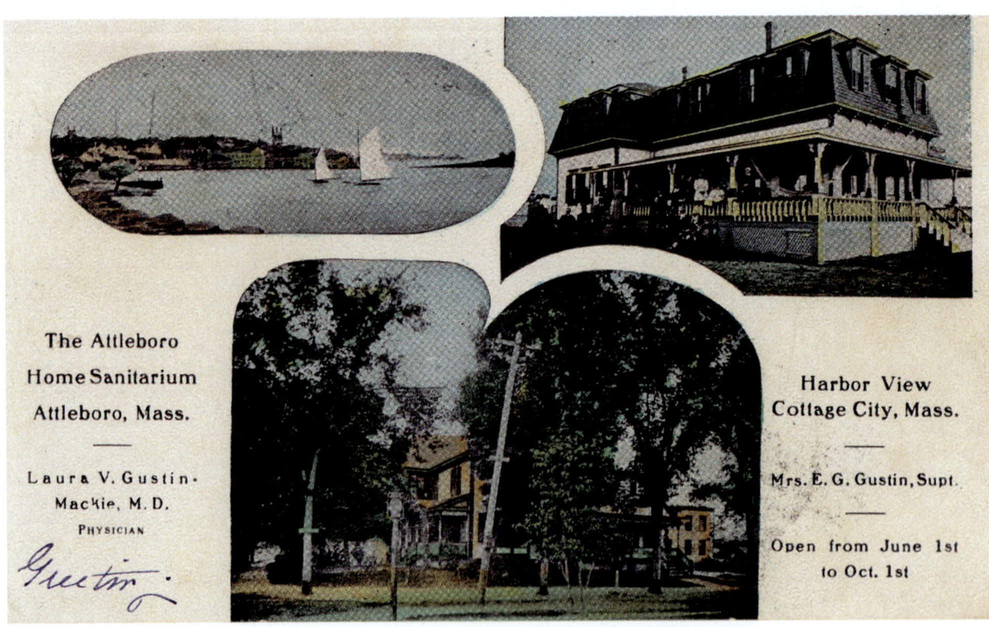

Figure 308

The New England Sanitarium and Hospital
Stoneham, Massachusetts

Several postcards (figures 309 and 310) show another private facility, the New England Sanitarium and Hospital at Stoneham, Massachusetts, a facility that was later called Boston Regional Medical Center.

The card in figure 311 shows the electrotherapy room at the sanitarium.

This facility later became the New England Memorial Hospital and the Boston Regional Medical Center. It was closed in 1999.

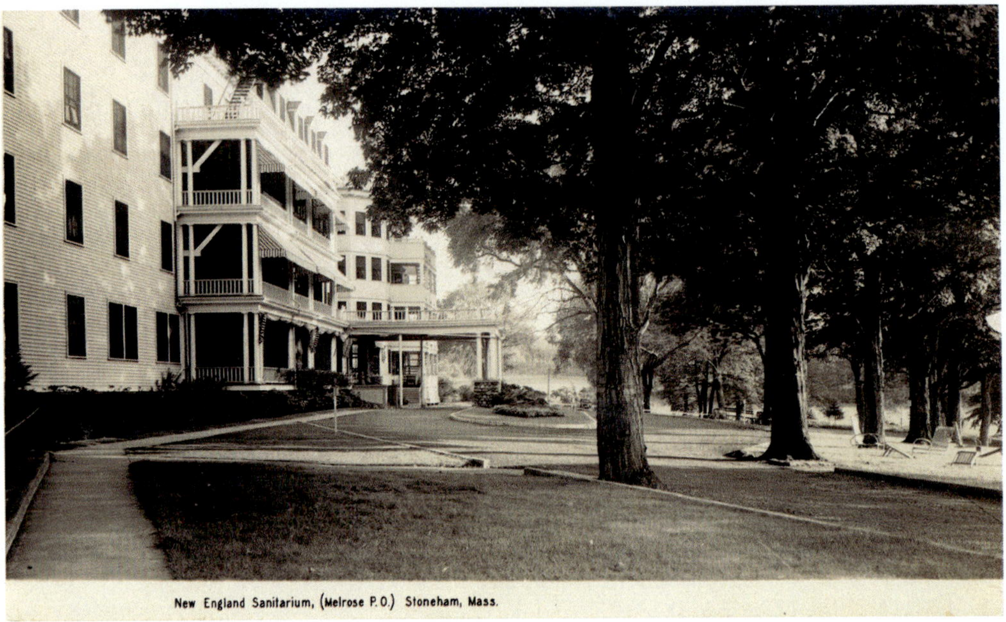

Figure 309

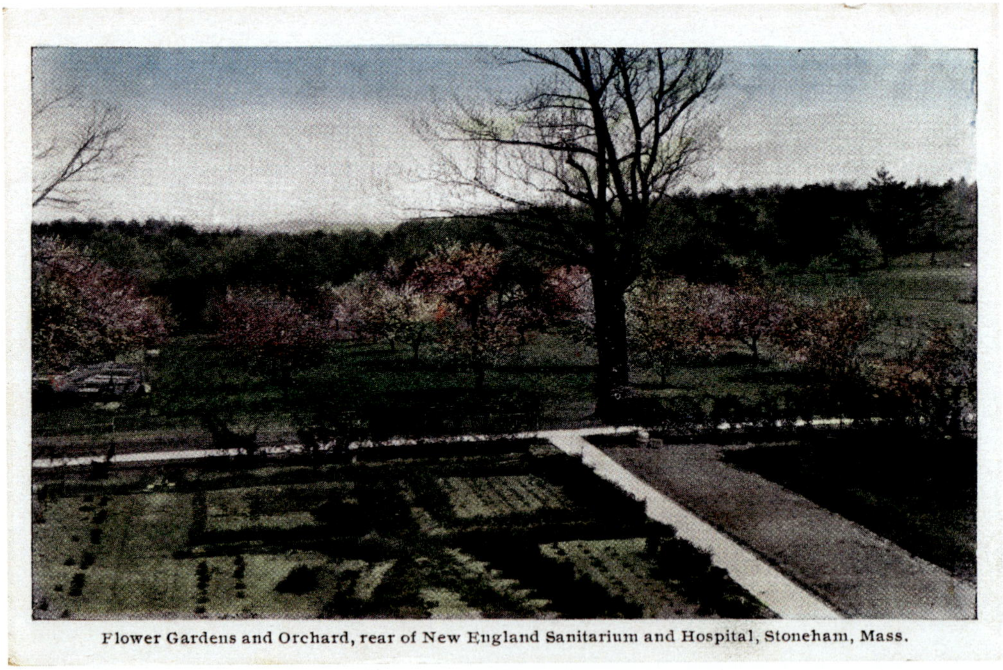

Figure 310

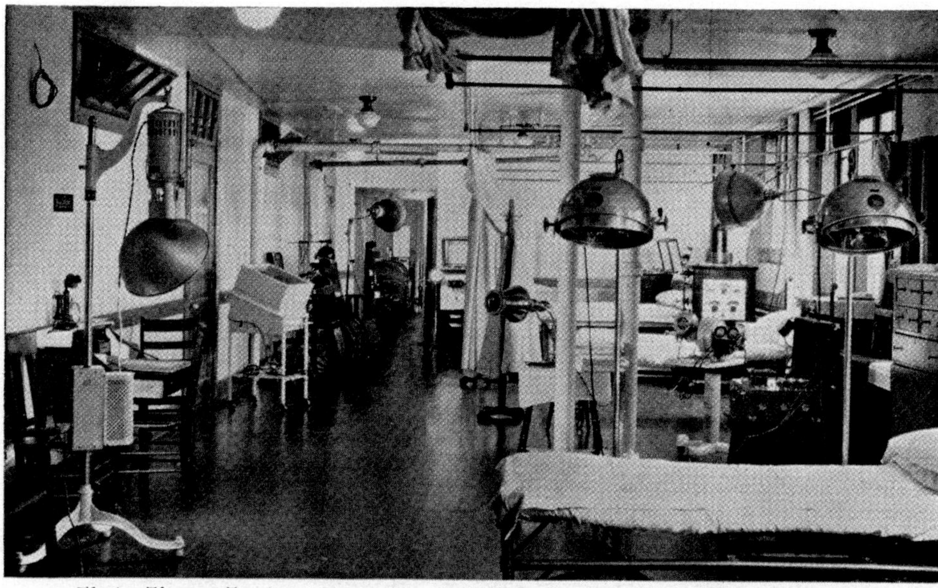

Electro-Therapy Treatment Rooms, New England Sanitarium and Hospital, Stoneham, Mass.

Figure 311

Conclusion

This book has provided the reader with a visual history of more than 100 institutions established between 1773 and 1898 to house and care for the mentally ill in the United States. These images of imposing administration buildings, inviting gardens, fenced in recreation yards, secluded tuberculosis quarters, and manicured tree-lined lawns provide a rare look at the history of asylum life in the United States. In many ways, they present the early American asylum as an inviting place, a calm and beautiful respite from the demands and chaos of urban life. In some respects, this is deceiving. As histories of mental health care in America have shown, the birth, growth, and dissolution of mental health care facilities has been and continues to be wrought with complications and controversies (Grob, 1983). Turn-of-the-century asylums were frequently overcrowded and underfunded and ideas regarding diagnosis and treatment have been wrought with conflict and controversy. A large body of historical research indeed demonstrates the scientific, political, and economic turmoil that served as the backdrop for these early institutions and for the development of mental health care more generally. Such histories seem almost contrary to the serene landscapes presented in the picture postcard.

Nonetheless, asylum postcards reveal as much as they obscure. For example, examining these cards reveals the image of the asylum that was most readily available to its contemporary public. Regardless of what occurred in these magnificent buildings, the public persona of the asylum is perhaps best represented by the picture postcard. The carefully curated images on these cards portray the asylum as a rationally designed, beautiful, and peaceful place, a place that would be perhaps ideal for the treatment of mental illness. It is important to note that this image was not curated by asylum officials and staff; the postcard images seem to have been produced by outside sources concerned primarily with the commercial value of the cards. In other words, there is little evidence to suggest that such cards were produced with the intention of portraying the asylum in a positive light in order to garner support for the institutions (Bogdan & Marshall, 1997). Nonetheless, in their attempt to sell as many cards as possible, postcard producers indeed provided the public with an idealized vision of the American asylum. An examination of these cultural artifacts therefore provides interesting and informative context for considering the public perception of asylum life.

Perhaps most importantly, these picture postcards provide a lasting image of the American asylum. As has been noted throughout this book, many of these structures have been repurposed, renovated, or demolished. Furthermore, the spaces that they occupied historically have been transformed dramatically over the last century. Asylums buildings that were once located in remote places far removed from the hustle and bustle of the city are now in the center of urban spaces that have expanded and taken over what were once the farms, grounds, and gardens of these asylums. Furthermore, the asylums also changed and grew in their own active lifetimes, sometimes starting out as single structures and growing over the years to add room for more patients, more staff, and more research and teaching facilities. Asylums appear in this book as works constantly in progress, with additions being made to some institutions nearly every year as funding became available and the need for more space grew pressing. Change in the physical structure of the asylum was also necessitated by the frequent fires in these early institutions, with such disasters often destroying facilities that were later rebuilt. In many cases, the history of the changing architecture of these facilities is most evident in these picture postcards. Although such images were often retouched or altered by the artists who created them (Bogdan & Marshall, 1997), they still provide a relatively faithful view of each facility's architectural history.

These picture postcards also provide a clear sense of just how large these facilities were and how much activity occurred within them on a daily basis. The asylum was a community unto itself, replete with farms, dairies, and gardens; dance halls, bowling alleys, and billiard rooms; laboratories, training schools, and pathology departments; and exercise quarters, Turkish baths, and hydrotherapy rooms. Viewing these images encourages us to view the asylum as a society, as a place where people lived, worked, played, and learned rather than just as a place for diagnosing, treating, and housing the mentally ill. The very multifaceted nature of asylum life comes into clear view as one examines postcards representing the asylum.

Although we have portrayed only the picture side of the postcards in this book, we should also note that the other side of these cards is as fascinating as the imagery.

Approximately 35% of the cards in the collection contain written messages. The content of these messages ranged from descriptions of personal travel and mundane communications between family and friends to descriptions of the facility pictured and impressions of its residents and operations. Some are penned by casual passersby, others by institution staff, and yet others by patients or visitors. Such written remarks provide yet another look at public perceptions of the asylum and of mental illness more generally. And, as is the case with all postcards, they also provide a personal look at the day-to-day life and musings of American citizens in this time period.

These images and the brief accounts that accompany them do not by any means constitute a complete or even a partial history of the American asylum. Indeed, we have largely left the images to speak for themselves. The material presented in this book suggests that a complete history would be a difficult undertaking, given the considerable diversity evident in early asylums in regards to size, capacity, architecture, and treatment philosophies. In many respects, the images displayed in this book raise more questions than they answer and in doing so, they encourage future explorations of the multifaceted nature of the asylum and the lives of its inhabitants. Combined with other images of the asylum, these postcards serve as the visual record of an important and intriguing part of American history.

References

Bogdan, R., & Marshall, A. (1997). Views of the asylum: Picture postcard depictions of institutions for people with mental disorders in the early 20th century. *Visual Sociology*, *12*(1), 4–27. doi: 10.1080/14725869708583772

Bogdan, R., & Weseloh, T. (2006). *Real photo postcard guide: The people's photography*. Syracuse, NY: Syracuse University Press.

Deese, A. W. (1994). A Study in Heideggerian Hermeneutical Methods, Workshop at the University of Wisconsin, Madison, WI, unpublished.

Deese, A. W. (2012). *Kentucky's first asylum: A saga of the people and practices*, Bloomington, IN: IUniverse.

Fourth Report to the Kentucky State Board for Charitable Institutions, 1909–1911. (1911) Frankfort, KY: Kentucky State Journal Publishing.

Grob, G. N. (1983). *Mental illness and American society, 1875–1940*. Princeton, NJ: Princeton University Press.

Hook, S. A. (2005). You've got mail: Hospital postcards as a reflection of health care in the early twentieth century. *Journal of the Medical Library Association*, *93*(3), 386–393.

Miron, J. (2011). *Prisons, asylums, and the public: Institutional visiting in the nineteenth century*. Toronto, ON: University of Toronto Press.

Morrissey, J. P., & Goldman, H. H. (1986). Care and treatment of the mentally ill in the United States: Historical developments and reforms. *Annals of the American Academy of Political and Social Science*, *484*, 12–27.

Report of the Fourth Kentucky Lunatic Asylum For the Year Ending November 28, 1873. (1873) Frankfort, KY: Printed at the Kentucky Yeoman Office.

Rogan, B. (2005). An entangled object: The picture postcard as souvenir and collectible, exchange and ritual communication. *Cultural Analysis*, *4*, 1–27.

Rosenberg, C. E. (1985). The therapeutic revolution: Medicine, meaning, and social change in 19th century America. In J. W. Leavitt & R. L. Numbers (Eds.), *Sickness and health in America* (pp. 39–53). Madison, WI: University of Wisconsin Press.

Thirty-Seventh Report of the Central Kentucky Asylum for the Insane. Lakeland: KY.

Yanni, C. (2007). *The architecture of madness: Insane asylums in the United States*. Minneapolis, MN: University of Minnesota Press.

Zwelling, S. S. (1985). *Quest for a cure: The public hospital in Williamsburg, 1773–1885*. Williamsburg, VA: Colonial Williamsburg Foundation.